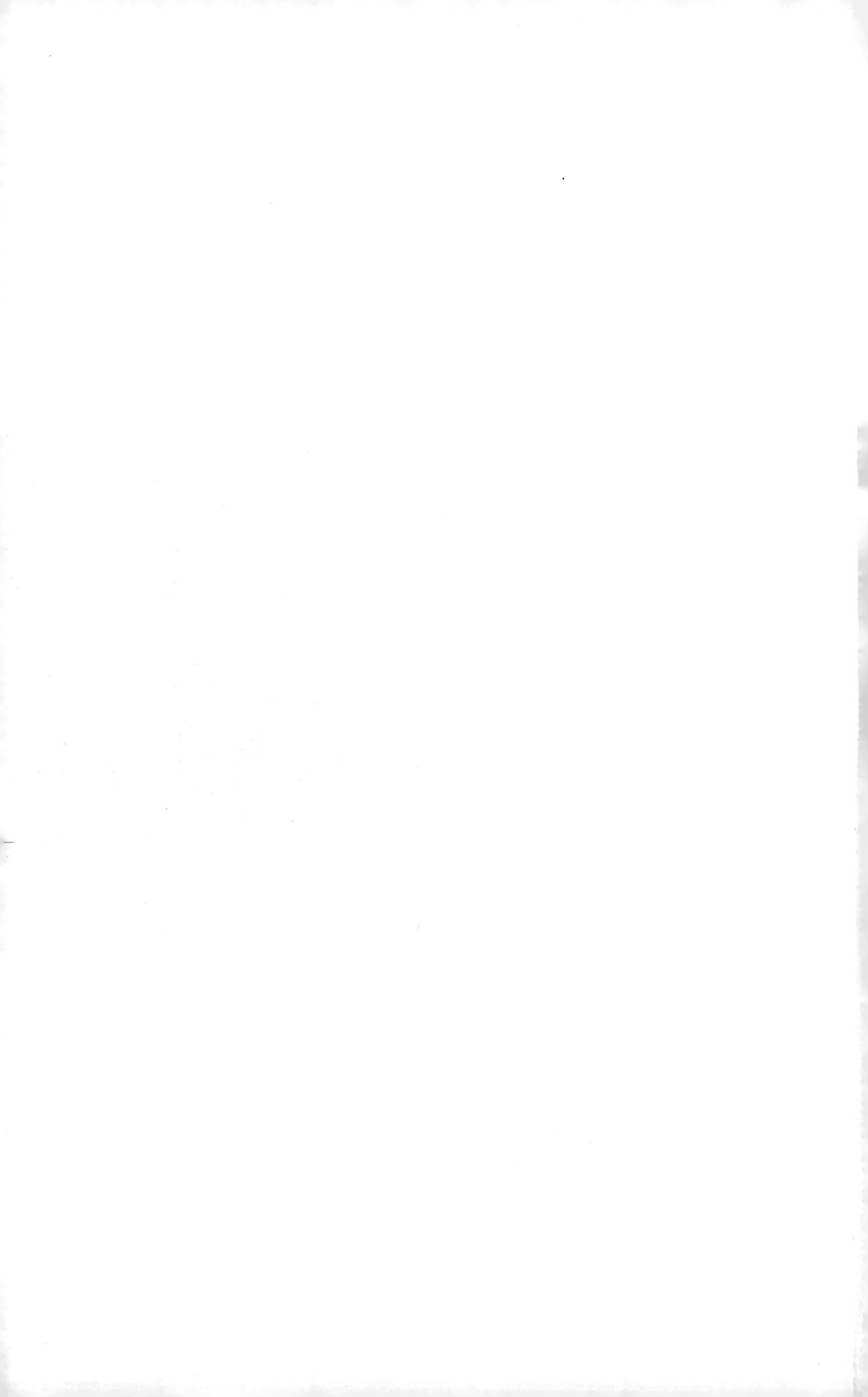

Springer Biographies

The books published in the Springer Biographies tell of the life and work of scholars, innovators, and pioneers in all fields of learning and throughout the ages. Prominent scientists and philosophers will feature, but so too will lesser known personalities whose significant contributions deserve greater recognition and whose remarkable life stories will stir and motivate readers. Authored by historians and other academic writers, the volumes describe and analyse the main achievements of their subjects in manner accessible to nonspecialists, interweaving these with salient aspects of the protagonists' personal lives. Autobiographies and memoirs also fall into the scope of the series.

More information about this series at http://www.springer.com/series/13617

Adrian Thomas • Francis Duck

Edith and Florence Stoney, Sisters in Radiology

Springer

Adrian Thomas
Faculty of Health and Wellbeing,
School of Allied and Public Health Professions
Canterbury Christ Church University
Canterbury, Kent, UK

Francis Duck
Formerly University of Bath
Bath, Somerset, UK

ISSN 2365-0613　　　　　　　ISSN 2365-0621　(electronic)
Springer Biographies
ISBN 978-3-030-16560-4　　　ISBN 978-3-030-16561-1　(eBook)
https://doi.org/10.1007/978-3-030-16561-1

© Springer Nature Switzerland AG 2019, corrected publication 2019
This work is subject to copyright. All rights are reserved by the Publisher, whether the whole or part of the material is concerned, specifically the rights of translation, reprinting, reuse of illustrations, recitation, broadcasting, reproduction on microfilms or in any other physical way, and transmission or information storage and retrieval, electronic adaptation, computer software, or by similar or dissimilar methodology now known or hereafter developed.
The use of general descriptive names, registered names, trademarks, service marks, etc. in this publication does not imply, even in the absence of a specific statement, that such names are exempt from the relevant protective laws and regulations and therefore free for general use.
The publisher, the authors, and the editors are safe to assume that the advice and information in this book are believed to be true and accurate at the date of publication. Neither the publisher nor the authors or the editors give a warranty, express or implied, with respect to the material contained herein or for any errors or omissions that may have been made. The publisher remains neutral with regard to jurisdictional claims in published maps and institutional affiliations.

This Springer imprint is published by the registered company Springer Nature Switzerland AG.
The registered company address is: Gewerbestrasse 11, 6330 Cham, Switzerland

We wish to dedicate this book to our wives, Di Duck and Johanna Thomas, and for their unfailing support and encouragement without whom this book would never have been written.

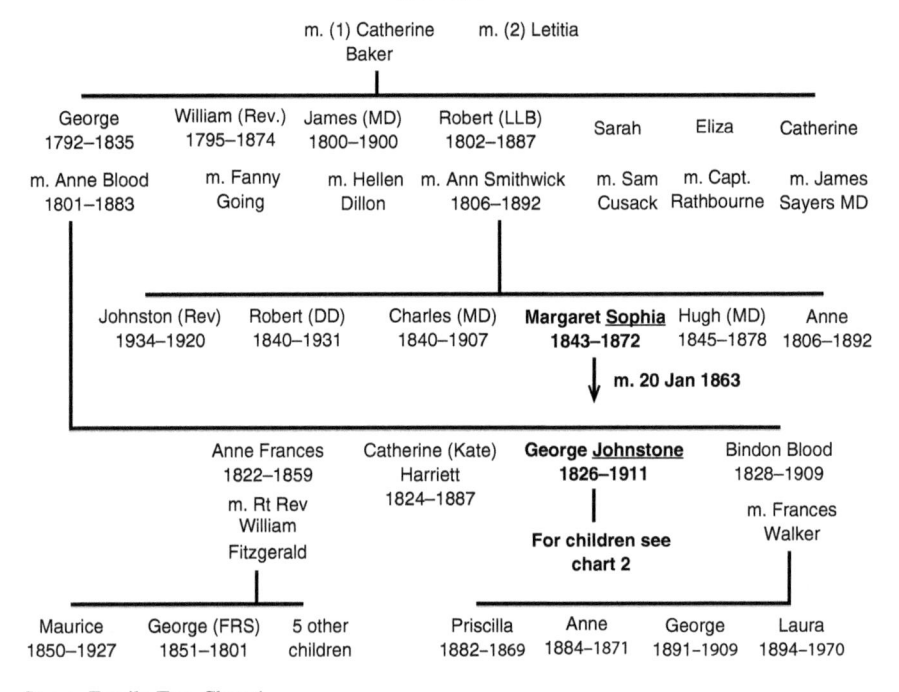

```
                          James Johnston
                             Stoney
                            1759–1824

                    m. (1) Catherine    m. (2) Letitia
                           Baker
```

George	William (Rev.)	James (MD)	Robert (LLB)	Sarah	Eliza	Catherine
1792–1835	1795–1874	1800–1900	1802–1887			
m. Anne Blood	m. Fanny	m. Hellen	m. Ann Smithwick	m. Sam	m. Capt.	m. James
1801–1883	Going	Dillon	1806–1892	Cusack	Rathbourne	Sayers MD

Johnston (Rev)	Robert (DD)	Charles (MD)	**Margaret Sophia**	Hugh (MD)	Anne
1934–1920	1840–1931	1840–1907	**1843–1872**	1845–1878	1806–1892

m. 20 Jan 1863

	Anne Frances	Catherine (Kate)	**George Johnstone**	Bindon Blood
	1822–1859	Harriett	**1826–1911**	1828–1909
	m. Rt Rev	1824–1887		m. Frances
	William		**For children see**	Walker
	Fitzgerald		**chart 2**	

Maurice	George (FRS)	5 other	Priscilla	Anne	George	Laura
1850–1927	1851–1801	children	1882–1869	1884–1871	1891–1909	1894–1970

Stoney Family Tree Chart 1

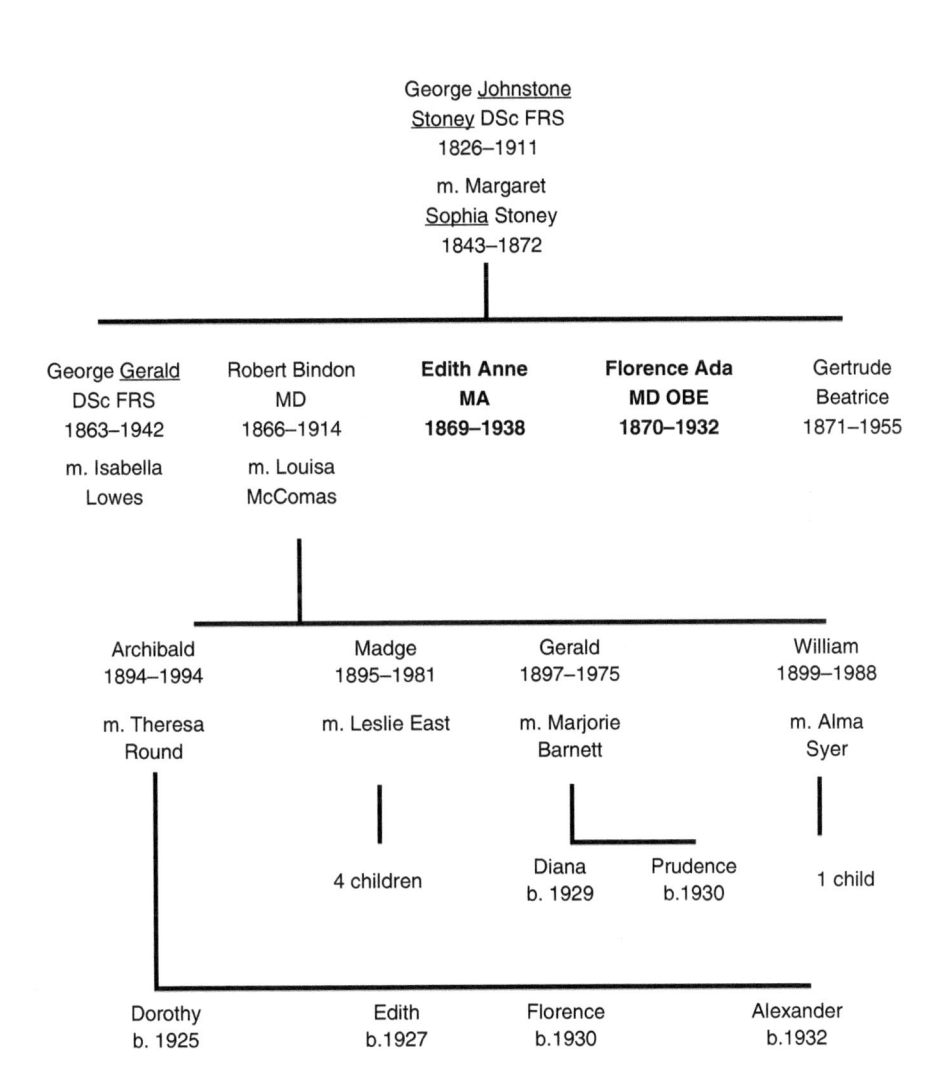

```
                    George Johnstone
                     Stoney DSc FRS
                        1826–1911

                       m. Margaret
                       Sophia Stoney
                        1843–1872
```

George Gerald	Robert Bindon	**Edith Anne**	**Florence Ada**	Gertrude
DSc FRS	MD	**MA**	**MD OBE**	Beatrice
1863–1942	1866–1914	**1869–1938**	**1870–1932**	1871–1955
m. Isabella	m. Louisa			
Lowes	McComas			

Archibald	Madge	Gerald	William
1894–1994	1895–1981	1897–1975	1899–1988
m. Theresa	m. Leslie East	m. Marjorie	m. Alma
Round		Barnett	Syer

	4 children	Diana	Prudence	1 child
		b. 1929	b.1930	

Dorothy	Edith	Florence	Alexander
b. 1925	b.1927	b.1930	b.1932

Stoney Family Tree Chart 2

Preface

This book is the true story of two remarkable sisters. One became a radiologist, and the other became a medical physicist. Their lives moved from their unusual upbringing in Dublin, to higher education in which they both excelled, and into careers in medicine that eventually resulted in deep involvement in the use of X-rays to manage the wounded soldiers during the First World War. Edith and Florence Stoney were pioneers and can lay claim to notable firsts. Florence was the first woman to practice radiology in Britain, both diagnostic and therapeutic. Edith was the first woman to practice medical physics. She was also the first woman to be awarded the M.A. degree from Trinity College Dublin. Florence was the first woman doctor to be employed in a British Military Hospital. These were all remarkable achievements. Florence Stoney's name emerged as the only woman in the otherwise purely male world of early radiology. In both cases, what little we learned of these two set them apart and made their lives and work worthy of investigation.

We, the authors of this book, are a radiologist and a medical physicist. Our interest in the histories of our own subjects led us to come across the two sisters quite independently from one another. In one case, during research for a book on the history of medical physics, an entry for E. Stoney in *The Lancet* as a lecturer in physics in 1899 opened a door to the older sister Edith and her extraordinary life. In the other case, an interest in early radiology necessitated an acquaintance with a remarkable woman radiologist. There is also the memory of a dear friend, the late Jean M Guy, MD, FRCR, DHMSA (1941–2012), and the many hours spent discussing the radiology pioneers in general and the Stoneys in particular [1]. Jean was a recipient of the Johnstone and Florence Stoney Travelling Studentship at Newnham College for 1963 and 1964.

Our search has led us to visit the leafy Victorian suburbs of Dublin, the grand portals of the old Royal Free Hospital in Gray's Inn Road in London, the ancient colleges of Cambridge and the exclusive medical practices of Harley Street. We followed them to Antwerp and back, to Cherbourg and back, to Serbia and Salonika and the final battles in France during the summer of 1918. The impact of the First

World War on their lives was such that almost half of the pages in this book are devoted to this period in history with its profound impact on all who lived through it.

The title of the book is slightly misleading. Certainly Florence and Edith each made their own contributions to radiology as it emerged as a distinct medical specialty during the first decades of the twentieth century. But the use of X-rays, for both diagnosis and treatment, was only one of a wide range of electrical technologies that were being developed at the same time. Florence was a Medical Electrician when she first used X-rays at the Royal Free Hospital in London. At one time or another, both sisters treated patients with electrical currents of a variety of forms from batteries and mains electricity; they used high-frequency oscillators and diathermy and treated patients with infrared and ultraviolet radiation. They used electric stimulation to test for nerve injury. In order to use these technologies effectively, they needed a clear understanding of the underlying science and a logical rationale for their clinical uses. The combined talents of Edith and Florence ensured these were in place.

The search for evidence has taken us to archives in London, Southampton and Glasgow, in Dublin and Cambridge and in Bournemouth and Royaumont. Many archivists have been enormously helpful in our search for evidence, and the archives that we have used are acknowledged at the end of the book. Such records are often limited to official documents, summaries of what happened, bereft of personal detail. We are particularly grateful, therefore, to several members of the extended Stoney family who have given us access to private family papers and pictures. In particular, Alex Stoney, their great nephew living in Australia, allowed us access to his complete digital archive of family papers, from which we could gain greater understanding of their Irish ancestors. These papers also included transcriptions of letters from the sisters to their Australian nephew during the 1920s and early 1930s. These letters have allowed us to soften, and to make more personal, the story of a period in their lives that might otherwise have been limited by evidence in more formal sources. It was a delight that Edith McKinnon (née Stoney), their great niece, was able to recall Edith's visit to Australia in 1934, with the help of her daughter Frances Smith.

Nearer home, but more distantly related, we have been greatly helped by Claire Keohone, whose great-grandmother's cuttings book held several fascinating and informative items about Edith and Florence and the Stoney ancestors. Sincere thanks are due to these members of the Stoney family for sharing their private family records.

Edith and Florence Stoney lived together, travelled together and worked together. They supported one another during the turbulent decades at the beginning of the twentieth century as the world they knew as children shifted and fractured. They were born in the United Kingdom of Great Britain and Ireland. By the end of their lives, the city of their birth, Dublin, was in another country, and their Protestant background was being consigned to history. Home Rule for Ireland polarised opinion as profoundly as Brexit.

The First Word War caused the conditions that created radiology as a distinct medical specialty, and they were actively a part of that. During their lives, radio waves were discovered and harnessed for communication, man took to the air, atomic structure was revealed and atoms were split, radioactivity was discovered, the roads filled with cars and lorries and moving pictures recorded action and entertained. X-rays were discovered in 1895, and this was the particular scientific discovery that drew the physicist Edith and the doctor Florence together.

In writing this double biography, it became clear that there was a third person who was always there, and whose influence on the sisters' lives was profound. This was their father, George Johnstone Stoney. It is not possible to approach an understanding of their drives and motivations without having some appreciation of his work and broader influence and his philosophical and political views. They absorbed much of their own world view from his, and his influence on them reached to the end of their own lives and beyond.

This book may be viewed most simply as a chronological biography of the lives and achievements of these two Irish sisters, during a time of enfranchisement for women. But in addition the narrative follows several intertwined themes as experienced by the sisters during their lifetimes. Their upbringing influenced by their liberal-minded scientist father set the tone for both lives. Irish independence fractured their family heritage. Educational possibilities for women opened. Their professional experiences, fulfilling for Florence as a qualified doctor, but often frustrating for Edith as a Cambridge-educated scientist, mirrored those of other aspiring women at this time. The suffragist movement expanded and women's lobby groups were formed. Their remarkable friends and colleagues were the new professional, educated women, exploring ways to contribute to society in their own right. But ultimately this is the extraordinary story of two sisters and their abiding love and support for one another. Independent yet bonded throughout life, they cooperated and shared in one another's successes and were always protective and supportive of each other in times of trouble.

Canterbury, UK Adrian Thomas
Bath, UK Francis Duck

Reference

1. Guy JM. Edith (1869–1938) and Florence (1870–1932) Stoney, two Irish sisters and their contribution to radiology during the World War 1. J Med Biogr 2013;21:100–7.

Acknowledgements

We have drawn on a wide range of sources in writing this biography. Our own collections of books, papers and ephemera formed the foundation for our research. Digital libraries were essential, especially the British Library Newspaper Archive and Gallica. Wikipedia always offered a first port of call for a previously unknown person or historical fact. The website devoted to the memory of those who served in the Scottish Women's Hospitals during the First Word War is filled with detail. The family history sites Ancestry and Findmypast have been used to access individual personal information. We have also drawn on documents held in various archives that are, as yet, not digitised. In London, these have been at the British Library, the Wellcome Library, King's College Library, the London Metropolitan Archives, the Science Museum Library, the Women's Library at the London School of Economics and the Royal Holloway Library. Outside London, the papers of the Scottish Women's Hospitals, held in the Mitchell Library in Glasgow, provided an extensive resource of original papers and letters, including many from Edith Stoney, which opened a window onto her wartime experience. Thanks are due to Jane Claydon for her assistance with information and advice on the life of Madame Österberg and her Training College. We would also like to note our appreciation to Anne Thompson, archivist at Newnham College, Cambridge, for her particular helpfulness. Other archives visited were at Winchester University, Cheltenham Ladies' College, Trinity College Dublin, University College Dublin, Queen's University Belfast and the Rosse Archive at Birr. The staff were universally helpful and considerate. We would like to note our particular thanks to Francis Tailleur, historian at Troyes, and to Nathalie Le Gonidec, archivist at Royaumont Abbey, whose generosity in giving access to photographic records from the war years was invaluable.

Personal thanks are given to Prof. Neil McIntyre for his advice and support and to his indefatigable work in recording the story of the Royal Free Hospital, the London School of Medicine for Women, and the fascinating and inspiring story of how British women became doctors.

Particular thanks must be extended to members of the Stoney family who have most generously given access to private family records. It has been a delight to be in touch with Alex Stoney, Edith and Florence's great nephew in Australia, who made available his whole Stoney family archive; also his sister Edith McKinnon (née Stoney), who could recall the visit that Edith, her great aunt, made to Australia in 1934; and also Frances Smith who inherited the bicycle. Closer to home, Claire Keohane's hospitality was made the greater from the opportunity to browse the Stoney family scrapbook and letters.

Andy Duck's editorial guidance is gratefully acknowledged.

Particular picture credits are indicated in parentheses at the end of each figure legend. The pictures are an important part of the book and whilst some may appear indistinct are representative of the originals, which were often printed on poor quality newspaper or under difficult wartime conditions.

Contents

1	**Dublin**	1
	Cycling for Ladies	2
	Early Education	8
	A Career in Medicine	12
	Examination Failure and Success	17
	References	22
2	**Oakley Park**	25
	Oakley Abandoned	29
	Parsonstown	32
	Queen's College, Galway	36
	Return to Dublin	37
	References	42
3	**Newnham College, Cambridge**	45
	Newnham College	45
	The Mathematics Tripos	51
	A Student in Cambridge	55
	Newnham College Astronomer	61
	References	66
4	**Cheltenham**	67
	Mathematics Teacher	68
	X-Rays and Astronomy	70
	New Opportunities	75
	References	77
5	**The London School of Medicine for Women**	79
	The London School of Medicine for Women	79
	Florence Moves to London	82

	The New Hospital for Women	88
	The Victoria Hospital for Sick Children, Hull	91
	The Anatomy Demonstrator	95
	Madame Bergman Österberg's Physical Training College and Women's Health and Education	97
	References	101
6	**Florence and X-rays**	103
	Pioneer Radiology	103
	Radiology and Anatomy	105
	The Royal Free Hospital Röntgen Ray Department	106
	Radiology at the New Hospital for Women	110
	Graves' Disease	112
	X-ray Notes from the United States	113
	Professional Life	116
	The Association of Registered Medical Women	117
	References	119
7	**Teaching Physics**	121
	The Stability of Marine Turbines	125
	Graduation at Last	127
	Becoming an Educationalist	130
	References	132
8	**Challenge and Loss**	133
	Visitors to Chepstow Crescent	134
	The Death of Johnstone Stoney	137
	Reynolds Close	139
	A Developing Crisis	141
	References	144
9	**Action and Reaction**	147
	The British Federation for University Women	148
	Militant Suffragettes	151
	Irish Home Rule	153
	References	154
10	**Florence's War**	155
	The Great War	155
	The War Office and Sir Frederick Treves	156
	Mabel St Clair Stobart and Antwerp	158
	The Anglo-French Hospital, No. 2, Le Château Tourlaville, near Cherbourg	164
	Fulham Military Hospital, Hammersmith	167
	Soldier's Heart or DAH	171
	References	174

Contents xvii

11 Chateau de Chanteloup..................................... 177
    The Scottish Women's Hospital for Foreign Service............... 178
    Chateau de Chanteloup, Troyes................................ 183
    Orders to Move... 190
    Off Towards Serbia... 196
    References.. 198

12 Serbia and Salonika....................................... 199
    Evacuation from Gevgheli.................................... 201
    Electrotherapy in Salonika................................... 203
    Conflict with Edinburgh..................................... 206
    Summer by the Mediterranean................................ 209
    Home and Rest... 211
    Return to Salonika.. 214
    Appendix.. 221
        LIST OF X_RAY GOODS............................ 221
    References.. 222

13 Mobile Radiography...................................... 225
    The Royaumont X-Ray Ambulance............................ 226
    The Edith Cavell X-Ray Van.................................. 232
    References.. 240

14 Villers-Cotterêts.. 243
    Back to France... 244
    Agnes Savill... 247
    Radiology at Villers-Cotterêts................................ 251
    27–31 May 1918... 257
    References.. 263

15 Royaumont Abbey.. 265
    Vera Collum.. 266
    Radiation Safety.. 270
    Planning Ahead.. 274
    The Closure of Royaumont.................................. 277
    References.. 282

16 Return to Civilian Life.................................... 285
    Awards and Decorations..................................... 285
    The British Association Meeting in Bournemouth, September 1919... 287
    Votes for Women... 289
    Florence Moves to Bournemouth.............................. 290
    The British Medical Association.............................. 294
    The Wessex Branch of the British Institute of Radiology........... 295
    Edith Returns to Education................................... 297
    Women and Engineering..................................... 301
    References.. 302

17	**Family, Retirement and Travel**	305
	Life in Retirement	305
	Edith Retires	307
	Florence in Retirement	309
	More Distant Travel	309
	Heliotherapy and Osteomalacia	311
	Edith and Women's Issues	313
	The Death of Florence	314
	References	316
18	**Legacy**	319
	Benefactress	322
	References	327

Correction to: Edith and Florence Stoney, Sisters in Radiology C1

Appendix: Wartime Uses of Radiology and Medical Electricity 329
    Radiography: X-ray Diagnosis of Gas Gangrene 329
    X-ray Localization of Foreign Bodies 333
    Electrotherapy 340
    Electrodiagnosis of Nerve Injury 343

References 347

Index 349

Abbreviations

Used in the Text

ARMW	Association of Registered Medical Women
ASGBI	Anatomical Society of Great Britain and Ireland
BAAS	British Association for the Advancement of Science
BARP	British Association of Radiology and Physiotherapy
BEF	British Expeditionary Force
BFUW	British Federation of University Women
BIR	British Institute of Radiology
BMA	British Medical Association
BMJ	British Medical Journal
BNSS	Bournemouth Natural History Society
BS	Bachelor of Surgery
DAH	Disordered Action of the Heart
DMRE	Diploma in Medical Radiology and Electrology
EGAH	Elizabeth Garrett Anderson Hospital
FMH	Fulham Military Hospital
LMSSA	Licentiate in Medicine and Surgery of the Society of Apothecaries
LSMW	London School of Medicine for Women
MB	Bachelor of Medicine
MD	Doctor of Medicine
MSR	Member of the Society of Radiographers
MWF	Medical Women's Federation
NHW	New Hospital for Women
NUWSS	National Union of Women's Suffrage Societies
OBE	Officer of the Most Excellent Order of the British Empire
RAMC	Royal Army Medical Corps
RFH	Royal Free Hospital
RFHSMW	The London (Royal Free Hospital) School of Medicine for Women
RSM	Royal Society of Medicine

RVWHH	Royal Victoria and West Hants Hospital
SWH	Scottish Women's Hospitals for Foreign Service
UK	United Kingdom
VAD	Voluntary Aid Detachment
VHSC	Victoria Hospital for Sick Children (Hull)
WES	Women's Engineering Society
WNSL	Women's National Service League
WSPU	Women's Social and Political Union

Used in the Reference List

AS	Alex Stoney. Private collection of Stony family papers
CK	Claire Keohane. Private collection of Stoney family papers
Crofton	Crofton E. The Women of Royaumont. East Lothian: Tuckwell Press; 1997
Fara	Fara P. A Lab of One's Own. Oxford: OUP; 2018
LMA	London Metropolitan Archives
ML	Mitchell Library, Glasgow
WL	Women's Library, London School of Economics

Chapter 1
Dublin

They were all very proud of Gerald. Not even their father had ever published his own book, in spite of his scientific eminence. The critic in the Irish Times was very complimentary: 'Their work rests on the best foundations—that of experience—and the only wonder is that the same gentlemen have never thought of issuing such a splendid specimen of joint authorship before'. Richard Mecredy and Gerald Stoney were both only in their mid-twenties, so they would have been hard put to have prepared a book on the topic much earlier, especially in such a rapidly changing area. The Art and Pastime of Cycling (1888) was 'a guide to the popular recreation of cycling', and 'no two men in Ireland know more about cycling in all its most attractive and practical features both on the track and on the road' [1, 2].

The men formed an ideal combination. Both were graduates of Trinity College, Dublin. Mecredy was the sportsman. In the 1886 Irish Cycling Championships, Mecredy had won the 1-mile, 2-mile and 4-mile track events. This needed athleticism, certainly, but it also needed the best equipment, and Gerald Stoney provided the technical support. He designed Mecredy's bicycle to be as efficient as possible, as fast as the solid tyres allowed, making their shared enterprise much more effective. He learned his engineering from his father, Johnstone Stoney. In what must be amongst the first papers in sports science, they reported detailed experiments to determine the energy expended in propelling a bicycle. It was published in the Transactions of the Royal Dublin Society [3], of which Johnstone was a vice president. They used Gerald's 'Xtraordinary Challenge' penny-farthing bicycle, riding above its 52-inch driving wheel, measuring its rotation as they coasted to a halt or using a pencil attached to spring-loaded pedals, later calibrated using weights. He pedalled outside their home along the gravel surface of Palmerston Park, past the mill on Dartry Hill and the 1-in-17 hill at Milltown Station. In a second publication, Gerald and his father described gears for his smaller-wheeled, 'Facile', machine (Fig. 1.1) designed to make it easier to climb Classon's Bridge Hill beyond the River Dodder, south of the narrow packhorse bridge. Uninterested in profiting from their inventions, they declared that 'it may be of advantage to communicate these three contrivances to the Royal Dublin Society, with a view to rendering them incapable of

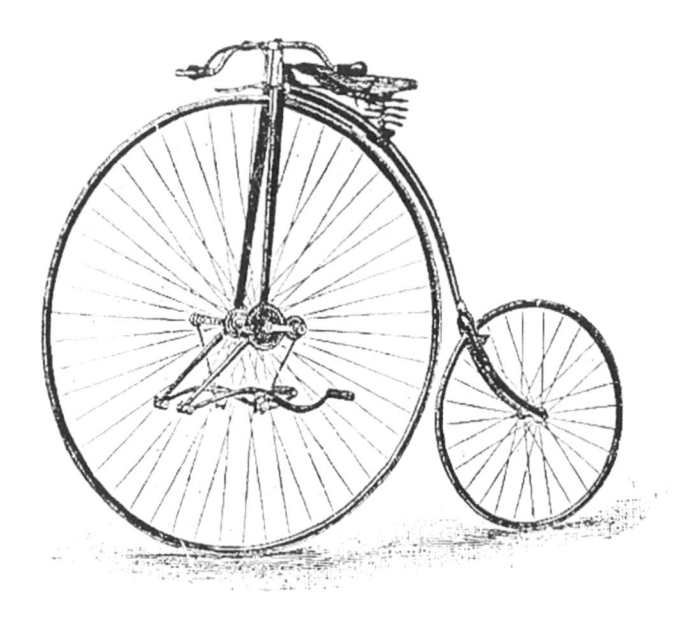

THE GEARED FACILE BICYCLE.

Fig. 1.1 A geared 'Facile' bicycle

being the subjects of patents' [4]. Eventually he placed an advertisement in the paper to sell his old penny-farthing for 'say £6'.

Edith and Florence Stoney grew up in this family, embedded in an open-minded world of science and technology. They watched and learned as their brother and father worked on their bicycles in their home workshop. Gerald had a wooden boneshaker when he was 13 and then his penny-farthing bicycles. As soon as safety bicycles became available in the second half of the 1880s, they, too, joined the family cycling trips, alongside the peat-brown water of the River Dodder, past its weirs and mills to Bushy Park and Templeogue. Or, going south over the valley towards their old house in Dundrum, where their mother had died, they crossed the cobbled surface of old Classon's Bridge. Here, they were told, bodies washed down the Dodder at the height of the famine in 1847 were wrapped in winding sheets at the inn before burial in a nearby mass grave.

Cycling for Ladies

Bicycles for both ladies and gentlemen could be obtained from Booth Brothers 63, Upper Stephen St., Dublin. Edith was 14 years old when the gearing paper was published, 16 when safety bicycles were introduced, and 19 by the time Gerald's book was published, with its chapter on 'Cycling for Ladies'. The male authors declared that 'It is with a feeling of awe and nervous dread that we approach the all-mysterious subject of dress'. Sensibly they recruited 'a lady cyclist of considerable experience' to help: could this have been Edith or Florence? She advised that 'A strong, cheap, rather coarse material is best' for the cycling costume and that:

> brown or grey heather mixtures will show the dust and oil stains less than anything else . . . . . for if one has to send a dress to be cleaned every time the oil stains become too perceptible round the end of the skirt it will cost a small fortune.

The undergarment should be wool, and a corset, if worn, should be loose. A woollen Tam-o'-shanter works well for headgear in the winter. Two short pieces of narrow elastic, clipped between the hem and the shows on each side, will keep the skirt in place in windy weather or when pedalling fast. Glycerine or vaseline, rubbed into the face, will prevent burning from the wind and sun: lemon juice and milk if the 'mischief has already been done'.

Edith loved cycling throughout her life. She was as fascinated by the engineering as from the enjoyment of riding and understood the advice to the lady cyclist that she should 'be sure to carry in your tool-bag wrenches to fit all the nuts, also oil, copper wire, a pneumatic repairing outfit, and some spare nuts'. By the time she left Dublin, she understood some of the physics: how the energy generated by the leg muscles was transformed to kinetic energy in the bicycle's movement. Later, Edith even followed her father's explanations of the forces that held her upright as she cycled along. She was stimulated by the exhilaration of the speed and the excitement of control. Above all, it was the freedom to be independent and to be confidently in charge with no artificial constraints on her actions, other than those from engineering design and natural forces. When they were on their bicycles, Edith and Florence were the equal of anyone.

Cycle rides gave them space and could be lengthened at weekends to reach the beach at Bray or the edge of the Wicklow Mountains, each within a dozen miles or so. Gerald's book also included a description of a mixed camping trip. The ladies tent was pitched 'round a convenient bend, where the undergrowth was thick', 150 yards from the gentlemen, and where it was understood that none of the male campers could go. There were six ladies, chaperoned by the wife of one of the gentlemen. After supper and singing round the camp fire, they retired at 11.30 pm, sleeping on clean straw with thick blankets for bedding. It does not matter whether the sisters went on this particular expedition. Their world included such weekend trips, and cycling was part of their lives.

There was, naturally, a male backlash to lady cyclists. A contemporary correspondent, writing to The Irish Times, pointed out that 'When cycling was first introduced, the male sex imagined that it was intended exclusively for their own enjoyment . . . . . . Their surprise and also indignation was great when they discovered that the weaker sex had encroached upon their lawful right'. He was replying to an earlier letter from a William Douglas who had written 'I have always used my influence to get young unmarried ladies to ride because it would give me a grand opportunity of flirting'. One is left feeling that if William had ridden up alongside the Stoney sisters, he might have finished up in the ditch [5].

Although Florence was a delicate child, cycling also allowed her to explore the area to gather insects and plants, which she could later examine at home under her microscope (Fig. 1.2). Her most likely reference book was *The Microscope, or Descriptions of Various Objects of Especial Interest and Beauty Adapted for Microscopic Observation* by the Irish scientist Mary Ward. This book had become extremely popular after it was first published in 1858, and by the time Florence was a teenager, it had reached its fifth edition [6]. From this book, Florence learned how to use her microscope, select a lens of the correct magnification, mount the specimen and illuminate the slide. Following the book's exquisitely detailed coloured illustrations, she observed the structure of the wings of earwigs, butterflies and moths, the scales of fish and insects, the structure of hairs and feathers and the detailed anatomies of the eyes of many creatures (Fig. 1.3). Biology was not a subject that her father was particularly familiar with, and so her knowledge must have been largely self-taught. Florence's best discussions about what she saw were with her brother Robert who, like her, was thinking of a future in medicine. One may

Fig. 1.2 Florence's Leitz 1a microscope (1888). The Leitz 1a microscope was a top-of-the range instrument at the time, with three eyepieces, four objective lenses and numerous attachments. The microscope box is marked J. Robinson & Sons Dublin, and it was bought second hand. The date and place suggests that it was used by Florence when she started her medical studies. Edith gave this microscope to her great-nephew Archie Stoney on her visit to Brisbane in 1934. (Frances Smith)

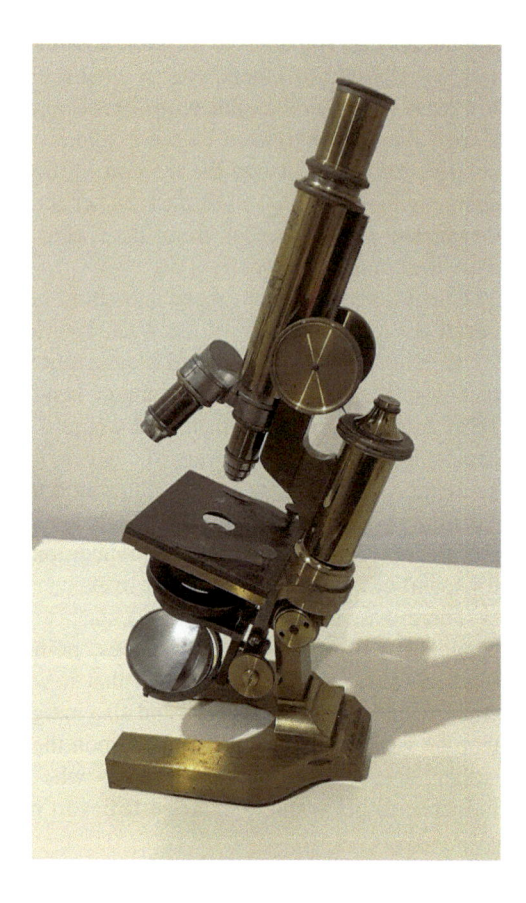

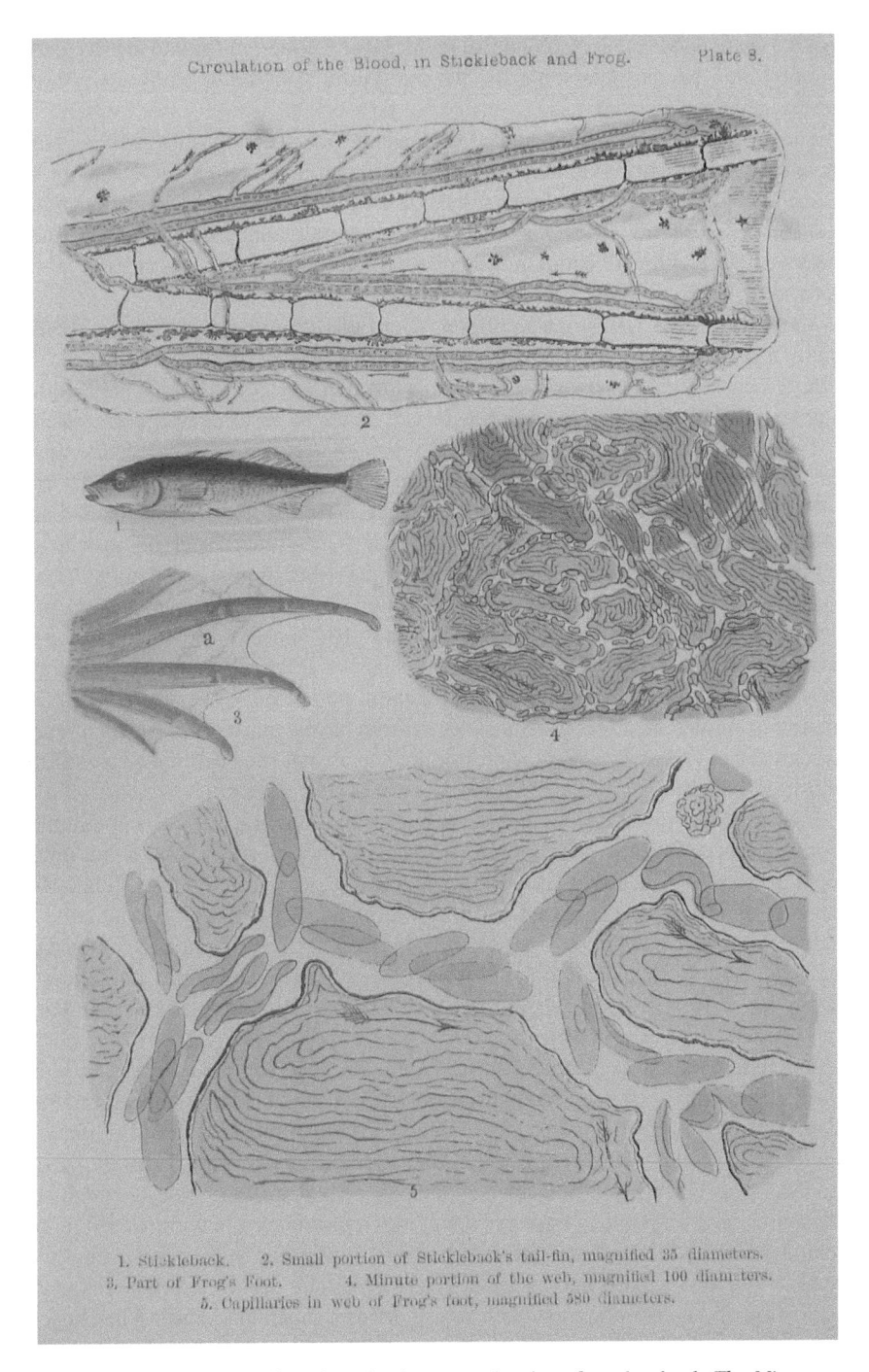

Fig. 1.3 One of Mary Ward's coloured microscope drawings from her book *The Microscope*, showing the circulation of the blood in a fish and a frog

imagine sister and brother catching fish in the River Dodder, or finding insects on the common land beyond Classon's Bridge and returning home to study then on the kitchen table.

The girls thus grew up surrounded by practical science. Not only did they learn bicycle mechanics from Gerald; they watched as he helped their father mount his 12-inch reflector telescope in their garden. On clear nights, he introduced them to the wonders of astronomy. They were introduced to photography, setting the exposures correctly and learning all about the chemistry of photographic processing [7]. It was that sort of family.

The youngest of Johnstone's children, Gertrude, was never going to make her future in science. But, like Edith, she had inherited another of her father's skills, an ability to draw. These two girls could go off together to sit quietly near the Dodder, to observe, draw and paint the tree-lined river, its weirs, its bridges and its wildlife.

Their mother had died in 1872, when they were very young. Their father never remarried, and so they were never challenged with the difficulty of sharing his love with a stepmother. The family moved from Dundrum to No 9 Palmerston Park, Rathmines in 1878.[1] It was a new, wide-fronted, three-storey, brick house with six bedrooms and two bathrooms, facing a quiet semicircular recreational park (Fig. 1.4). This new development had been built following the construction of a tramline that terminated round the corner from their house at the southern end of Palmerston Road, giving easy access to the centre of Dublin. The park itself is now enclosed, with a notice that says 'No ball games, no cycling', but when the Stoney family first moved in, it was possible to enter from the pavement opposite their house through the mixture of conifers and deciduous trees that screened their view of the recreational space beyond.

Johnstone was on a high enough salary to employ domestic staff, as was common in middle-class families at this time, so the cooking, cleaning, and some child-minding were looked after. The girls sometimes helped in the kitchen. Edith later remarked that their 'excellent cook could not read and had to get a small child to spell out a recipe from a book if needed' [8]. In an age before the internal combustion engine, the family coachman took the growing girls between the family residences in Rathmines and Ballsbridge, where Johnstone's brother Bindon lived on Elgin Road with his wife Frances and their cousins.

A severe setback was in store that, for their father, was the most distressing of his whole professional career. It also had a major impact on the family finances. In 1882, Queen's University, the organisation to which he had devoted much of his life, was closed. 'At a stroke of the pen, I beheld the labour of nearly thirty years of my life annulled' [9]. Edith placed the blame squarely on the Conservative Government, displaying her own political colours [10]. It was replaced by a new organisation, the Royal University. Their father continued to refer to himself as the 'late secretary of Queen's University' well into his older years, a measure of the affront he felt at the destruction of the institution to which he had devoted much of his life. When he left,

---

[1]The house was renumbered from No. 3 to No. 9 not long after they moved in.

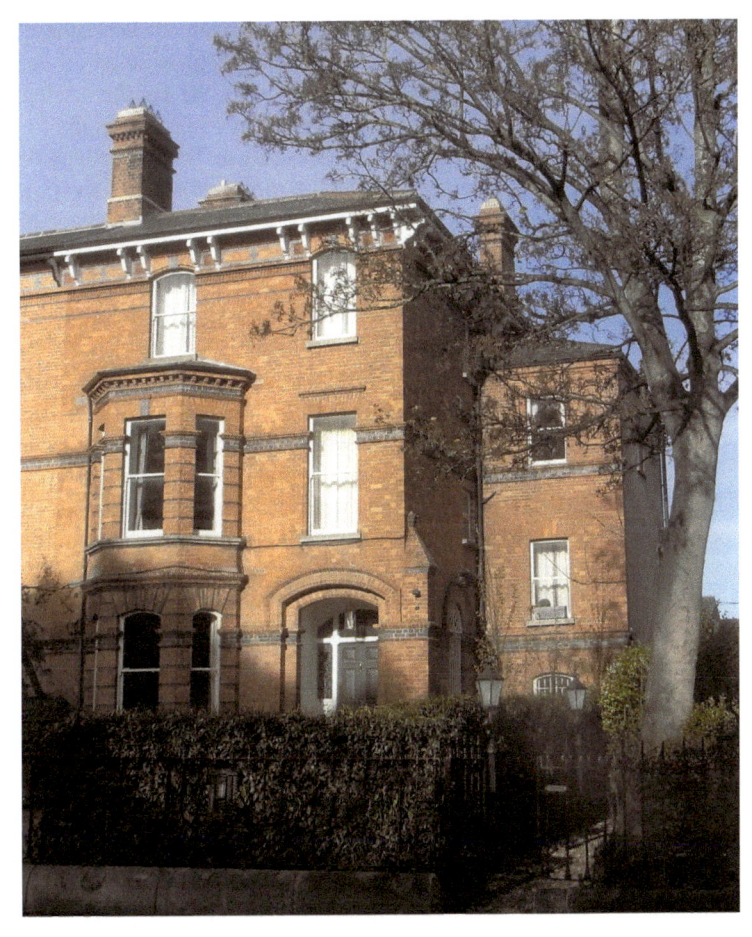

Fig. 1.4 9 Palmerston Park, Rathmines, the home of Johnstone Stoney and his family from 1878 to 1895

he was authorised to take with him many of the documents and papers relating to Queen's University, including the sealed charter signed by Queen Victoria on 3 September 1850. These artefacts stayed with him until his death, when they passed to his daughters. Greatly to his credit, Johnstone Stoney continued to make valuable contributions to the Royal University for several years through his experienced advice at Convocation meetings.[2]

His income, required to support the education of his growing family, reduced considerably. Nevertheless he retained his appointment as Superintendent of the Civil Service Examinations in Ireland, at a salary of £250 per annum.

---

[2]Queen's College Belfast remained independent of the Royal University and became Queen's University Belfast, which remains to this day.

The home education of Gerald and Robert was maintained. When he was only 13 years old, strictly too young to be eligible, Gerald registered as an occasional student at the Royal College of Science for Ireland (RCSI) for the academic year 1876/1877, taking a course in practical physics [11]. In 1882 he was the first of the siblings to start at university, gaining entrance to study at Trinity College. When he graduated with an engineering degree in 1888, he took first place in every group of subjects and gained three special certificates. For a year he worked for his uncle Bindon, who was by then chief engineer of the Dublin Port and Docks Board. He then moved to Northumberland to be apprenticed to Clarke Chapman and Co, commencing an extended association with the engineer and entrepreneur Charles Parsons, youngest son of Lord Rosse of Parsonstown.

Robert was always somewhat in Gerald's shadow. Moreover, he was not as fit as the others, having contracted tuberculosis during his youth.[3] When he entered Trinity College in July 1883, he boldly asserted his intellectual independence by declaring himself as an agnostic. His studies were put on hold when he emigrated to South Africa and then to Australia, arriving there in 1886 when he was 20. There was a link between Sydney University and Trinity College, which allowed him to complete his medical examinations back in Ireland during a brief 6-week visit in 1891 [12]. He did not stay in Ireland, however, and returned to Australia where he married and raised a family [13]. Later, both Gerald and Robert would re-enter the lives of their sisters.

Early Education

After 1882, when he lost his post at Queen's University, their father had time to devote more attention to the upbringing and education of his children. The date is important: Edith, Florence and Gertrude were, respectively, 13, 12 and 11 years of age. His educational ideas were well formed, and he applied his concept of a broad liberal education to his children. He chose not to send his daughters to Alexandra College, a girl's school that was established just before Edith was born [14], and instead decided to have his daughters educated at home, as he had arranged for Gerald and Robert, probably under the general supervision of a governess.

Johnstone's three daughters grew up in this middle-class social environment. Educational expectations for girls at this time included basic literacy and numeracy, with special skills in art, musical appreciation and needlework, supported by some knowledge of modern languages and history. However, educated at home as they were, they were buffered from the social pressures to conform to this norm.

Once the family had settled in Palmerston Park, Edith commenced classes at the Metropolitan College of Art in order to extend her home education. This was the new

---

[3]Tuberculosis often ran in families, and at least one of their cousins also died of the disease. This was before the days of contact tracing.

name given to the Royal Dublin Society's School of Drawing when it was taken over by the Science and Art Department in South Kensington, London in 1877. Her father had led the delegation that had proposed this development, which gave government support to an institution previously dependent on public donation. It was always open to both male and female students. There, Edith attended classes in geometry and perspective, as well as in freehand drawing, modelling and architectural drawing. She continued to attend these classes from the age of 13 until she was 19 [15]. All three sisters attended the prize giving on 9 January 1886 when Edith was presented by the Countess of Carnarvon with one of the third-grade prizes for work sent for examination to South Kensington. Her father took an active part in the proceedings, giving a short speech and recounting how the origins of the College of Art made it the oldest in the United Kingdom.

Edith got her prize for a picture of a foot. Such depictions were a normal part of art training, incorporating draughtsmanship, surface anatomy and antiquity into a single work. It must have been drawn to a very high standard, but it was still only a foot and a cast of a foot at that [16]. It was a safe but uncreative selection, an allegory for Edith's character, seeking perfection in detail, not too concerned with the whole. It also suggests the tension that may be seen throughout her life, a tendency to aim for perfection within each comfort zone, followed by abrupt, insecure, leaps into the unknown. This transition was imminent.

Edith enjoyed Art College. For the next couple of years, she took her youngest sister Gertrude along, and, when Edith left, Gertrude continued to study art until her final departure from Dublin 7 years later. She had greater skill as an artist than her older sister, later making some fine portraits of her father. A newspaper report noted that her chalk drawing from life of the head of a child was 'extremely natural and spirited'. Edith's precisely accurate depiction of the cast of a foot was not in the same league.

Music was also part of every young woman's rounded education, although there is no evidence that they had any particular musical talent. Much later, Edith referred scathingly to 'the strumming of a piano by every girl however unmusical' [8]. This was before the days of readily available recorded music. If you wanted music at home, you made it yourself. But they could take advantage of their father's interest in music and acoustics, accompanying him to the chamber concerts that he initiated at the Royal Dublin Society. It is surely not a coincidence that his four papers about music and the piano were published at exactly this time [17].

Dublin was an intellectually stimulating and vibrant city in which to grow up. The literary environment nurtured W B Yeats and James Joyce. Many wives and daughters amongst the intelligentsia of Dublin society attended the wide spectrum of public lectures and exhibitions that were on offer. The Stoney family were no exception. One family letter mentions their grandmother making a visit to view 'The Death of Chatterton', an oil painting by Henry Wallis, when it was exhibited in Dublin in 1859 [18]. By the time the sisters were growing into adulthood, scientific and technological interests were also being catered for. The Dublin Mechanics Institution members had 'power to introduce a lady' to free lectures on a wide range of scientific topics. Public lectures, open to all, were also given at the Royal

Dublin Society, where they might have listened to Dr. Kane speaking about the steam engine, rural philosophy or sources of industry in Ireland.

The world of science brought to them through their charismatic and caring father was obviously influential in opening their eyes to careers in medicine and science, but it was far from inevitable that this would be their life. Their uncle Bindon's three daughters showed no such tendencies. Bindon had a similar upbringing, education and early career to their father and was, by this time, the Chief Engineer for the Port of Dublin, a position of considerable status and responsibility. Like their father, he married late, in 1879 when he was over 50, and to a much younger woman, Frances Walker. They lived not far away so the families had the opportunity to see quite a lot of one another. But none of his three daughters, Priscilla, Anne and Laura, went on to higher education. The society in which they lived expected them to find an eligible husband with prospects, from a suitable family, and all three followed this convention.

The expectation to find a good husband was not as strong in Johnstone's family as it was in uncle Bindon's. Without a mother in their home, there was no maternal role model through which to imagine their own future. A modern equivalent of having Johnstone Stoney as a father would be as the daughter of a physicist who was contributing to the study of quantum gravity and the meaning of time, who at the same time could make deep concepts accessible and had a very broad view of education. In the 1880s he could only tell them about what was later known as classical physics, even though he himself was beginning to see beyond it. He could describe stars in nebulae but not black holes or the big bang. He was exploring electrons in atoms but knew nothing of their free existence or of atomic structure. He could explain that light could be understood as electromagnetic radiation, without having to add that it could also behave as quanta of energy. He was able to tell his daughters how to follow the flow of energy starting from the sun, transported by radiation, to be trapped as chemical energy in plants, to be later released as heat and work in their own muscles. Heat was, he told them in the words of his compatriot John Tyndall, 'a mode of motion'. When they asked about the source of the sun's energy, he told them that Lord Kelvin said that came from meteorites crashing into the surface, releasing their kinetic energy as radiation. Understanding thermonuclear reactions was decades away. But, deeply knowledgeable about spectroscopy, he may have speculated about the origin of the lines in the sun's spectrum indicating an unknown substance they called helium, which would later become part of the story of radioactivity. He insisted on using his own physicists' word ultraviolet, and not the chemists' term actinic, for radiation beyond the blue end of the optical spectrum. He could tell them nothing about X-rays, yet to be discovered, which would play such a key role in the lives of both the sisters.

During their formative teenage years, their father was developing his own philosophy of the unity of the universe. He presented one of his ideas at a lecture that he had been invited to give at the Royal Institution in London on 6 February 1885. He gave it the title, 'How thought presents itself among the phenomena of nature'. The only record of this lecture lies in an unattributed abstract [19]. Unlike most of his work, this was never fully published, mentioned only in his later, fuller, paper on metaphysics.

This idea lasted in their minds long after he died. In her later years, Florence recalled this work, intrigued by his thesis that thought arose from 'motions' [20]. Her strong recall suggests she knew about it by being there, sitting in the steeply tiered wooden seats in the historic lecture theatre in Albemarle Street. Her father's hypothesis was that motions existing in nature were also the underlying mechanism of human thought. The first sentence sets the theme: 'Every phenomenon which a human being can perceive may be traced by scientific investigation to motions going on in the world around him'. He remained unspecific as to what was in motion, mentioning as examples sound and electromagnetic waves and the random motion of molecules. It may be remembered, however, that he had already postulated a unit of electricity on the basis of its motion during electrolysis, and he had worked on the spectra of light, postulating that it was emitted from molecules in vibration. He was convinced that what happened in the living brain was fundamentally no different from what happened in the rest of the universe and controlled by the same set of fundamental laws of nature. More, he linked the external world to the processes of thought through a necessary, though complex, series of cause and effect, from external world though our senses and nerves to our thoughts. There was no need or possibility for an independent 'vital force' that was unconstrained by natural laws. He even extended his thesis to imply the existence of subconscious as well as conscious thoughts, his 'motions' occurring naturally throughout all areas of the brain. So general was his conception of the equivalence of the motion of all matter and thought that he extended the principle to say that the external cause whose final effect was our thought was also thought itself. Whilst this metaphysical/theological idea allowed him to reject harsh, atheistic Victorian materialism, it is not one that could be sustained as the biophysical and biochemical basis for neuronal action became clearer.

Johnstone eventually developed his metaphysical ideas in a long paper read to the Royal Dublin Society in 1890 [21]. He declared that he intended to find out 'in what way the scientific study of nature is related to the actual existences and events of the universe'. He concluded that natural science can only reach what he called shadow laws and that 'the real laws of the universe of which these are shadows are beyond its grasp'. Finding himself at the edge of knowledge, he wrote 'If Nature, the mere shadow, is wonderful past all searching out, WHAT MUST THE GREAT ORIGINAL BE!' (His capitals). His ideas were discounted at the time, but the sisters remained true to his underlying ideas throughout their lives. Recalling her father's metaphysics in an interview in 1934, Edith said 'He really forestalled the work that Sir James Jeans is doing on what we might call the Great Mind of the Universe, but he never wrote in a popular form'[22]. Jeans was a mathematician and astronomer with agnostic views, who strongly opposed Victorian materialism and considered that mind and matter, if not proved to be of similar nature, are at least ingredients of one single system.

Today, the action of the brain is understood in terms of an unbelievably complex interconnecting electrical and chemical network, operating through the controlled flux of charged ions through ion channels and activating biomolecular agents. 'Everything we think, feel and do is governed by electrical and chemical events taking place in our nerve cells' [23]. As Johnstone Stoney told his audience at the Royal Institution that Friday night in 1885, as his daughter Florence repeated to her nephew when she wrote to him in 1922 and as today's neurophysiologists believe, thoughts really are formed from motions.

The sisters were surrounded by Fellows of the Royal Society: their father and uncle Bindon were Fellows, as was their cousin George FitzGerald. George and his brother Maurice were nearly 20 years older than they were. George was by this time Fellow of Trinity College and was becoming a leading member of the British physics community. In 1883, they heard about his latest work. FitzGerald was one of the few men who could understand the mathematics of James Clerk Maxwell's theories of electromagnetism. He had already informed the Royal Dublin Society, in 1880, of his prediction that waves could be generated by electric forces [24]. In August 1883, he described to his colleagues at the meeting of the British Association in Southport how an oscillating current through a resistance might produce electromagnetic waves 'of as little as 10 metres wave-length, or even less' [25]. As his predictions of radio waves matured from the first demonstrations by Hertz and Lodge 6 years later, through Marconi's first wireless communication across the Atlantic in 1901, to the emergence of broadcast radio and even television before they died, it must have been a huge pleasure to recall being there at the start of it all. George FitzGerald is better known for his conjecture that if all moving objects were foreshortened in the direction of their motion, it would account for the null result of the Michelson-Morley experiment. The FitzGerald-Lorentz contraction was a precursor for Einstein's special theory of relativity. He also shared with his uncle an interest in the applications of physics to medicine. From 1885 until his early death in 1901, he gave the physics lectures to medical students at Dublin University. He was one of many who tried and failed to give a purely physical explanation for muscular contraction: his was based upon surface tension [26]. It would be decades before a biomolecular explanation based on the interaction between myosin and actin emerged.

This scientific excellence throughout the Stoney family was achieved through a combination of expectation, ability, determination and confidence. Edith and Florence were endowed with all four and were on a par with the other achievers within their family.

A Career in Medicine

Yet the options for educated women were narrow. The traditional life was to marry, for which an endowment and an education were advantages, but not mandatory. This had been their grandmother's life. It also carried the hazard of childbirth, as they knew only too well. Another option was to be the family carer: their aunt Kate's life. Alternatively, an educated unmarried woman from a middle-class family could find employment as a governess, in nursing or as a teacher, depending on their education, inclination or circumstance.

By the time that the young women were planning their future, a new opportunity had emerged: to become a doctor. Several of their male uncles and cousins were doctors, particularly through their mother's side of the Stoney family, including uncles Charles and Hugh and cousins Richard and George. The Medical Act of 1858 had excluded from medical practice any who had not undergone approved courses of training and obtained qualifications to practice. Laudable in aim, a side effect had been to exclude women, since both the medical schools offering training and the medical colleges licensing practice were open only to men. Unknown to Edith and Florence, changes were occurring in the 1870s that would open doors closed to those born earlier. A timetable of some events in the Stoney family set against events affecting women's general and medical education is shown in Table 1.1. The first chink had occurred in 1865, before either of the sisters was born. On 28 September, Elizabeth Garrett had passed the examinations of the Society of Apothecaries to become the first British woman Licentiate of the Society. The following year her name was added to the Medical Register, eligible to practice medicine.[4] The Universities of Bern, Geneva and Paris were the first to open their academic doors to women students, and Elizabeth Garrett became the first woman to graduate from Paris with a medical degree in 1870. Other pioneering British women such as Sophia Jex-Blake followed. Nevertheless, the British medical colleges such as the Royal College of Surgeons in London held that a foreign degree was not equivalent and that, as was the case for men, this did not allow licence to practice in Britain.

Not all medical colleges were so stubborn, and the tide was turning. The first institution to allow women who were educated abroad to take their licensing examination was the King and Queen's College of Physicians in Ireland. Thirty years later, when Florence found out that she was still not permitted, as a woman, to sit for the London College of Physicians membership examination, her father told her that he had supported this earlier change in Irish medical practice.[5] On 10 January 1877, Eliza Louisa Walker Dunbar (Zurich 1872) became the first woman to qualify with a medical licence from a medical academic institution in the United Kingdom [27]. Four more, including Sophia Jex-Blake, followed that year and four more the next.

The legislation that changed things had been passed on 11 August 1876. Edith was 7 and Florence was 6. The Medical Act prohibited the exclusion of women from

---

[4]The first woman Licentiate of the Society of Apothecaries was the American Elizabeth Blackwell, whose name was entered on the Medical Register in 1859.

[5]The Dictionary of National Biography 1912 supplement entry for G Johnstone Stoney states 'it was mainly through his exertions that women obtained legal medical qualifications in Ireland before they were able in England or Scotland'. Florence Stoney's obituary in 'The Vote' says 'His position as Secretary of the old Queen's University of Ireland gave him the opportunity to press his views, and through his influence, the first medical licence was opened to women'. Nevertheless, the King and Queen's College records do not mention Stoney's involvement, so his influence seems to have been indirect.

Table 1.1 A timetable of some events in the Stoney family set against selected events affecting women's general and medical education

Year	Some relevant events in the education of women	Selected Stoney family events
1864	Cambridge local higher examinations opened to women	
1865	Elizabeth Garrett admitted as a Licentiate of the Society of Apothecaries, so eligible to practice medicine	
1866	Alexandra College, Dublin, founded	
1867	Royal College of Science for Ireland opens, continuing the acceptance of women inherited from the Museum of Irish Industry	
1868	University of London admits women	
1869	Trinity College Dublin allows women to attend	Edith Stoney born
1870		Florence Stoney born
1872		Sophia Stoney dies
1875	Newnham Hall, Cambridge opens	
1874	London School of Medicine for Women opens	
1876	The Medical Act prohibits exclusion of women from universities and medical schools	
1877	First women licentiates of the King and Queen's College of Physicians of Ireland	
1877	Metropolitan School of Art formed	
1878	University of London conceded degrees to women	Stoney family move to 9 Palmerston Park
1881	Cambridge University allows women to be admitted to the Tripos examinations London University awards first Bachelor of Science degrees to women	
1882	Royal University of Ireland opens, allowing access to women	Edith commences classes at the Metropolitan School of Art Dublin, until 1888
1883	Women admitted to lectures at Owens College Manchester	
1888	First woman admitted to Queen's Belfast Medical School	
1889		Edith and Florence attend courses at the Royal College for Science for Ireland: Gain first class in Cambridge Higher Examinations
1890		Edith enters Newnham College Cambridge
1891		Florence enters London School of Medicine for Women, London
1897	Women graduated from Victoria University (Leeds, Manchester and Liverpool) except in engineering and medicine	

(continued)

Table 1.1 (continued)

Year	Some relevant events in the education of women	Selected Stoney family events
1898		Florence awarded MD from LSMW
1904	Trinity College Dublin allows women to graduate	Edith awarded BA and MA from Dublin
1910	First women licentiate of the Royal College of Physicians, London	
1948	Cambridge University allows women to graduate	

medical courses at universities and medical schools. During the subsequent decade, by slow degrees, opportunities emerged that would allow career planning for young women with ability to include medicine as an option, knowing that pioneering women such as Jex-Blake and Elizabeth Garrett-Anderson had pushed the door ajar. It did not swing open quickly. It was another 10 years before the Royal College of Surgeons of Dublin admitted women and 1910 before the Royal College of Physicians in London accepted its first women licentiate.

Before reaching that hurdle, any aspiring woman doctor had to gain access to training at university level in order to be awarded a medical degree or to satisfy the requirements for application to one of the medical colleges. Trinity College Dublin, the natural option for all the bright (and not so bright) boys of middle-class Irish families, did not graduate women students until 1904. Attendance at lectures was open to the sisters, since Trinity College had opened its doors to women students in 1869, but the University only awarded a certificate, not a degree, to successful women examinees. This was of no use to a woman with serious aspirations, and only a few young women used this means of higher education. As early as 1874, their father had been part of a deputation to the Lord Lieutenant, encouraging the government to commit more funds for the higher education of women but without success [28]. The three Colleges of Queen's University, at Cork, Galway and Belfast, did not award degrees to women either until, in 1882, they came under the regulations of the Royal University.

This did not prevent women, in principle, from attending lectures, however. In 1876, just after the Medical Act was passed, Johnstone Stoney received a letter from Mary Edith Pechey, addressed to the Senate of Queen's University, requesting permission to take examinations for the MD degree. This was not the first time that Miss Pechey had written on the same topic. In 1873, following an earlier application, the senate, split on the matter, sought legal opinion and was advised to reject the application. Now that the Medical Act had been passed, senate approved her application and advised her to approach the colleges to gain entry. Her letter to Queen's College Galway asked permission to attend four classes in order to comply with the regulations for attendance. She even offered to pay to cover any additional costs if the classes had to be spilt into two, one male and the other female. Queen's College Galway responded that it could foresee 'such grave difficulties' in admitting women to the college that they 'declined to avail themselves of the act'. Senate decided not to interfere. Replies from Cork and Belfast were similar. Belfast's first woman medical student was finally admitted in 1888, Cork's in 1890 and Galway's, eventually, in 1902. Thus, when Florence, and perhaps Edith too, was considering how to enter medical training in the 1880s, the opportunities for doing so in Ireland were very narrow.

Johnstone Stoney had taken a strong interest in medical education. In particular he was concerned that the Queen's University medical curriculum was too specialised and proposed that parts of the B.A. degree course should be merged so that medical studies became part of a more liberal education. He set out his views in a memorandum placed before the Senate of Queen's University in May 1874 [29]. Of particular interest here is his proposal that

> 'physics and chemistry—sciences which admit of direct application in medical practice—are abundantly provided for in the present scheme. Fortunately these studies are not only of constant use to the practicing physician, but stand in a different educational category from his other professional studies, and are therefore admirably suited to help to render his education liberal'.

Even before he came to Dublin, when he was still Professor of Natural Philosophy at Queen's College Galway, he had set MD students questions in their Natural Philosophy examinations such as 'Point out why, if there be an enlargement on a blood-vessel, there is more pressure there tending to burst it than elsewhere' and 'By what experiment may it be shown that the eye is blind at the *punctum coecum*?' [30].

Their father's view of the place of the basic sciences in medical education was more aligned with practice in continental Europe at that time than in the rest of Britain or indeed in the United States. At the time that Stoney was preparing this memorandum, Jean Gavarret, Professor of Physics at the Faculty of Medicine in Paris, had already published his monograph '*Les phénomènes physiologiques de la vie*' exploring the application of the new principle conservation of energy to physiological processes [31]. However laudable was Stoney's view, he understood that there was not enough time in the students' timetable to include everything, so some part of the curriculum would have to be curtailed. In his view '*Materia Medica*'[6] consists of a vast accumulation of particulars with but little connexion that the mind can lay hold of', so 'from an educational point of view, it is a study which it is desirable to minimize'. He failed to appreciate that medical training set authority and accumulated knowledge more highly than analysis and investigation. Not surprisingly, senate did not accept his plan.

---

[6]Materia medica refers to the body of knowledge and beliefs about the therapeutic properties of all substances used to treat illnesses and ailments.

Examination Failure and Success

By 1887, Florence and Edith may both have been thinking about becoming doctors. If they were to embark on a career in medicine, they had to bring themselves up to a sufficient standard to expect to gain high marks in any entrance examination for a university place. The first step in this direction was to prepare for the Cambridge Higher Local Examinations. These examinations had been established in the 1850s for young women 18 years or older who wished to establish their academic ability and perhaps apply for higher education in a college or university. Although the Cambridge Highers had been opened to men in 1873, the candidates remained predominantly female, and by 1889 only 3% of the 898 candidates were male. The examinations were held in a number of centres around the United Kingdom, in December and June each year.

There was, though, a question of cost. The fee to enter for the first time was 40 shillings. If this resulted in a pass in arithmetic or in any three in one group of subjects such as languages, natural sciences or classics, any subsequent entry fee was reduced to 20 shillings. It was quite common for candidates to spread out their examinations over several sittings, gaining experience, resitting following failure to pass or from a wish to gain a higher mark. The official emphasis on arithmetic needs comment. A priority was placed on girls' ability to calculate, in order that they could manage their own domestic and financial affairs. In this Victorian capitalist age, control lay in the hands of those who managed money, and it was a deliberate objective of the early suffrage movement to give girls necessary skills in budget management. The arithmetic examination was intended to examine numeracy, testing whether the candidate could calculate accurately and quickly.

Once Edith had reached her 18th birthday, her father agreed that she could have a go at the examination to see how she got on. There was no arrangement to take the Cambridge Higher examinations in Dublin, so, in December 1887, she set off on the 8-hour crossing by ferry to Liverpool. As she left Dublin's deepwater port, she passed the huge quay walls, built of 300 ton concrete blocks, that formed the northern boundary of the tidal basin. She was inspired by the thought that her uncle Bindon had designed most of the new quays she passed, contributing to the growth of the port that now handled almost 2 million tonnes of shipping each year. Could a woman do as much?

The arithmetic examination was a short, 2-hour test of practical numeracy. It included questions such as 'If 4.80 dollars exchange for £1, how many articles of which 13 cost £28. 16s. 10½d. can be bought for 213 dollars?' and 'How much must be invested in 2¾ per cents. stock at 96¾ to produce an income of £550 a year ?' [32]. These questions, easy in principle, were made deliberately difficult by the selection of the numeric values. In another question the candidate was required to either know, or to work out, the cube root of 1.331.[7]

---

[7] The cube root of 1.331 is 1.1.

Edith failed. She was one of the 16 out of 57 who did so at this examination. Somehow her preparation had been quite insufficient to reach the expected standard. Was this because she thought she could sail through without study? Or was their German governess simply not up to the job?[8] If her aspirations were not to be thwarted, then she needed to learn from her experience and try again. Undaunted, she paid a further 40 shillings fee and took the boat to England again the following June, this time sitting the examinations in Manchester. To her relief the results were a bit better, an outcome that gave her confidence that, if she worked, success should follow. It wasn't wonderful though: she passed in arithmetic, chemistry and botany, but the aggregated score in these Group C subjects only gave her a third-class grade. She still needed to work harder, study more deeply and do better, if she had any chance of getting in to any form of higher education. Her selection of subjects, omitting physics, suggests that she was still considering medicine at this stage. At least further examination entries would only cost 20 shillings a time.

In December, Florence took her first examinations, travelling with her now experienced sister to Manchester. Like Edith the previous year, she took arithmetic. Like her sister, she failed. Florence took German also, which she passed. Edith went on to improve her mark in mathematics, at last demonstrating where her true ability lay. She really was not interested in the difficult sums that had constituted the rather pedantic arithmetic paper but give her a few mathematical puzzles, and she was in her element. The mathematics papers were spread over 4 days. The questions were broadly similar to those set for modern advanced level mathematics papers, although the examinations themselves were longer. The first, a 2-hour examination on 'Differential and Integral Calculus' on Monday 17 December, was followed by 3-hours on Tuesday on 'Statics, Astronomy and Dynamics', a 3-hour examination on 'Algebra and Trigonometry' on Wednesday afternoon and the following morning by 14 questions on 'Euclid and Conic Sections'. Edith gained a distinction.

If they were to enter medicine, however, they also needed to demonstrate excellence in botany and biology. Women were permitted to study at the Royal College of Science for Ireland (RCSI), a principle that had been established from its founding in 1867. The RCSI, in St. Stephen's Green, was the first higher education college in Britain to admit women as students to its courses, laboratories and examinations. Edith and Florence registered together as occasional students on 8 April 1889 to attend two laboratory courses, special biology and special botany. The record of attendance is identical for both sisters, and they stopped before the end of term, attending only 12 of the 20 biology sessions and slightly more for botany. Their purpose was a form of revision before taking the Cambridge Higher Examinations in June. Florence went back 2 years later, registering for laboratory courses in zoology and physics as she prepared herself to sit the London Matriculation and preliminary science examinations, requirements for entry to the London School of Medicine for Women [33].

---

[8]The 'German governess' is a plausible invention. That Johnstone Stoney employed a governess to look after the education of his three daughters is highly likely, in line with common practice in many middle-class families at the time. That she was German is suggested by the successful entry of both Florence and Gertrude in the Cambridge Local German examination.

Attendance by women at the RCSI was allowed, but the evidence suggests that relatively few young women were taking advantage of the educational possibilities that this offered. Women attendees at the Museum of Irish Industry, the RCSI precursor, have been estimated as about 15% of the total [34]. This level of attendance was not sustained. The register of associate (full-time) students for the period 1867/1868 up to 1904/1905 lists only eight who can be definitely identified as women. Amongst the occasional (part-time) students, there were more, but still only accounting for about 5% of the total. Undated photographs of the laboratories and lecture theatres from the beginning of the twentieth century tell a similar story. There are only 2 women in a physics class of 28, 2 out of 26 in a mechanics laboratory and only one in the physics laboratory accompanied by 26 young men. Many of the students were also studying medicine, adding courses in the basic sciences to underpin those in clinical medicine, and a higher proportion of women appear in, for example, the photograph of the advanced zoology laboratory. Nevertheless, higher education in the sciences for women was still to take hold in the minds of the majority [35].

The summer Cambridge Higher Local Examinations commenced on Monday 17 June 1889, and once again both Edith and Florence went to Manchester to sit them. They had encouraged one another, tested one another's knowledge and revised together and now understood what was required of them. This time they excelled. Within a year they had transformed their examination performance. Edith's marks were much better than the previous year, outstanding even. Those for Florence equalled those of her sister revealing herself to be a talented academic student, a confident scientist of considerable ability. Both emerged as being amongst the most able young women in science of the whole nation. Only 22 women took the natural sciences group of subjects that year. A mere six were awarded firsts, and this number included both Edith and Florence. There were no other firsts awarded to Irish women candidates in any subject. Florence was the youngest of the six. Edith passed chemistry and botany again, presumably with higher marks this time, and gained distinctions in a general studies 'elementary' paper and, notably, in physics. Florence passed in arithmetic, chemistry and the elementary paper and gained a distinction in botany. Florence added a further success the following year, sitting the mathematics examination again and gaining a first, an action suggesting that she was considering following her elder sister into academic rather than vocational higher education [36]. Young Gertrude also took the examinations in 1889, passing in German and gaining a third class in the languages group of subjects [37].

The sisters had made their first important step towards their careers. Stopping for a moment, we can judge whether this made success inevitable, by considering what happened to the other four women, their peer group who also gained firsts in the Cambridge Highers in Natural Science that year. Did their lives, too, continue to shine brightly? Two, Annie Armstrong and Mary Millard, became schoolteachers. Helen Bowers became a nurse. Mary Williamson remained without a career, identified in 1901 as the partner of Bertha Martinvale, the head of a small school in Weston-super-Mare. One, Mary Millard, eventually married. These outcomes give a fair sampling of the actual lives of promising young women scientists of their times.

Fig. 1.5 Edith Stoney c. 1893. Werner & Son, 39 Grafton St, Dublin. (Newnham College, Cambridge)

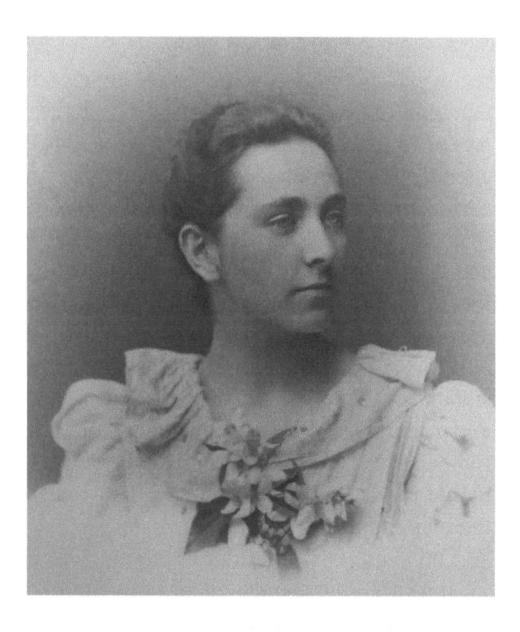

Fig. 1.6 Florence Stoney as a medical student

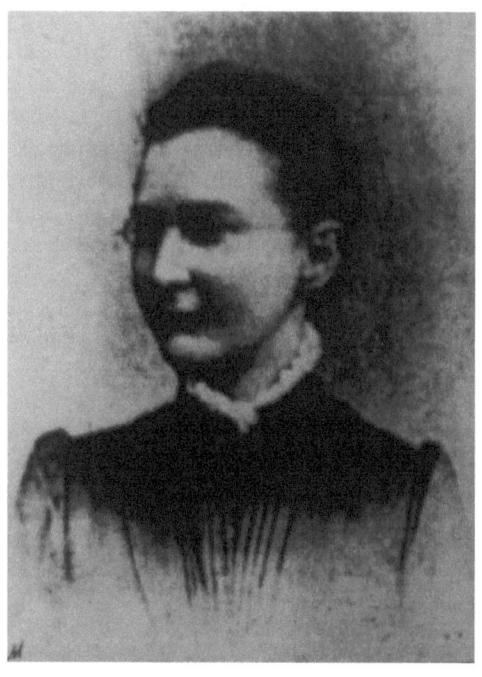

Emerging into Dublin society, all three sisters were admitted as associates of the Royal Dublin Society once the examination results were announced. Photographs of them as young women show them modestly dressed, earnest, serious and calm (Figs. 1.5, 1.6, and 1.7).

Fig. 1.7 Gertrude Stoney as a young woman (Claire Keohane)

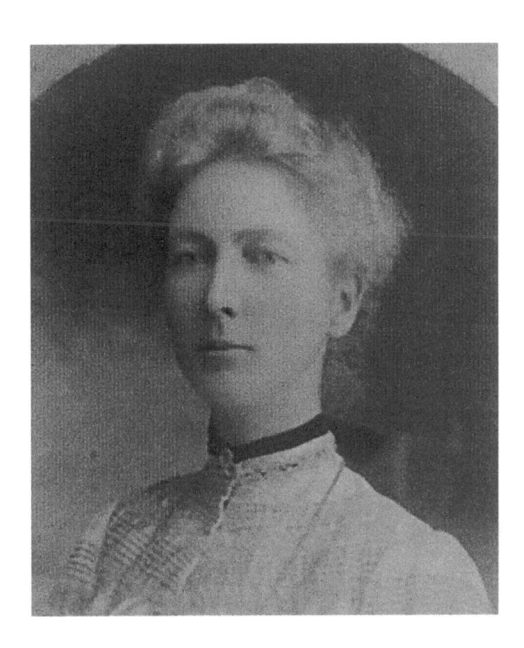

Ten years later, in a commentary on the opening to women of the Catholic University Medical School in Dublin, comparison was made between acceptance of women doctors to that of lady cyclists:

> A very little time ago the sight of a lady on a bicycle caused not only surprise but consternation, and drew all eyes and all tongues on the fair rider. How a few short years have changed all this! How thoroughly we have been accustomed to, and how warmly we approve of, the lady cyclists. So it is with other departures. In like manner, though perhaps with not such striking rapidity, our views have changed on the subject of professions for women. Twenty years ago well educated and well-to-do young girls never dreamt of a profession, or if they did they were looked on in amazement by all their friends, and worried until the idea was shamed out of their heads. In those days a lady doctor was a dreadful anomaly, a thing almost unheard of, and to be avoided. Again, how all of this, too, is changed. How many fair and gentle and womanly women—as well, no doubt, those of the more stern and manly type—may now be found in these countries amongst the ranks of the medical profession! [38]

Lives turn on small events. There was little to separate the abilities and examination performance of these two brilliant sisters. Had Edith gained a distinction in biology like her sister, perhaps she would have become a doctor. Florence's distinction in mathematics could have led to high academic honours in the Cambridge Maths Tripos. Family expectations and educational opportunities had formed the vigorous springboard that had launched Edith and Florence Stoney into their new lives. On a minor difference in one examination, their lives separated, yet they remained bonded forever.

References

1. Mecredy RJ, Stoney G. The art and pastime of cycling. Dublin: Irish Cyclist and Athlete; 1888.
2. The art and pastime of cycling. The Irish Times. 1888 Sept 20.
3. Stoney GJ, Stoney GG. On the energy expended in propelling a bicycle. Trans R Dublin Soc (Ser 2). 1883;1:307–17.
4. Stoney GJ, Stoney GG. On gearing for bicycles and tricycles. Proc R Dublin Soc. 1885;4:20–4.
5. 'Charlie'. Should ladies cycle?. The Irish Times. 1892 Mar 26.
6. The Hon Mrs Ward. The microscope or descriptions of various objects of especial interest and beauty adapted for microscopic observation. 5th ed. London: Groombridge; 1880.. (First published 1858)
7. Dowson R. George Gerald Stoney 1863–1942. Biogr Mem Fellows R Soc. 1942;4(11):283–196.
8. Stoney EA. Thermometers and heat-control in domestic appliances. Women Eng. 1931;3(7):111–2.
9. J.J. (John Joly). George Johnstone Stoney, 1826–1911. Obituary notices of fellows deceased. Proc Roy Soc Lond. 1911;A86:xx–xxxv.
10. Stoney EA. Newnham College Letter. 1904. p. 37–43.
11. Royal College of Science for Ireland, Register of occasional students 1876/7. Archives of University College Dublin.
12. A.J. Stoney interviewed by Edith McKinnon. AS. p. 180.
13. AS. Personal communication.
14. O'Connor AV, Parkes SM. Gladly learn and gladly teach Alexandra College and School 1866–1966. Dublin: Blackwater Press; 1966.
15. Dublin Metropolitan School of Art. College Student Registers. www.nival.ie.
16. Metropolitan School of Art. Dublin Daily Express. 1886 Jan 11.
17. These include 'On musical shorthand' (1882) and 'On equal temperament, and on the cause of the effect of piano music produced by the key in which it is set' (1883).
18. Letter from Charles Stoney to his mother. Undated c.1859. CK.
19. Stoney GJ. How thought presents itself among the phenomena of nature. Nature. 1885 Mar 5:422 and 1885 Apr 9:529.
20. Letter from Florence Stoney to Archie Stoney. 1922 Apr 4. AS.
21. Stoney GJ. Studies on ontology, from the standpoint of the scientific student of nature. Sci Proc R Dublin Soc. 1890;6:475–524.
22. Miss Edith A. Stoney. Melbourne Argus. 1934 Jan 17:15.
23. Ashcroft F. The spark of life, electricity in the human body. London: Penguin; 2013. p. 256.
24. FitzGerald GF. On the possibility of originating wave disturbances in the ether by means of electric forces. Trans R Dublin Soc (Ser 3). 1880 Feb;1 and 1880 Nov.
25. FitzGerald. On a method of producing electro-magnetic disturbances of comparatively short wave-length. Report of the 53rd meeting of the BAAS. 1893. p. 405.
26. FitzGerald GF. On the superficial tension of fluids and its possible relation to muscular contractions. Trans R Dublin Soc Ser 2. 1878 Dec;1:95–9.
27. Kelly L. 'The turning point in the whole struggle': the admission of women to the King and Queen's College of Physicians in Ireland. Women's Hist Rev. 2013;22:97–125.
28. The higher education of women. The Freeman's Journal. 1874 Dec 15.
29. Stoney GJ. Memorandum on the Medical Curriculum of the Queen's University. May 5 1874. The Queen's University of Belfast Archive. QUB/2/1/12/3(5).
30. Science papers set by Professor Stoney for BA, MA, Civil Engineering and Agriculture in the Years 1855 and 1856. Natural Philosophy Honors M.D. Adrian Ryder. An Irishman of Note George Johnstone Stoney. Appendix I. 2012. Private publication.
31. Duck FA. Physicists and Physicians: a history of medical physics from the renaissance to Röntgen. York: Institute of Physics and Engineering in Medicine. p. 203.

References

32. Cambridge Local Higher Examinations: Group C: Arithmetic. 1888 Dec 18. Cambridge: Cambridge Assessment Archives.
33. RSCI register of Occasional Students for 1888/89 and 1890/91. University College Dublin Archive.
34. Cullen C. Laurel's for fair as well as manly brows. In: Mulvihill M, editor. Lab Coats and Lace. Dublin: WITS; 2009. p. 13.
35. Royal College of Science for Ireland. Registers of occasional students, and of associate students, from 1867/8 to 1904/5, and undated photographs. Dublin: Archives of University College.
36. Manchester Courier. 1890 Aug 16.
37. Successful Irish students in Cambridge Higher local examinations. Belfast Newsletter. 1889 Aug 19.
38. The Medical Profession for Women. The Freeman's Journal. 1898 Aug 18.

Chapter 2
Oakley Park

On 1 April 1911, Edith sat down at her desk at home in Chepstow Crescent Kensington, took up her pen and, with a heavy heart, considered how to word a letter to her father's old friend John Joly. She knew that their father could not live much longer, and she wished to ensure that his legacy was not forgotten. With Gerald's encouragement, she had

> 'jotted down some facts of my father's history which might help anyone to write a notice about him who had not known him. These notes are far too intimate and long for publication, but I thought a general knowledge of his private life, tho' not used publicly, might help to understand and so put down better the things which should be given publicly' [1].

The letter remains, but her notes have been lost: the family history must be reconstructed from other evidence.

We dip back, with Edith, into these distant memories. It was approaching Christmas 1833. George and Anne Stoney, Edith and Florence's grandparents, were on a visit to Edinburgh. They had gone to see Anne's father Bindon Blood and her stepmother for the festive season, taking some of their children with them. Anne loved to browse through her father's antiquarian book collection. It made her feel safe, away from the discontent in Ireland.

While they were away, their house at Oakley Park, King's County, was broken into. At home, George Johnstone Stoney, always known as Johnstone, would be eight next birthday. Bindon was only 5 years old. They had been left in the care of Granny Letitia, who had married George's father James after their own grandmother had died. They had returned from the evening service at the ancient church of Seirkieran. It was mid-November, and, before bedtime, they warmed themselves before the evening fire. Suddenly they heard voices, loud hammering on the front door, then a crash, as a bedroom window was broken open, followed by sounds of looting. The gang soon left empty-handed. They were not looking for food or money, but for arms, and the gang's size suggests they were from Breaghmore, families of George Stoney's largely Catholic tenants [2]. The break-in was a significant turning point in George's life and, with him, the rest of his family.

Fig. 2.1 The Stoney family arms

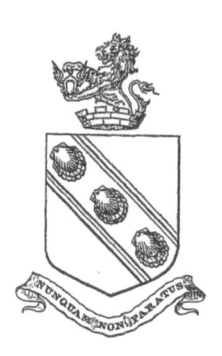

George Stoney (1792–1835) had inherited the 1500 acre estate of Oakley Park on his own father James' death in 1824. It was in the Barony of Ballybritt in King's County at the western foot of the Slieve Bloom Mountains in central Ireland. James had gained a lease from the Ecclesiastical Commissioners for three lives (generations) to develop it as a country estate and farm. He was part of an extended family descended from Thomas Stoney (1675–1726), an emigrant from Kettlewell in North Yorkshire who had acquired property in Tipperary, distributed by King William shortly after the Revolution of 1688. The Stoney family motto was *Nunquam Non Paratus* (Never be unprepared) (Fig. 2.1).

The church where they worshipped had been built on the site of the fifth-century monastery of Seirkieran. Ballymoney Castle, now a ruin in the trees to the south of the main house, was built by the Celtic chieftain family of O'Carroll around 1622, the same family who had built the Castle in nearby Parsonstown.[1] It was one of the smaller estates in Ireland. The house had a dining room, large drawing room, breakfast parlour, seven bedrooms and offices (Fig. 2.2). The servants lived in the basement. The butler, John Walsh, was assisted by a coachman, a cook, a kitchen maid, a housemaid, a child's maid and a groom [3]. Outside there were orchards and a walled garden. George spent a lot of money to improve the 'demesne', adding a large ornamental lake and a deer park (Fig. 2.3).

There were 750 acres of fertile land in the estate, with five or six farms and some woodland. George Stoney also owned about 1700 acres of farmland to the east, lying around a tributary of the Little Brosna River, on which about 50 tenant families lived, mostly Catholic labourers and farmers. The nearest town was Parsonstown, about 5 miles to the east, where some of George's relatives lived.

The Stoney family had been a relatively wealthy landowning family, gaining income from rents and produce. At the other end of the social scale, 54% of families in Ballybritt depended on manual labour. In a country characterised by social divisions, the separation between haves and have-nots was not so extreme here, and the Stoneys of Oakley Park had been able to share some of their good fortune

---

[1]A note on place names. The Irish county is now Co. Offaly. At the time it was called King's County. The local town, now called Birr, was called Parsonstown. The names King's County and Parsonstown are used here as they better represent the social culture in the country at that time.

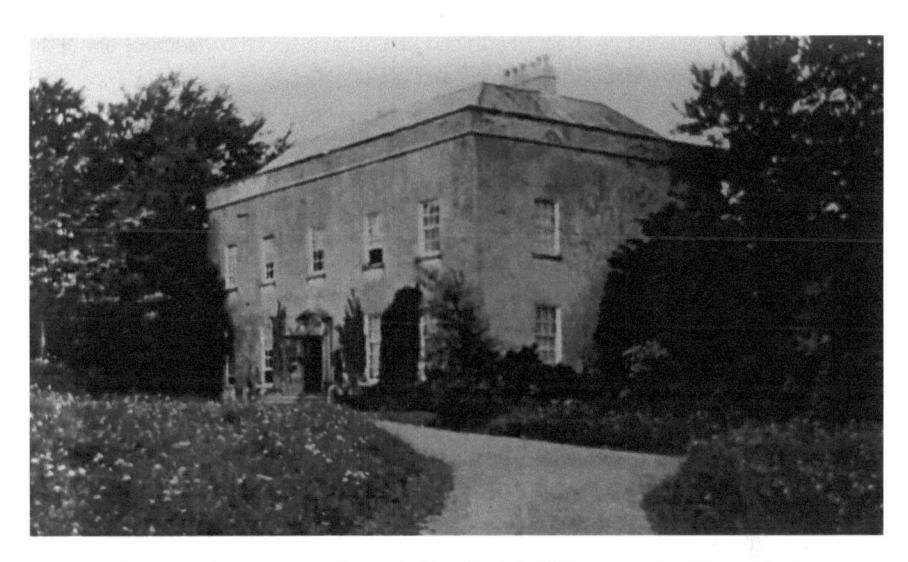

Fig. 2.2 Oakley. Almost none of the Oakley Park buildings remain. The main house was demolished in 1956: there is now a woodyard in one of the outhouses. The pentagonal wall that surrounded the 2-acre enclosed garden is still in place. (Claire Keohane)

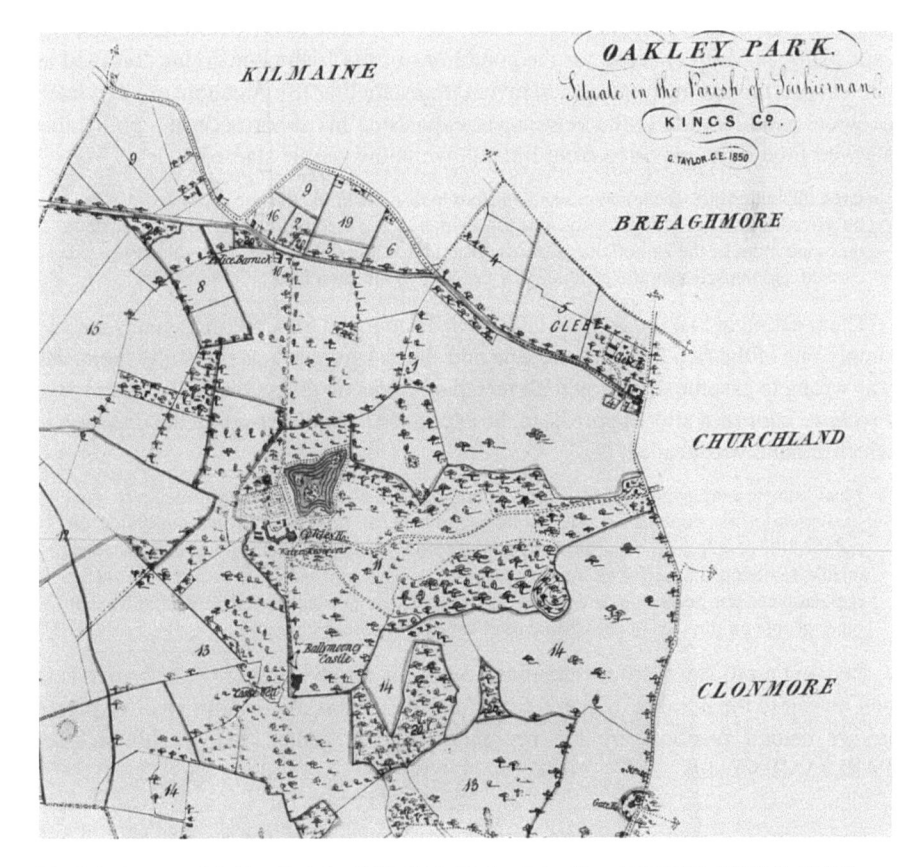

Fig. 2.3 A map of Oakley Park in 1850. (Irish National Archives IRE-LEC-4506849-00452)

with those who depended on their wealth and to exhibit a social conscience about the broader inequalities of their country [4].

When George inherited Oakley, the farms were not doing as well as they had during the wars with Napoleon, when the need for Irish produce to feed the army and Irish linen to clothe it conferred an artificial value on home produce. Irish property values fell during the post-war period after 1815. George was keen to create new jobs and unsuccessfully tried to develop a woollen mill, advertising in England for an investor [5]. But the potato harvest, on which the poor on his estate depended for food, failed in 1815–1817 and again in 1821–1822. When it failed again in 1830, many poor were unable to feed their families or pay their rent. They were also unwilling to pay the tithe to the Church of Ireland, and some became violent. George's advertised claim that it was 'a peaceable county' was already looking like a bit of Irish blarney. Nevertheless, he 'expended large sums of money adorning with all the diversities of water and landscape his mansion here, and in doing that which, in a public point of view, is still more creditable, namely, giving employment to the labouring classes' [6].

He also joined in political debate. The Irish Reform Act, intended to do something about the system of church tithes in Ireland, had just been thrown out by the House of Lords. He spoke out at a King's County Reform Meeting at Tullamore in December 1831, supporting a strongly worded motion against the system of tithes. He also publicly supported his tenants against the vicar of Seirkieran, Rev. James Lynar [7], expressing his deep concern for the conditions of the Irish poor, living 'on food as wretched as human ingenuity could invent to sustain life' [8]. A couple of years later, he wrote another letter to the newspaper, expressing his abhorrence of a policy that allowed food to be exported from Ireland, while the people starved.

> Even the buttermilk, the labourer cannot afford to drink with his potatoe ... because it must be given to the pig fatting for the English market .... Travelling last summer over three thousand miles of the United States of America, I have found the slaves infinitely better fed, clothed and housed than the generality of the poor of our own land.

The break-in at Oakley was the last straw. To many of his Catholic tenants, he was simply one of the rich landowners, who had stolen land that was rightfully theirs. He was wrong to assume they would all feel that he was on their side. In his letter to the *Freeman's Journal* after the break-in, he expressed his concern about the direction in which Ireland was headed.

> I had hitherto employed as many, if not more, of the labouring population than any other gentleman in my country, in ornamental improvements, and have always advocated the rights of the people ..... when I consider the disorder consequent on a powerful population, unable to obtain the pitiful earning of six-pence a day, it is absurd to expect that such a population can be peaceable, and my only surprise is that they have so long endured what no other people on the face of the earth would have suffered.

He went on to say that for the protection of his family, 'my only alternative is to add myself to the number of absentees until such time as my country shall be placed in her natural position, by the restoration of her gentry, her wealth and her PARLIAMENT' [9].

He was an ardent and patriotic Irish nationalist and opposed to the loss of Irish autonomy that had resulted from the act of Union that brought Ireland into the United Kingdom in 1801/1802. He saw Ireland as his own country, not to be ruled from Westminster but by its own parliament in Dublin. He was part of the Protestant Ascendency, defending the rights of the landed gentry to run Ireland as they had since the end of the seventeenth century. He was also very sympathetic to the needs of the rural population who were, largely, Catholic. Nevertheless, it was impossible to separate religious allegiance, Catholic against Protestant, from the social positions associated with each church. It was a conflict that he could not resolve.

Oakley Abandoned

So the family abandoned the country of their birth and moved to London. They took a house where they could see the trees in Regent's Park, 12 Blandford Place, in a terrace on Park Road. George Stoney, Florence and Edith's grandfather, became an 'absentee landlord', one of those on whose shoulders history has placed the deeper miseries still to befall Ireland.

He knew that beneath the continuing strife in Ireland lay the fundamental problem of religion. He had been brought up a Protestant but opposed the imposition of tithes. He was deeply engaged with finding a way to deal with the poverty of the largely Catholic underclass. Moving to London gave him an opportunity to distance himself from these difficult challenges and to start again. He and his family joined the Irvingite church, joining the growing numbers of disaffected Protestants and Catholics who were challenging their church establishments.

On 30 March 1835 his children, Anne, then aged 12, Kate (11), Johnstone (9) and Bindon (6) were all baptised at Newman Street Catholic Apostolic Church in St Marylebone. The Catholic Apostolic Church was one of a number of independent religious movements and sects that were emerging at that time, and it aspired to recover the spiritual heritage of first century Christianity, unsullied by later sectarian division and creed. It appealed to George as a possible counter to the embedded antagonism between Irish Catholics and Protestants that he had experienced back in Ireland.[2]

Their stay in London was to be very brief. When George died later that same year, Anne took her children back to Ireland. There is a gap in the detailed genealogical record where George's death should be. Such a gap asks to be filled, even speculatively, by a biographer. The fact that there is a gap, in an otherwise detailed family record, suggests either that he disappeared or that the manner of his dying was in some way an embarrassment, a matter to be kept unrecorded. The former is unlikely:

---

[2]The father of the eminent physicist Lord Rayleigh, John James Strutt the second Lord Rayleigh, also followed the Rev. Irving.

Anne quickly declared herself to be a widow as soon as she returned to Dublin.[3] A clue to the latter explanation lies in the record of a non-conformist burial of a 43-year-old George Stoney in Boulogne in August 1835. Northern France was a common place to escape creditors at this time, and, given later events, one explanation is that George was avoiding imprisonment for debt. Within a few years, Oakley Park was subject to a court order because of its financial state. There is thus strong circumstantial evidence to suggest that George had another reason to absent himself from Ireland and that his creditors had finally caught up with him in London. Death released him from his own responsibility but left his wife with a financial problem that remained unresolved throughout much of her children's upbringing.

Widowed Anne took her four children back to Ireland. It was unsafe to return to Oakley Park. She took a house in Dublin at 2 Camden Street. She drew a jointure from the Oakley estate, £200 a year, which was sufficient to pay the bills. She did not marry again. There is circumstantial evidence that she retained her connection with the Catholic Apostolic Church, since their house was located close to the two addresses associated with the Dublin branch of this sect.[4] At a time when most middle-class families attended church, joining this new church in a strange city would have given Anne and her children welcome security and support.

The estate management of Oakley Park was taken over by George's younger brother Robert, a solicitor. The law on tithes changed in August 1838, now requiring the landlord to be the tithe collector on behalf of the church, instead of the occupier paying the tithes directly. Rev. James Lynar soon demanded payment for the 3 years of unpaid tithes since George had died. What followed was of sufficient interest to be reported as far away as London. The Attorney General ordered Anne to indicate why these tithes had not been paid. A rumour rapidly spread that the tenants were to be evicted and a huge crowd congregated at Bellhill, part of the Breaghmore area, swollen by others from as far away as Tipperary and Queen's County. They came prepared: 'Those of sufficient age were carrying weapons of all shapes and forms—reaping-hooks, scythes mounted on poles, pitchforks, and bludgeons of the most formidable size'. It took all of Chief Constable Cummins' negotiating skills to assure the crowd their tenancies were safe, although he still was obliged to protect Rev. Lynar from attack [10].

The tithe question was only one aspect of the continuing problems with an estate that was falling increasingly into debt. Finally, in about 1840, and apparently by mutual agreement with a 'friendly creditor' William Greene, Robert Stoney decided to take the matter to court for it to be resolved there. This was a lawyer's solution.

---

[3] In October 1835, Anne Stoney offered an 11-year let on Oakley Park during the minority of her son George Johnstone Stoney. The local arrangements were placed in the hands of George's brother Robert, who was a lawyer in Parsonstown. The property was let to Sandford Palmer of Roscrea.

[4] A few months before they returned to Ireland, Edward Hardman, an Irish Protestant minister of independent views, had himself returned from London to set up a new Irvingite assembly in Aungier Street. In 1863, when his church had become well established, it opened a new building, St Finian's Church in Adelaide Road. Both were within a 10-minute walk of the Stoney home at 2 Camden Street.

Unfortunately the conflict was impossible to resolve, and it dragged on until the final sale of the estate in 1850.

There were other causes than tithe collection that resulted in the financial collapse of the Oakley estate, when others survived [11, 12]. George incurred debts in part 'as the result of lavish hospitality'. George had spent too much on park improvements and entertainment as the land values and estate income contracted. Trips to America and rebuilding the demesne did not come without cost.

The agreement between George's brother Robert, now in charge of the Oakley affairs, and William Greene removed both the responsibility and the authority from Robert's shoulders. However, one unforeseen outcome was that the jointure of £200 from the estate that had been paid each year to James Stoney's second wife Letitia was frozen. Without discussion with her stepson Robert, Letitia Stoney acted independently, endangering his whole strategy [13]. She arranged to bring armed bailiffs to seize stock from one of the tenant's farms and sell it at a local market. Robert managed to intervene at the last minute and returned the stock to its owner. In due course he reached a reasonable compromise with his stepmother.[5] Nevertheless, he took the view that legally she had been in her right to confiscate the stock, even though the tenant had fully paid his rent. Such imbalances of rights were endemic in Irish land management and clashes of this sort proliferated.

Living in Dublin, Anne and her children were somewhat protected from the worst effects of the great Irish famine. In 1845, the potato harvest, essential for life for the bottom tier of the Irish rural poor, failed again. This time the potato blight was much more widespread, destroying the crop over much of Ireland [14]. Outside aid was slow in reaching King's County, because the Government thought that it was rich enough to look after itself. It was not, and deaths in King's County from the famine continued to rise until 1850 when the worst of the blight was over. Violent action, always in the background, escalated. In September 1846, Lord Rosse reported that 'armed bands are beginning to go about at night to organise resistance to rent'. During the next month, attacks on corn convoys stopped shipments out of King's County by canal.

The repeal of the Corn Laws, in 1846, made things much worse. The bottom dropped out of the grain market, causing any residual viability of Oakley to evaporate. The market price for wheat in the nearby town of Tullamore plummeted. It was 28–32 shillings per hundredweight in 1845. By 1848 it had dropped to 10 shillings per hundredweight and went on going down. The same thing happened to oats and barley [4]. For an area such as Ballybritt, economically dependent on grain, this was nothing short of a disaster. With insufficient income to feed themselves, Oakley's tenant farmers could not afford to pay the rent. Further financial pressure resulted from the increase in poor rate during the famine that 'completed the ruin of many Irish families in those districts where the unfortunate tenants stood

---

[5]There was no mention of Anne's jointure as a liability on the estate in the financial statement of the sale of Oakley in 1850. This suggests that Robert supported his sister-in-law for the intervening 6 years.

most in need of the landlords' assistance'. Estate finances collapsed, with no funds to pay taxes, tithes or staff. The population of King's County fell by 23% in a decade [15].

Anne continued to be allowed to draw a sufficient income from the estate, and this was enough to pay for tutors for Johnstone and Bindon, even financing violin lessons [16]. It was difficult, but in spite of the catastrophic finances of Oakley Park, the boys were expected to enter university before following a career. Even then it was assumed that Johnstone would take over Oakley, whilst Bindon would have to find a professional calling for himself. In past generations, the eldest inherited the family home, while the remaining sons entered the army, the law, the church or medicine, depending on their interests and ability. Of Johnstone's three Stoney uncles, Robert was a lawyer, William entered the church and James became a doctor. Anne's half-brother, William Bindon Blood, became a civil engineer. There was therefore plenty of choice of career in the family precedents. Johnstone gained entry to Trinity College Dublin, shortly followed by Bindon. As they could not afford the fees, they both earned their way through Trinity as pupil teachers.

Kate stayed at home and looked after her mother. Anne found a nice young man, the Rev. William FitzGerald, and they were married on 23 April 1846.

Parsonstown

Johnstone Stoney became 21 years old in February 1847 at the height of the famine. The next year he gained his B.A. degree from Trinity College, but he still had no clear idea what to do about the bankrupt estate that he had inherited. Johnstone could now reach Oakley from Dublin using the Great Southern and Western Railway that had just been completed as far as Limerick. He had three good reasons to travel west. First he needed to visit his Uncle Robert in Parsonstown to discuss with him the financial problems of the estate. Johnstone learned that there was still no resolution in the courts. Oakley remained a liability and not an asset, so he needed to find another source of income. Secondly it was good for him to meet and spend time with his much younger cousins. The twins Robert and Charles were now eight. Their sister Sophia was fun to be with too, although Johnstone could never have imagined that this little girl would later become his wife.

Finally, he knew about the new Parsons telescope at Birr Castle and hoped to make a visit there. Robert was in a position to introduce him to William Parsons, the third Earl of Rosse in the Castle in Parsonstown. It was not uncommon for bright young graduates to find employment as tutors to the children of the aristocracy, and Parsons saw an opportunity to educate his first son Lawrence, now 8 years old, by employing Johnstone, this son of a local landowner who had fallen on hard times. Parsons was also looking for a scientific assistant, and this opportunity was much more exciting. He had an unquenchable interest in astronomy, and his wife Mary had brought with her sufficient funds to allow him to indulge this interest. He had finally completed the 'Leviathan of Parsonstown', with its 72-inch reflector, and it had

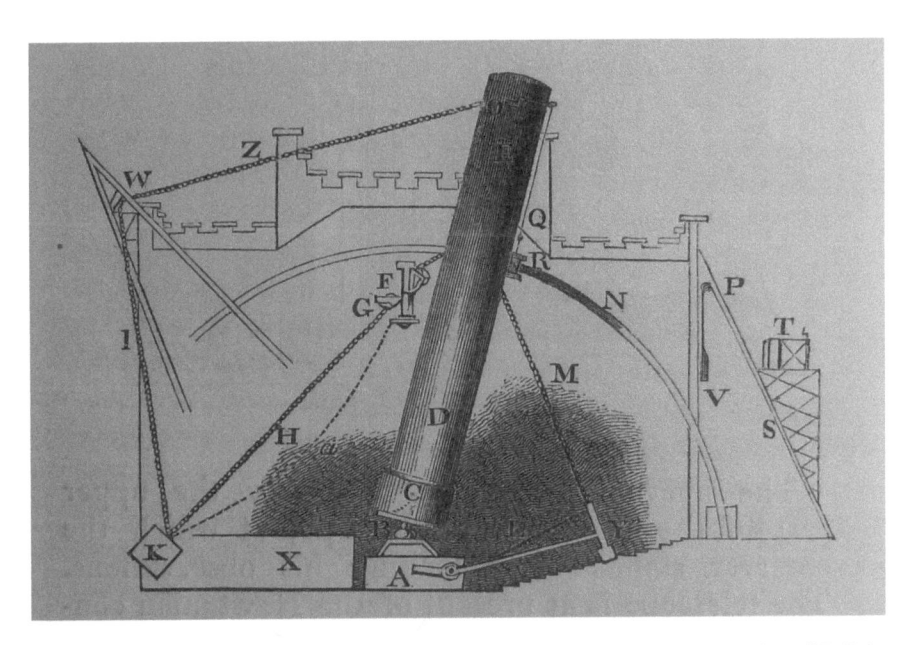

Fig. 2.4 The Leviathan of Parsonstown, showing A,B the universal joint mounting, C,D,E the telescope. The remaining letters indicate the chains, pulleys and weights, lever, handle and windlass used to adjust the position of the telescope (From the appendix of Thomas Dick, The Practical Astronomer, London, Seeley. 1845.) The name 'Leviathan' has been attributed to Sir James South

begun regular use in the spring of 1845 [17] (Fig. 2.4). This telescope would remain the most powerful in the world for many decades, and Parsonstown (later renamed Birr) became the international Mecca of astronomy, attracting famous astronomers and public figures to inspect the wonders of the heavens that it revealed.

The Leviathan had been completed just as the potato blight first appeared, and the Earl's other public responsibilities during the next few years meant that he was not able to work with the new instrument as much he had intended. Late in 1847 his friend and fellow astronomer, Rev. Thomas Robinson, Director of the Armagh Observatory, brought his nephew William Rambaut with him to be trained in astronomical observations and to act briefly as Parsons' assistant, while he completed his degree at Trinity. The vacancy when he left in June 1848 was, for Johnstone, a heaven-sent opportunity to become not only Lawrence's tutor but also to take over as William Parsons' astronomical assistant, a dream research post. He stayed for 2 years, until June 1850, during which time he made numerous original observations of star clusters and nebulae, with a resolution that had never previously been achieved [18].

He made his first observation, of the Nebula H.2098, on the night of 23 October. After that, whenever the night was clear enough, more nebulae were observed. Each observation involved a team of four men to work with him. He climbed high up to the observing gallery, where the telescope eyepiece was located. Two of the men worked the winches that positioned the telescope, another to move the observation

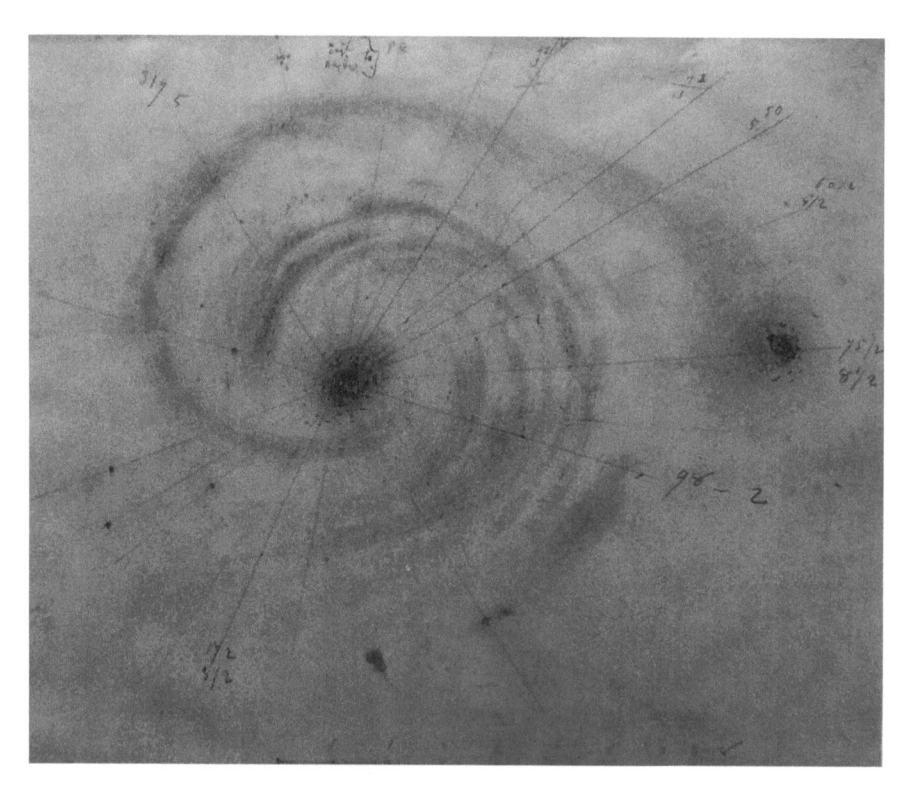

Fig. 2.5 Johnstone Stoney's micrometrical measurements of M 51 in Canes Venatici

platform and a fourth to attend to all other matters. Whilst the concentration needed during observation was extremely tiring, it only happened infrequently. Cloud cover or moonlight meant that the opportunities for good observation were quite infrequent. As a result, as pointed out by Robert Ball, a later astronomical assistant for Lord Rosse, 'Diligence at the telescope was, therefore, not incompatible with tutorial duties in the day'. On the night of 22 December 1848, Johnstone made his first observation of a previously unrecorded nebula, NGC 258. Three more were discovered during January. By the end of his time at Parsonstown, they had discovered some 50 new nebulae, largely as a result of his own observations. His other major project during this time was to measure accurately the positions of the visible stars within the Whirlpool galaxy H.1622 (Fig. 2.5).

At least Oakley was close by, so it was possible to deal with the problems of the estate more directly. It was a thankless task being a landlord in the famine, unable to stem the flow of funds haemorrhaging from the estate, nor to effectively protect his tenant farmers or staff from its effects. Johnstone was finally relieved of his nightmare by a piece of legislation about which Gladstone later commented that it had been passed with 'lazy, heedless uninformed good intentions' and 'its effect was disastrous': though not, in the event, for the Stoney estate. This was the Encumbered

Estates Acts, 1848 and 1849, legislation that allowed the sale of Irish Estates whose owners, because of the collapse of the Irish agricultural economy during the famine, were unable to meet their financial obligations. It was intended to enable English investors to buy Irish estates and thereby replace what was considered to be uneconomic farming practices in Irish agriculture with efficient 'English' farming practices.

Oakley was offered for sale by auction on Friday 13 December 1850 in Dublin. Robert was named as the receiver. The petitioners included William Greene and his wife, to whom the estate now owed a great deal of money. All of the family were parties to the sale, including Bindon, Kate and Anne, together with Anne's new husband, the Rev. William FitzGerald. The law did not allow a married woman to hold property in her own right, so Anne's inheritance had passed to her husband's control [19].

The Oakley land was divided into two lots, offered for sale separately. The first lot included the main house and grounds together with a number of cottages and farms. With 773 acres of land, the house was described as being 'ornamentally planted, and by a small expenditure on the Mansion House, would form one of the most desirable residences in Ireland'. This disguised the fact that the house was already falling into a state of disrepair. But no one was interested. No English purchaser appeared. So it was bought back into the Stoney family for £400 by the one bidder, George's old stepmother Letitia Stoney, now 80 years of age. There was no bid for the second lot of 1670 acres, the agricultural land of Braeghmore farmed by Catholic tenants, so quite failing in the purpose of injecting English capital into the Irish agricultural economy [20].

Of course, old Letitia was not in a position to run the estate. Further negotiations followed and, not long afterwards, the estate was taken over by a local landowner George Winter, who moved in to the main house and took over most of Oakley Park, leaving the Lodge House and about 120 acres of land still leased to Robert [21]. This left the larger lot of the Breaghmore farmland, unsold at the auction. Within a couple of years, almost all of this land was in the hands of William Greene, the original protagonist whose case against the Stoney family was never resolved in the court. The resale of the house and estate, together with the sale of the farmland, raised about £14,000, and Anne regained welcome financial security.[6] It was really the best outcome that they could have hoped for, and Johnstone had been able to dispose of a property that he could never again have made profitable. George Winters gained a country house and estate that he wanted, at a bargain price. William Greene became the new landlord of an extensive acreage of farmland.

---

[6] In John Joly's obituary of Johnstone Stoney, he mentions that the estate was sold for about eight times the reduced rental, which was given as about £1700 gross in the particulars of the sale.

Queen's College, Galway

Johnstone needed now to consider his own career. Bindon had just graduated from Trinity, and he was happy to accept William Parsons' offer to replace his brother as tutor and astronomical assistant in Parsonstown, which allowed Johnstone time for further study. During the next 2 years, he shared his time between Dublin and Parsonstown, studying at Trinity College during the week and, weather permitting, working with Bindon on the Leviathan at the weekends. In 1852 he gained an M.A. from Trinity, again paying his way through college by coaching other students. He also took second place in the Trinity College Fellowship examination, still conducted in Latin at that time.[7]

On his visits to Dublin, he stayed with his sister Anne in her new home in Lower Mount Street, where he got to know her husband William. Several people, including William Parsons, recommended that he should apply for a professorship at one of the new Queen's Colleges, which had been recently opened in Cork, Galway and Belfast. In July 1852, he applied for the Natural Philosophy post at Queen's College, Galway. William Parsons wrote a glowing testimonial. So did his brother-in-law William FitzGerald, who was by then chaplain to the Lord Lieutenant of Ireland and to the Archbishop of Dublin and Professor of Moral Philosophy at the University of Dublin. He wrote

> 'He has a singularly clear judgement and much firmness and resolution combined with great gentleness of manner & disposition & a temper which it is not easy even to ruffle. I have never met with any one who is so zealous, patient and successful in imparting information' [22].

There were four on the short list for the post, including the famous Irish physicist John Tyndall. Johnstone was successful, and, at the end of October, he was offered the post as Professor of Natural Philosophy at Queen's College Galway with the generous annual salary of £250.

By 1855 he was Dean of the Science Division and examiner in Natural Philosophy for all three Queen's Colleges. Following his initiative, the engineering course was extended from 2 to 3 years. There was insufficient student accommodation, so Johnstone proposed that halls of residence should be established. He was committed to making university-level education more relevant to the wider community and more accessible to young men from all backgrounds.

Johnstone took a particular interest in Robert's children, who grew up in the part of Oakley Park that their father had retained. Robert, Charles and Sophia were young teenagers when Johnstone went to Galway, and Charles spent several years at school there, living with him in Shires House in the Galway suburb of Shantalla [23].

---

[7]In recognition of Johnstone and Bindon Stoney's astronomical contributions, a 45-km-wide crater on the far side of the moon has been named Stoney, and, in 1973, one on Mars at longitude 138.49° and latitude −71.35° was also named Stoney Crater.

Return to Dublin

Johnstone had been at Galway for only 5 years when the possibility opened to move back to Dublin. The three Queen's Colleges were run from a central office in Dublin, where the Secretary, Dr. Robert Ball, took overall charge. When Ball died suddenly in March 1857, Johnstone, by then 31 years old and still unmarried, applied for the vacant position. Soon he was back in Dublin, leaving the lecture room and teaching laboratory behind him. He had gained one of the most influential posts in Irish higher education. His salary was £600 a year.

Johnstone moved in with his mother and sister at 89 Waterloo Road. He arrived just a year after his brother Bindon, who had secured the position as Assistant Inspector of Works at the Port of Dublin. Bindon's initial salary in Dublin was £250 per annum, so at last the family were again very comfortably placed. They had enough room in Waterloo Road for young Charles Stoney, finished with his schooling in Galway, now pursuing his studies to become a doctor at Trinity College. Johnstone took the role of mathematics tutor with lessons on Euclid, 'from 6 till breakfast'. In a letter to his mother, Charles expressed pleasure to be part of Johnstone's telescopic demonstrations of the moon, which he called his '*demonstralis sancta*'. He also reports a bit of coded gossip, that 'Johnstone came up regularly done up from overwork which includes royal progresses with Margaret and Hugh (another brother)' [24]. Johnstone's chaperoned courting of his cousin Margaret Sophia was clearly considered hard work by her brother. Charles gained his MB degree in 1863 and became a Licentiate of King and Queen's College of Physicians in Ireland the same year.

During the next 25 years, Johnstone worked from the Queen's University offices in Dublin Castle. As Secretary of the Queen's University of Ireland, he oversaw a unique federation of the three nondenominational provincial colleges in Cork, Galway and Belfast. Queen's had been established by the Queen's Colleges Act in 1845 to establish Colleges 'in order to supply the want, which has long been felt in Ireland, of an improved academic education equally accessible to all classes of the community without religious distinction.' But, right from the beginning, there was a lot of opposition and the nickname 'godless' stuck, taken up by opponents of all religious persuasions. In particular, Pope Pius IX unleashed a broadside condemning the Colleges as detrimental to religion and proposed the foundation of a Catholic University. The Irish Bishops concurred, setting up The Catholic University in 1851. Catholic parents were strongly discouraged from sending their sons to any of the Queen's Colleges.

Johnstone's employment at the Queen's University head office was not full time. Once his administrative responsibilities were complete, he could spend time thinking about physics. He established contact with other British scientists by becoming a life member of the British Association for the Advancement of Science, attending their annual meetings and contributing to their committees. The British Association gave him the forum to present his own work and to discuss it with and learn from other senior scientists of his day. At the same time, he became a member of the Royal Irish

Academy and the Royal Dublin Society and often spoke at their meetings. He was honoured when the Royal Society of London elected him to become a Fellow in June 1861 on the basis of his contributions to physics, including astronomy, wave theory, molecular, crystal and general physics.

Being Secretary of Queen's University of Ireland, he also met people in the upper echelons of Irish Civic Administration. He was frequently called to the House of Commons to give advice on educational matters pertaining to Ireland. In 1868 he was even approached with a view to becoming Under-Secretary for Ireland on the retirement of Sir Thomas Larcom. When the Lord Lieutenant, Lord Mayo, sounded him out, he declared his support for Gladstone's Irish Church Disestablishment Bill. The Bill, which came into force on 1 January 1871, finally did away with the church tithes that had caused so many people so much distress. He knew that Lord Mayo was vehemently opposed to the Bill when he made his views known, but he could not pretend anything other, even when he knew that it would lead to his inevitable rejection as a candidate.

It was a disappointment that his married sister Anne FitzGerald moved to Cork in 1857, just as he came back to Dublin from Galway. They were delighted, of course, that her husband had been made Bishop of Cork and impressed that Anne was now living in a palace. In addition to being the mother of six children, Anne had played an essential role in her husband's literary career, and large portions of the original manuscripts of his *Lectures on Moral Philosophy* and *Ecclesiastical History* are in her handwriting, either from her own composition or taken down from his dictation [25]. Tragically, Anne died a couple of years later, probably in childbirth. Later, when their sons George and Maurice FitzGerald were older and came back to study at Trinity College, the family became closer again.

Charles Stoney's letters home to his mother and sister make it clear that Margaret Sophia was much loved by her brothers, not only by Charles himself but also his serious twin brother Robert, by now becoming well established as a minister in the Church of Ireland, and his younger brothers Hugh and George. There were several opportunities for Sophia to meet Johnstone, both on her visits to Dublin and on his visits to meet Lord Rosse in Parsonstown. Their flowering romance was met with family approval, in spite of their considerable difference in age, and they were married in Parsonstown on 20 January 1863. She was yet to reach her 20th birthday, and he was approaching 36 years old (Fig. 2.6).

The new couple set up home at 40 Wellington Road, a short walk from Waterloo Road. Bindon moved in next door. Their first son, George Gerald, who was always known by his second name, was born on 28 November 1863, followed by Robert Bindon on 28 June 1866, Edith Anne on 6 January 1869 and Florence Ada on 4 February 1870. Little Gertrude Beatrice arrived on 19 May 1871. The family moved at about this time to the parish of Dundrum on the southern outskirts of Dublin where their uncle, Canon Robert Stoney, was now curate.

In August 1872 their father attended the British Association meeting in Brighton, where he acted as reporter for a small committee appointed to prepare catalogues of optical spectra arranged on a scale of wave number. This had been his own proposal. He was exploring numeric associations within spectral series, using harmonic

Fig. 2.6 Margaret Sophia Stoney (1843–1872) mother of Edith and Florence. (Claire Keohane)

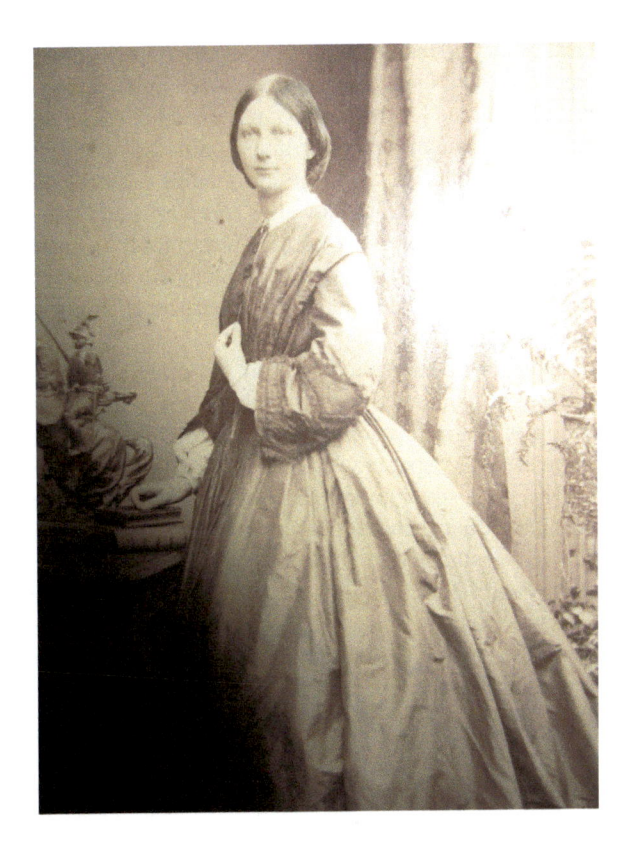

analysis to do so. This analysis was made easier by evaluating spectra by frequency rather than by wavelength. At the same time, he suggested the term 'ultraviolet rays', to replace the commonly used 'chemical rays' which had been used for much of the nineteenth century [26].

Sophia was expecting her sixth child. Shortly after Johnstone's return home, tragedy struck. Sophia died in childbirth on 13 October. Her body was laid to rest in St Nahi's Churchyard, next to Dundrum's tiny old church. Her brother, Canon Robert, took the funeral service. The inscription they chose for her grave, was 'Some men a forward motion love, but I by backward steps would move. For time, that gave, doth now this gift confound' from Henry Vaughan's *The Retreate* (c.1650).

Johnstone was left as a widower parent of six children under 10. Florence and Edith were only 3 and 4 years old: Gertrude was only 17 months. The newborn daughter only lived for a month. The next few years were ones of difficulty and instability. The strain started to take its toll, and their father suffered two severe illnesses, smallpox in 1875 and typhoid in 1877. Either disease could have been fatal, and the children were faced with the real possibility of becoming orphans.

Nevertheless, with domestic staff to maintain the household, they survived. Their home at Weston House, near Dundrum, was a spacious four-bedroom villa on the crest of the hill, set in about 5 acres of land, with views of the Dublin Mountains to the south. It was reached at the end of a long sweeping drive from Churchtown Road just as it turned left towards Dundrum church. The house is still there in its walled enclosure, though streets of houses now fill the estate where they played. Cows, mostly Ayrshires, cropped the surrounding pastures, described by a local as coloured with buttercups, daisies, cowslips and purple and white clover. Buffered from adult worries, there were many exciting places for the girls to explore, visiting cook in her kitchen and pantry, wandering through the wine cellar and vinery, talking to the coachman in the stables and coach house and helping the gardener in the orchard and vegetable plot.

Johnstone's scientific output all but dried up during these difficult years. Nevertheless, he continued to think about some fundamental problems in physics. A couple of years after Sophia died, at the 1874 British Association meeting in Belfast, he presented a paper in which he proposed an idea that would become the one that he has been mostly remembered for. His paper 'On the physical units of nature', postulated that there existed a distinct fundamental quantity of electricity, with a charge he estimated to be about 10–20 coulomb, one of three fundamental physical units. He called his fundamental quantity the 'electrine' [27].

It was soon after he gave this paper that Johnstone fell ill. But he went on thinking about the topic and, in 1881, presented his ideas again at the Royal Dublin Society and published them in the *Philosophical Magazine* [28]. He wrote:

> 'A charge of this amount is associated in the chemical atom with each bond. There may accordingly be several such charges in one chemical atom, and there appear to be at least two on each atom. These charges, which it will be convenient to call *electrons*, cannot be removed from the atom; but they become disguised when atoms chemically unite' [29].

He wrote these words before there was any conception about the internal structure of atoms. Whilst he was confident in his own truth, it was reassuring to learn that the prolific German physicist Herman von Helmholtz had reached a similar conclusion at about the same time [30].[8]

The family suffered another loss in 1883 when their grandmother Anne died aged 82. Edith and Florence were in their mid-teens. Anne was buried alongside their mother in Dundrum churchyard, the funeral procession slowly moving from Bindon's house in Elgin Road along the 3 mile journey south through Rathmines. They placed a text from the Psalms on her grave: 'Thy word is very pure; therefore thy servant loved it' [31]. As Edith and Florence grew into womanhood, they may have considered the lives that their grandmother and other women in the Stoney family had lived, wondering whether it would be their destiny to follow similar

---

[8]Their father's work on fundamental units has been identified as equivalent to that of Max Planck over a quarter of a century later, with his introduction of natural units into physics (John D Barow. Natural units before Planck. *Q J Roy Astr Soc* 1983;24:24–2). More recently it has been claimed that the 'Stoney Scale' is consistent with Einstein's theory of gravitational ether, in that it does not require gravitational and inertial mass to be equivalent in an electromagnetic setting. (Ross McPherson. Stoney Scale and large number coincidences. *Apeiron* 2007;14(3):234–265.)

paths. Their grandmother had been widowed at 35, never remarried, carrying the burden of responsibility for managing a household of four children on her own. Their Aunt Anne, who they never knew, followed the conventional pattern of marrying well and producing children. But she sacrificed her own life for it, as their mother did. Their Aunt Kate never married, taking the role of domestic manager for her mother and then her brother, until she, too, died in 1887. Her body was laid to rest beside those of her mother and grandmother.

Perhaps, as Edith and Florence planned their future lives, and their father wondered whether there were any female role models from his past life who he might tell them about, he remembered two women he had met in Parsonstown, whose positions in wealthy families allowed them to be active participants in science. Mary Parsons had married 'an aristocrat who himself had an open and enquiring mind providing her with opportunities for self-realisation that were available to few women of her time and class' [32]. Lady Parsons took an active interest in the building and use of her husband's telescopes and also developed a scientific hobby of her own. In 1850, photography was very new indeed, and William Parsons was starting to investigate it as a means to record his remarkable astronomical observations. Mary was creating her own photographs from at least 1853, shortly after Johnstone moved on to Galway, but he still made regular visits back to the Castle and kept in touch. In 1872, Mary asked for his advice about the design of a novel optical prism using glycerine and carbon disulphide as the refracting media, possibly for stereoscopic photography. He replied to her as an equal, considering her to be a competent and knowledgeable scientist [33].

The other woman scientist he met at Parsonstown was Mary Ward, almost exactly his own age. She was William Parsons' cousin, married to Hon. Henry Ward. Her particular skill was in carefully drawn images, particularly of insects, observed through a microscope. These drawings were published in a charming book that she wrote with her sister Jane, a book that would certainly have been available to Florence when she started using her own microscope. The new microscopes, such as those used by Florence and Mary Ward, took advantage of recent advances in lens design, the achromatic microscopes preventing the coloured distortion caused by earlier designs. Her other deep interest was in astronomy, and she was one of only three women on the mailing list for the Royal Astronomical Society, the others being Queen Victoria and Mary Somerville.

The lives of these women of Ireland, and others, form the backdrop to this story about Edith and Florence Stoney. There was the unnamed, unremembered majority, wives of cottiers and farmers, mothers of the next generation, struggling to survive. Sarah Larkin and Bridgit Hines, maids at Oakley Park, were surplus to requirements when the family moved out leaving Letitia Stoney, ageing annuitant from an earlier, wealthy time, to be a drain on an impoverished estate. Edith and Florence's widowed grandmother set the highest educational and moral standards for her children. Her daughter, Mrs. Anne FitzGerald, newlywed, lost control of her inheritance to her husband even before it was received, then obediently helped to co-author his religious tracts. The lives of the girls' aunt and mother, were both cut short by childbirth. Even so, their other aunt Frances, securely married, expected her daughters to do the same. At the top of the social scale, Lady Mary Parsons and the Honourable Mary Ward had the wealth, time and imagination to be hobby scientists. They were all part of the social fabric into which was woven the lives of two young women, growing into a new world of expanding opportunities.

References

1. Letter from Edith Stoney to John Joly. 1 April 1911. Trinity College Dublin Archives MS 2312/391.
2. George Stoney. Letter to the editor, The Freeman's Journal. 1833 Dec 7. (also The London Standard. 1833 Dec 10).
3. Ireland Census 1821 for Ballamoney (now Oakley Park), Seirkieran, Ballybritt, King's County.
4. O'Neill TP. The famine in Offaly, Chapter 20. In: Nolan W, O'Neill TP, editors. Offaly history and society, interdisciplinary essays on the history of an Irish County. Dublin: Geography Publications; 1998. p. 721.
5. Leeds Intellegencer. 1825 Sep 22.
6. The Dublin Penny Journal. 1834 Oct 11.
7. James Lynar. The Freeman's Journal. 1831 Dec 28.
8. George Stoney. The Freeman's Journal. 1832 Jan 16.
9. Stoney G. The Freeman's Journal. 1833 Jan 24;
10. The Morning Post, 19 December 1838.
11. J.J (John Joly). George Johnstone Stoney, 1826-1911. Obituary notices of fellows deceased. Proc Roy Soc Lond 1911;A86:xx–xxxv.
12. John RC. Plunket Joly and the great famine in King's County. Dublin: Four Courts Press; 2012.
13. Stoney R. Evidence taken before Her Majesty's Commissioners of Inquiry into the State of the Law and Practice in respect to the Occupation of Land in Ireland, Dublin; 1845. p. 583–584.
14. Woodham-Smith C. The Great Hunger, Ireland 1845-1849. London: Penguin; 1991 and Delaney E. The curse of reason – the great Irish famine. Dublin: Macmillan; 2012.
15. Breen GC. Landlordism in King's County in the mid-nineteenth century, Chapter 19. Nolan and O'Neill.
16. Ball RS, Johnstone Stoney G. A monthly review of astronomy. The Observatory. 1911;34(438):287–90.
17. Steinicke W. Birr Castle observations of non-stellar objects and the development of nebular theories, Chapter 7. In: Charles Mallon C, editor. William Parsons 3rd Earl of Rosse; astronomy and the castle in nineteenth-century Ireland. Manchester: Manchester University Press; 2014. p. 210–70.
18. Ryder AJ. An Irishman of note: George Johnstone Stoney. Privately Published; 2012.
19. Encumbered Estates Court. In the matter of the estate of George John Stoney Esq. and others. 13th December 1850. Dublin: Irish National Archives.
20. Incumbered Estates. Evening Mail. 1850 Oct 18 and The Freeman's Journal 1850 Dec 14.
21. Griffith R. General valuation of rateable property in Ireland, King's County. Dublin; 1854.
22. Ryder p 82, quoting from Queen's College Galway papers held at the National Archives, Dublin.
23. CK: Claire Keohane. Private collection of Stoney family papers.
24. Charles Stoney to his mother. Undated. CK.
25. Fitzgerald W. In: Fitzgerald W, Quarry J, editors. Lectures on ecclesiastical history. London: Murray; 1885. p. 26.
26. Turing S. Alan M Turing. Cambridge: Heffer; 1959. p. 7.
27. O'Hara JG. George Johnstone Stoney, F.R.S. and the concept of the electron. Notes Rec Roy Soc. 1975;29(2):265–76.

References

28. Stoney GJ. On the physical units of nature. Phil Mag. 1881:11(5);381–391 and Sci Proc Roy Dublin Soc. 1883;3(2):51–60.
29. Stoney GJ. On the cause of double lines and of equidistant satellites in the spectra of gases. Sci Trans Roy Dublin Soc 11th Ser. 1891;4:563.
30. Stoney JG. Of the "electron," or atom of electricity. Phil Mag Ser 5. 1894;38:418–20.
31. Ball FE, Hamilton E. The Parish of Taney. A history of Dundrum, near Dublin, and its neighbourhood. Dublin: Hodges Figgis; 1895. p. 44.
32. McDowell D. Alison Countess of Rosse, Davison D. Mary, Countess of Rosse (1813–85), Chapter 3. In: Mallon C, editor. William Parsons, 3rd Earl of Rosse. Manchester: Manchester University Press; 2014.
33. Letter from Johnstone Stoney to Lady Rosse. 10 May 1872. Rosse archives: Birr Castle K12.

Chapter 3
Newnham College, Cambridge

The letter that arrived for Edith from Newnham College, Cambridge in the late summer of 1889 was a very pleasant surprise. She and Florence had been delighted by their outstanding results in the Cambridge Highers, and they could now think about medical school. For Edith, the letter changed everything. Newnham College was offering her a Winkworth Scholarship, valued at £50 per year, to study at Cambridge. It was the most valuable of several scholarships offered by Newnham, operating over the full 3 years of her undergraduate study. It had been her 'distinguished success at the Cambridge Higher Local Examinations' that had brought her to the attention of Newnham, always on the lookout for young women who might be expected to do credit to the College.

It was too late to arrange to go up to Cambridge that year, and Newnham College was happy to postpone her entry until the Michaelmas Term of 1890. Florence was working to improve her mathematics, gaining outstanding results in the 1890 Highers, and perhaps Edith worked with her in preparation for her own anticipated challenge ahead. She later referred to a time when she worked as her father's laboratory assistant, and this 'gap year' offers the most likely space in her life for this to have happened [1]. Her father was continuing his work in interpreting optical spectra at this time, leading to the paper in which he stated his molecular electronic theory of the origin of spectra [2]. In this work, more than in his more theoretical studies, he needed spectroscopic experiments, and these required an assistant to set up the equipment and to record results, offering Edith vital experience in experimental physics.

Newnham College

Newnham College, where Edith was now headed, had been conceived in the same year as she had been born. Lectures for ladies were started in Cambridge in 1870. Students from a distance needed somewhere to stay. The following year, five

---

The original version of this chapter was revised. A correction to this chapter is available at https://doi.org/10.1007/978-3-030-16561-1_19

© Springer Nature Switzerland AG 2019
A. Thomas, F. Duck, *Edith and Florence Stoney, Sisters in Radiology*, Springer Biographies, https://doi.org/10.1007/978-3-030-16561-1_3

students were given accommodation in a house rented by the philosopher Henry Sidgwick, overseen by Miss Anne Clough, a Cumbrian schoolteacher, who became the first college principal. By 1875, sufficient funds had been raised to build Newnham Hall (now known as Old Hall).[1] Board and lodging was £20 per term of 8 weeks, less for those intending to become teachers. Wine and heating were charged extra. There was a lower age limit of 17 [3]. By 1878, Christ's College had opened its lectures in natural science to the Newnham students, as had King's College for history. In both cases it was necessary for Miss Clough to attend, as chaperone.

There was still the need for women to be officially accepted by the University. Initially there was an informal arrangement whereby women were allowed to enter for university examinations as a favour of private examiners. On Thursday 24 February 1881, at the University Senate meeting, 'Three Graces', or rules, were offered for vote, to agree a change in the rules of the university concerning women. These Graces were agreed by an overwhelming majority. As a result, women would now be admitted for the Tripos examinations, for which the residency certificates issued by Girton and Newnham would be accepted. In addition, examination class lists for the women would be published and 'those who were successful would receive certificates to this effect': not degrees, just certificates. One student, reflecting the female excitement of the occasion, observed 'When women get the Degrees (for this is only the thin end of the wedge) it will be nothing to this' [3, p. 4]. If she had known that it would not be until 1948 that Cambridge started to award degrees to women, she might not have felt so euphoric.

By 1890, when Edith arrived, the accommodation had grown, and there were now three students' halls, accommodating about 150 students in total. Newnham had become part of Cambridge university life. Some of the early pioneering spirit had become muted. No longer were the students 'pre-Raphaelite' in dress, with William Morris wallpaper in their rooms. The sense at the start was more of an academic finishing school than a centre of learning. By now, many intended to become teachers, focussed on studying hard in order to secure employment, as well as enjoying the broader university experience.

Why was Edith selected to be the recipient of the Winkworth Scholarship rather than any of the other high achievers of the 1889 Local Higher Examinations? Certainly it was important to select someone who had a good chance of being a credit to Newnham. Miss Bayne, the 1885 Winkworth Scholar, only managed a disappointing third in the Classics Tripos. Perhaps as a result, for the next few years, a Winkworth Scholar was selected who might be expected to read mathematics. There was status to be accrued from achieving honours in the Mathematics Tripos, which was accepted to be the most challenging examination set by Cambridge University. Those graded with firsts were called 'Wranglers': only the men, of course. But, by then, any women who had sat for the Maths Tripos examination

---

[1]The other Cambridge women's college at the time, Girton, opened in October 1873.

were given a position alongside them in the final list, such as 'between 4th and 5th Wrangler' or 'equal to the 20th Wrangler'.

In making the selection for the Winkworth Scholarship, the Newnham Awards Committee had access to the results of the Cambridge Higher Local Examinations. In Edith's year there had been 88 firsts, but only 13 were in mathematics or the natural sciences. This narrowed the field, but was there anything else that Edith was bringing to give her an edge over the others? One answer comes, naturally, through her father, although he could have had no direct influence over the decision. Nevertheless, he was well known to two influential women at Newnham, Anne Clough and Eleanor Sidgwick. Mrs. Sidgwick was one of the first students at Newnham, married to its founder Henry Sidgwick and was by then treasurer of the College. She knew Edith's father through the work of the standards committee of the British Association for the Advancement of Science. This long-standing committee had been established under the chairmanship of James Clerk Maxwell to determine more precise values for the electrical units, volt, ampere and ohm.

Edith's father was a member of this committee and had continued to be an active participant in the British Association electrical standards work. In this capacity he worked closely with Lord Rayleigh, another of the eminent members of the committee. Eleanor Sidgwick was Lord Rayleigh's sister-in-law.[2] Moreover, she had taken an active part in Rayleigh's scientific work. In particular, starting in 1881, she had worked with him in the Cavendish Laboratory on experiments to redetermine the ohm, the unit of electrical resistance, as part of the continuing work of the committee. She co-authored five of Lord Rayleigh's papers on the subject and was acknowledged as a participant in three others [4]. Johnstone Stoney's contributions to the British Society and his deep thinking on the fundamental problems in physics were well recognised by Lord Rayleigh.

Anne Clough's association with Edith's father was not as close and had arisen some time before she moved to Cambridge. She had written to him, on behalf of the Liverpool Ladies Committee, for advice about plans to set up in England the University Extension Lectures already established in Irish towns and supported by Queen's University [5]. This meant that she understood the position that Edith's father held in the Irish academic community and recognised the support that he could give Edith were she to be offered the scholarship. It would not have been difficult for Anne Clough and Eleanor Sidgwick to make a convincing case on Edith's behalf to their Newnham colleagues.

Edith arrived in Cambridge in October 1890, one of 46 freshers who arrived at Newnham that year. Edith had packed her large travelling trunk in Dublin, making the 3.5-hour voyage by ferry to Holyhead and then by rail to Cambridge. She stepped down onto the longest platform she had ever seen, 500 yards long, trains in each direction stacked up one behind the other. A mile by Hansom cab took her to the

---

[2]John William Strutt, third Baron Rayleigh, married Evelyn Balfour, in 1871. Her sister Eleanor Balfour married Henry Sidgwick in 1876. Their brother, Arthur Balfour, was the British Prime Minister from 1902 to 1905.

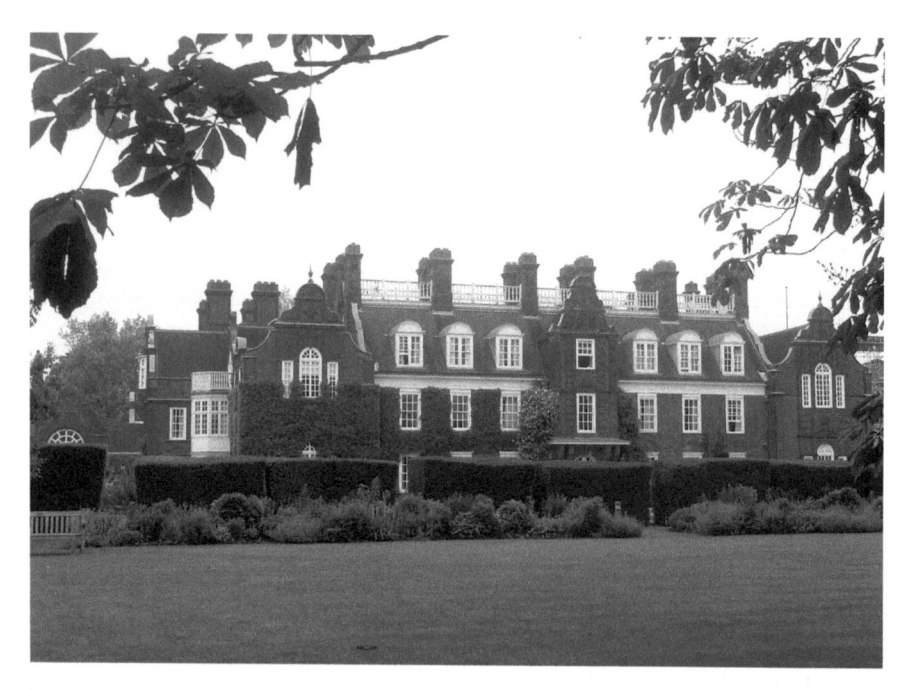

Fig. 3.1 Sidgwick Hall, Newnham College, Cambridge

centre of the town and then left over the River Cam on the cast-iron Silver Street Bridge. The route narrowed as Newnham College was approached. In Malting Street the walls were so close that it seemed impossible for returning carriages to pass. A couple more minutes' ride brought her to the red brick buildings of Newnham College, set in eight acres of grounds. Old Hall was to the left and Sidgwick and Clough Halls were on the right. There was countryside at the end of the path. Cambridge seemed small, provincial and rural almost, compared with her familiar Dublin with its bustling sophistication and culture.[3]

Edith was welcomed to 10-year-old Sidgwick Hall (Fig. 3.1) by its resident Vice-Principal, Helen Gladstone. A little younger that Edith's mother would have been had she lived, Helen Gladstone had been one of the earliest Newnham students. She was the youngest daughter of the Liberal Prime Minister, William Gladstone. Edith was aware of the changes that Gladstone had been able to effect in Ireland during his earlier premiership. Leading a previous government, he had managed to improve the rights of tenant farmers in Ireland and to disestablish the Church of Ireland, both acts aligned with the Stoney family view. Edith recalled how her father's open support for Gladstone's disestablishment bill lost him the opportunity to become the Under-Secretary for Ireland. Her father had also been deeply involved in Gladstone's

---

[3]The populations of Dublin and Cambridge in 1890 were approximately 400,000 and 35,000 respectively.

thwarted attempt to restructure Irish universities in the mid-1870s, though they were not necessarily in agreement. During Edith's time at Newnham, William Gladstone, now over 80, tried, once again unsuccessfully, to get an Irish Home Rule Bill passed through parliament, destroyed by massive opposition in the House of Lords. Helen was deeply involved with her father's political negotiations. A political opponent at the time, making reference to the Gladstone household, noted 'Mrs G. and Helen waylaying everybody, scheming this and scheming that, intercepting letters and almost listening at keyholes' [6]. With overlapping political interests, Edith was drawn to Helen Gladstone, who acted as her mentor and advisor for these five important years in her life. She acted as an effective counterweight to the expectation on her to succeed academically, and Edith responded to Miss Gladstone's sense of fun and the need to balance work with recreation.

Edith was approaching 21 years old when she arrived, older than many of the freshers, socially confident as a result of mixing with her father's academic and political contacts and friends from the highest strata of Dublin intellectual society. A few of the new students were still studying to take the Cambridge Highers, some for the 'Little Go', the more general examination that had to be passed before proceeding to study for any Tripos examination. The most able, including Edith, were identified as Tripos candidates on entry. At this time there were a total of 145 students at Newnham of whom 113 were studying for one of the Tripos examinations. Her room gave her a good space in which to gather her personal possessions, making the room that would be her termtime home for the next 5 years as comfortable as possible. She would study mostly during daylight hours, but when the nights drew in, especially during the Lent term, candles gave a background light, whilst oil lamps gave enough illumination to enable her to work in the evenings.

The ageing principal, Anne Clough, had always understood that a student's first arrival might be somewhat daunting. Life in College would be a quite new experience for Edith. She had no shared experience of the previous school life of most of the freshers, the dormitories, the school uniform and the teaching timetables of the secondary girls schools that they had attended. In spite of her relative maturity and confidence, Edith was pleased and surprised to be visited in her new room by most of the second and third-year students in Sidgwick Hall who, following Miss Clough's tradition, knocked on her door to introduce themselves and welcome her to her new home [7]. In due course, Edith discovered that there were several other students who, like her, were not from England, including a few Americans, a young woman from India who planned to enter medicine, and an older woman from Moscow [7, p. 31]. One friend, Melian Stawell, was from Melbourne, a brilliant classics scholar, the youngest daughter of Sir William Stawell, chief justice of Victoria, who was described in her obituary in *The Times* as 'perhaps the most remarkable member of a remarkable family' [8].

Likewise, it was a novel experience for Edith to find that her freedom of action was curtailed within her new home. She found that she was not allowed to be out after 6.30 pm during the Michaelmas and Lent terms, relaxed to 8.30 pm on Sundays and during the summer. She was expected to consult Miss Gladstone if she was invited to visit a friend in one of the other Colleges, or wished to make an excursion.

Such rules did not prevent her going out and she would have been given more leeway than some of the younger students, but it did limit her ability to visit her sister and father during termtime once they had both moved to London. And when her father came to visit, whilst she was allowed to entertain him to tea, she was not allowed to invite any other friend into her room to meet him. Most of her friends were happy to accept these rules, some even viewing life in college as being very free in comparison with their home life in restrictive Victorian families. Unlike them, Edith's upbringing had encouraged her to be independent in thought and action, her home ethos being set by her father, whose inclination was to set standards rather than rules.

There was one topic that filled the corridors and common rooms of Newnham College when she arrived. This was the astonishing success of the Newnham student Philippa Garrett Fawcett in the Mathematics Tripos examinations in the previous summer. She was only a year older than Edith when she had become the first women to achieve the highest mark in the Part 1 of the Maths Tripos, placed, in the terminology of the time, 'above the Senior Wrangler'. On hearing of her success, the Newnham College students lit a bonfire, illuminated the College grounds and sang 'She's a jolly good fellow', accompanied by some rowdy Selwyn College men who had broken through the hedge and trespassed on the sacred lawn of Newnham.

Philippa Fawcett's academic achievement set a target for Edith during her time in Cambridge. It was also further confirmation of Edith's belief, held throughout her life, that, given the opportunity, there was no inherent difference between men and women in what they could achieve.

Philippa Fawcett's success was lauded in widely circulated poem by an undeclared author:

> Hail the triumph of the corset
> > Hail the fair Philippa Fawcett
> > Victress in the fray
>
> Crown her queen of Hydrostatics
> And the other Mathematics
>
> > Wreathe her brow with bay.

After a few further verses, the rhyme ended:

> May she increase in knowledge daily
> > Till the great Professor Cayley
> > Owns himself surpassed
>
> Till the great Professor Salmon
> Votes his own achievements gammon
>
> > And admires aghast.[4]

---

[4] Arthur Cayley (1821–1895) Sadeirian Professor of Mathematics at Cambridge University and sometime chair of council of Newnham College: George Salmon (1819–1904) Mathematics Professor at Trinity College Dublin.

The inclusion of the Professor of Mathematics at Trinity College Dublin, who was undoubtedly well known to the Stoney family, makes a strong case that the unknown poet was Edith herself.

Philippa Fawcett remained at Newnham, placed in the top division of the first class in the Part II Tripos examination the following year, followed by a scholarship year of research into fluid dynamics. She was then appointed as a Newnham College lecturer, remembered by a former student for her 'speed, concentration and infectious delight in what she was teaching, and also her patience with students who were trying their hardest'.

Edith's previous world of contacts had been defined by her father. She was now entering a new world of influence of her own, intersecting with other intellectual families of political standing. Philippa's mother Millicent had co-founded Newnham College and, not long after Edith left Cambridge, became the President of the National Union of Women's Suffrage Societies (NUWSS), an organisation that would be of increasing significance in Edith's life as she engaged in the suffrage movement. Philippa's aunt, her mother's sister Elizabeth Garrett Anderson, proudly continued to use her family name throughout her life as pioneer woman doctor. Edith's and Florence's careers developed within the London medical college and hospitals that she created. Eleanor Sidgwick, sister of Arthur Balfour who became prime minister in 1902, was the first president of the British Federation of University Women, for which Edith would become the first treasurer. Edith was becoming part of a new female web of influence, and this web would continue to influence her life and activities long after she left Cambridge.

The Mathematics Tripos

Edith was steered towards the Maths Tripos, rather than natural sciences. She joined a group of six talented young women at Newnham with whom she would study the deepest aspects of mathematics during the next 3 years. Amongst her fellow students was Ada Johnston, who had been offered the Clothworkers' Scholarship following her performance in the 1889 Higher Examinations, one of only six who gained first class in the mathematics and arithmetic section. Ada came was from a modest background, living locally in Cambridge. Her father, Charles, was a cook and confectioner. Ada had gone to the local school, Mrs. Evans' Upper-Grade School for girls in Park Street, where her ability had been nurtured.[5] Edith and Ada were equal in ability, but from utterly different backgrounds: one, privately educated, whose grandfather was an Irish landowner, and the other, a cook's daughter who went to the local school. Ada and Edith became academic sparring partners,

---

[5] Another ex-pupil of Park Street School was Helen Chambers. After studying at Newnham and the London School of Medicine for Women, she rose to eminence as a radiation pathologist, and was one of the founders of the Marie Curie Hospital after the First World War.

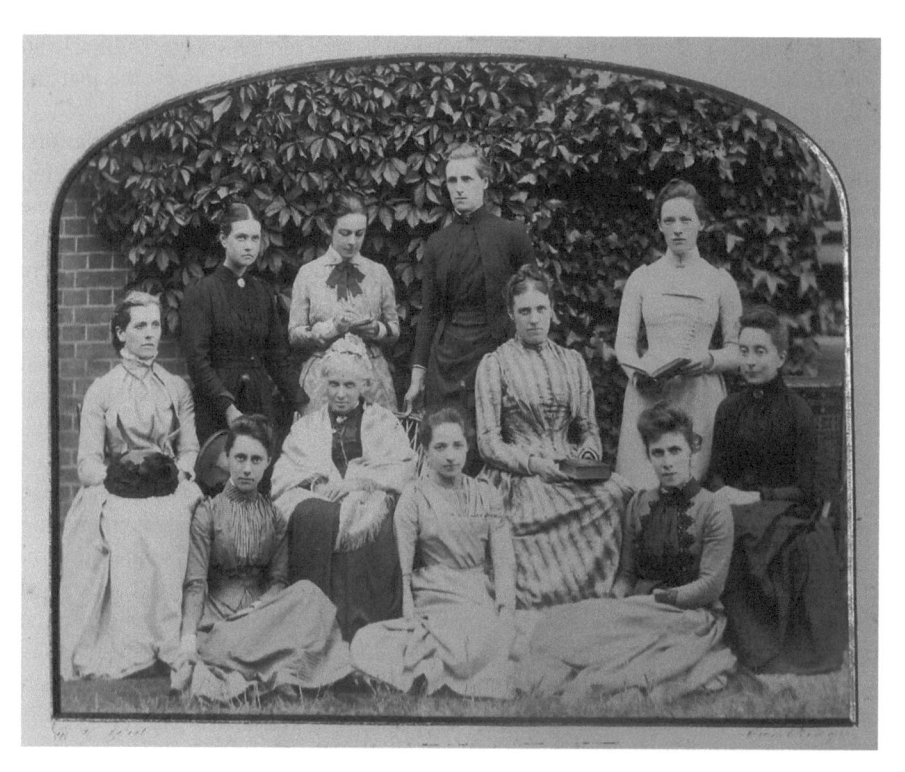

Fig. 3.2 Newnham College staff about 1890. Standing, Left to Right: A Gardner, BA Clough, ER Saunders: ME Rickett (physics lecturer), Seated middle row: H Gladstone (Vice-Principal of Sidgwick Hall), SJ Clough (Principal of Newnham College) K Stephen, L Lee. Front row: MJ Tuke, EM Sharpley, AB Collier (physics lecturer). (Newnham College, Cambridge)

brought together under the watchful eye of Anne Clough, the Sidgwicks and the other Newnham Staff (Fig. 3.2).

In addition to attending their college lectures, the Newnham mathematics group also attended lectures from the most eminent Cambridge mathematicians of their day, in the men's colleges: Henry F Baker at St John's; Arthur Berry, William E Johnston and Herbert W Richmond at King's; William H Young at Peterhouse; and, notably, Ernest W Hobson at Christ's College. Three of these men had been Senior Wranglers, so the standard set could not have been higher.

From the outset, Edith was one of Newnham's star students. She knew that she was the College's most expensive Scholar of her year and was under no illusions that she was expected to emulate Philippa Fawcett's brilliant performance. With Philippa now lecturing at Newnham, Edith was able to draw on her experience as she worked her way towards the challenges of the Part I and Part II Tripos examinations, inspired by her lead, following in her footsteps, dreaming of the same outstanding results.

The topics that Edith studied covered both pure and applied mathematics, overlapping with mathematical physics. Lectures in her second year included astronomy, optics and hydrodynamics as well as advanced trigonometry, hydrostatics and differential and integral calculus. Edith was not restricted to lectures only in mathematics and was free to attend those given to the natural science students also. Amongst these were a set of lectures by JJ Thompson, who by then was the Cavendish Professor of Physics and a highly gifted teacher. Newnham students who attended his advanced physics course conducted their own experiments in the upstairs laboratory in the College, where Professor Thompson visited from time to time to supervise and advise [7, p. 30]. It was just at the time when he was beginning to investigate the passage of electricity through gasses, but before his demonstration of the existence and characteristics of the free electron, the name that Edith's father had suggested for this smallest negatively charged particle. Edith knew that she would be quizzed by her father on the contents of JJ Thompson's lectures, so she was motivated to pay special attention.

As the final Tripos examination approached, Edith's studies were guided by Professor Ernest Hobson of Christ's College, an eminent mathematician who had been the Senior Wrangler in 1878. Hobson provided special coaching for high-flying undergraduates. He had modified his earlier opposition to higher education for women and had been persuaded to act as tutor for Philippa Fawcett as she prepared for her Tripos examinations. This experience seems to have altered his view about women students, because he subsequently agreed to coach Edith also. He made no special concessions to her as a woman, and she seems to have reacted well to his exacting standards. Edith could judge herself against a fellow student mathematician, George Manley, similarly coached by Hobson, who became Senior Wrangler that year.

The Tripos examinations were held over a period of 3 weeks, starting in the middle of May. The first six 3-hour examinations were held on three consecutive days. Edith left Newnham College through the newly built Clough gateway, under Pfeiffer Hall, still awaiting the arrival of the magnificent ironwork gates commemorating the principal who had welcomed her to the College when she had arrived 3 years before. By now, Eleanor Sidgwick had succeeded Anne Clough as the Principal of the College, following Clough's death in 1892.

A 15-minute walk took Edith and her cohort to the YMCA Hall where the examinations were held. The morning examinations started at 9.00 am. Edith was highly focussed, glancing only briefly at the legend around the ceiling which read 'If thou do well, the pain fades, the joy remains. If ill, the joy fades, the pain remains'. Edith knew that she was not expected to finish each examination: marks accrued depending on how many of the questions were answered and how completely. Each evening she returned to Newnham with her six Maths Tripos companions to a special table set up for them for their evening meal. After these examinations were over, they rested and revised for a couple of weeks before sitting six more examinations over a further 3 days. It was a gruelling, exhausting experience.

The Maths Tripos was widely accepted to be the highest challenge that Cambridge had to offer. A few examples from a Maths Tripos examination from the early 1890s give a feel for what Edith read as she sat down to take the examination. There was no set pattern, some papers having as few as nine questions, some twice that number. There were seductively easy-looking questions, for which it was extraordinarily difficult to gain high marks in the limited time available: 'Write a brief account of the methods of producing electromagnetic waves and the means employed to determine their wavelength', a question that, in a mathematics paper, required the student to have a detailed knowledge of the derivation of Maxwell's equations for electromagnetic wave propagation. There were ones demanding a deep understanding of mathematical terminology and meaning: 'Shew that any covariant of one or more quantics, which involves more sets than one of cogredient variables, may be expressed as an emanent of a covariant involving one set'. And there were the ones from applied physics and hydrodynamics, many including page-wide partial differential equations to analyse or derive. One from this topic asked the student to 'Shew that the motion of the liquid outside a certain surface surrounding a circular vortex ring the radius of whose core is small compared with the radius of its aperture, is the same as that due to the motion of this surface through the liquid with the velocity of the translation of the ring. Find the equation to this surface and the length of the axis of the ring intercepted by it.'

Edith did not disappoint her coach, nor Helen Gladstone, nor the senior staff of Newnham College who had awarded her the Winkworth Scholarship. A combination of innate ability and hard work was crowned with success, and she gained a first. When the list of women's examination marks was read out, after the list of the men's results, hers was announced as equal to that achieved by the 17th Wrangler. Ada Johnston had done slightly better: her mark placed her between the 5th and 6th. Six further women passed with second class, including three from Girton and another two at third class.

These were remarkable results. Some in the national press considered their achievements to be as significant as that of Philippa Fawcett 3 years before, suggesting that Newnham College might throw another celebratory party as they had done in 1890. More seriously it was noted that 'these successes in great examinations are doubly flattering to women, because they imply as much force of character as intellect. Only a cool hand can hope to win them'. A second article added

> How much longer will the universities refuse to admit women to the degree they have earned? The present system of exclusion is absurd. These ladies take high rank in the tripos, yet they are not in the tripos at all. Their numbers simply mean that, if they had been men, they would have had their reward. The day will come when the present attitude of our leading Universities towards women will be regarded with the same contemptuous surprise with which we now regard the barbarisms of the Middle Ages [9]

Newnham did well overall in the Tripos examinations of 1893, with a total of 36 students passing, one-third of these being in maths and natural sciences. For most of them, this ended their time in Cambridge, and they went down for the last time at the end of the May term. Four of Edith's maths companions soon found posts as teachers in girls' secondary schools, on Merseyside, in Winchester, in Chester and in Hertford. Then, as now, able mathematics teachers were in high demand.

For Edith and Ada, their results were sufficiently good for them to continue their studies and sit for the Maths Tripos Part II examinations the following year. There were only six examinations this time, held over 3 days, but the questions were more challenging. Ada did equally well as in 1893, her mark placing her in the top band of the first class. Edith did creditably, but not as well as the previous year, achieving second class in band 2. It is as though she was paying less attention to the expectations of Eleanor Sidgwick, and more to the broader world view of Helen Gladstone, taking her foot off the pedal marked 'academic excellence' and changing gear slightly to refocus on her life-work balance.

A Student in Cambridge

Edith did not restrict herself to only academic studies during her first 3 undergraduate years at Newnham. When she arrived in the autumn of 1890, she found that there was a bewildering array of societies to join, more than enough to fill any free time. The Political and Debating Societies and the Historical, Classical, Literary and Scientific Societies were all available to her to join. The Debating Society was the most prestigious, and most of the students, Edith included, became members. It was in Edith's nature to take charge, and she was appointed as the President of the Debating Society in the Michaelmas term of 1893, leading it during the whole of her fourth year. Edith and her committee needed to put together an interesting programme of debates for the coming year. An animated debate followed the motion 'that women do not take sufficient interest in their food', proposed by Edith's tennis partner, Florence Davies, which failed by three votes. Other motions, 'that no great cause can succeed without fanaticism' and 'That Puritanism has been injurious to the English nation' were both lost. The Newnham women were largely from serious establishment backgrounds. A most lively debate followed the proposal 'that humour, like salt, should be in every dish', strong feelings being expressed on both sides before the proposal was defeated by 82 to 72. The total number of votes cast indicates not only the popularity of the debates for Newnham students but also those students who attended from other colleges, notably from Girton. There was also a lively debate for the motion 'that strikes are productive of more good than evil', a subject of considerable interest at the time. The May Term motion proposed 'that the decline of patriotism would be disastrous to the world at large', eloquently debated, with a clear majority of 75 feeling proud to be British.

Judging by the opposition to the motion 'that the influence of fashion is injurious both to society and the individual', Edith was not alone amongst the students in having a sense of dressing well. This was not taken from Eleanor Sidgwick's lead, whose limited and practical dress sense was widely known. She once criticised a student for packing a dressing gown when taking a trip, advising her that she, Mrs. Sidgwick, used her mackintosh coat when she needed to visit the bathroom. The photograph of Edith from this time shows her to have a consciously feminine view of her appearance (Fig. 1.6). We have the College Debating Society to thank for this picture: it is included in an album of photographs of the Presidents of the Debating Society, such were their special position at Newnham. Philippa Fawcett, an earlier president, is there. The photographs of the other presidents show them dressed in unadorned formal clothes, mostly darker shades and with very high collars. By contrast, the photograph of Edith, made by Werner and Son in Dublin, shows her in a relaxed informal white blouse with slightly puffed shoulders and neck uncovered, and at her throat, there is a posy of lilies held in a clasp. This is a deliberate choice of a woman confident enough to dress as she wished.

The second forum in which the young women expressed their opinions to one another was in the Political Society. This was structured to mimic the House of Commons, and each year a prime minister was elected, who then chose her cabinet. Party support was evenly split. In Edith's fourth year, the numbers of students associating themselves with each party were the following: conservatives 44, liberals 46 and liberal unionists 44. There were 12 independents, quite possibly those with socialist and radial views yet to coalesce around a political party. Here in a nest of female emancipation, fledgling politicians exercised their wings, learning techniques that they hoped soon to engage in the public arena. The liberal 'Prime Minister', Miss Skeat, introduced a bill for female suffrage that was, unsurprisingly, carried by a large majority [10]. Any opposition seemed very odd to Edith, whose property-owning grandmother had the right to vote in Irish local elections from a time before Edith was born. These young women were sufficiently well informed to know that, on 19 September 1893, New Zealand had given women the right to vote in national elections and were excitedly anticipating that similar developments would occur soon in Britain. In 1894, there was a small legislative step in Britain towards female suffrage. The Local Government Act was extended to allow married women to participate as voters and councillors in rural and urban districts. By 1900 there were about 200 women parish councillors. Any momentum towards full national emancipation slowed, however, hopes dying as progress stalled. The wait would test their patience, some turning to militancy in frustration as women failed to gain the right to a national vote. Throughout the next decades, both Edith and Florence continued to engage with the suffrage movement but equally opposed the Suffragettes' policy of violence to achieve votes for women.

Other bills were debated in the Political Society, with outcomes representative of the group opinions of these young female students. A bill for the abolition of the House of Lords was rejected by a majority of ten; a call for the disestablishment of the Church of England was likewise defeated, as was a private member's bill protesting against state interference with the hours of adult labour. Under a liberal unionist 'government', a bill for the establishment of a 'System of Retail Sale of Intoxicating Liquor by an Authorised Company' passed easily [11]. These were knowledgeable, opinionated, confident young women, testing the strength of their ideas within the safety of the College debating chamber, preparing to engage in the wider world ahead.

In the Lent term 1894, there was another heated discussion when the Irish question was debated. Balfour's policy at the time was to 'kill Home Rule with kindness' [12]. Edith was one of the few in Newnham with a family experience of the situation in Ireland and its history. She was only too well aware of the simmering tensions in her home country and followed with acute and personal interest the actions in Westminster to develop Ireland's farming through the Land Acts of 1887 and 1891 and the creation of jobs using new infrastructure projects. Edith was deeply

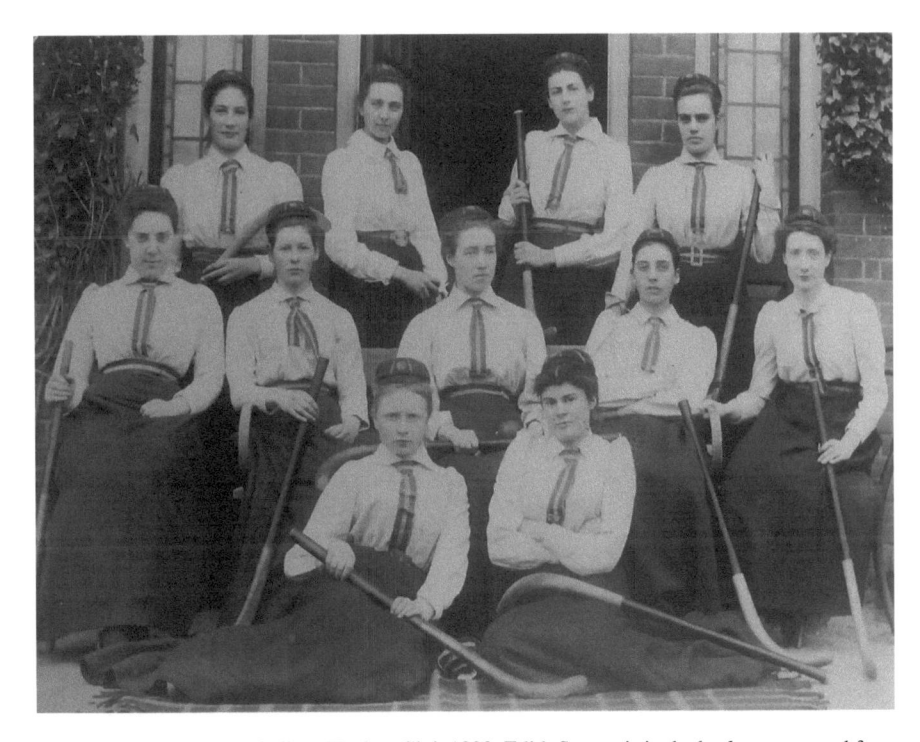

Fig. 3.3 The Newnham College Hockey Club 1893. Edith Stoney is in the back row, second from the left. Isabella Jameson, second row, second from the right, studied with Edith, and gained a third in the Maths Tripos. She went on to teach at Winchester High School and was co-founder of the All-England Women's Hockey Association in 1896 (Newnham College, Cambridge)

aware of her father's failure to sustain his Queen's University against concerted opposition, not least from the Catholic Church, and understood, even then, that the tide of history was leading Ireland towards eventual home rule. She was aware of the potential for violence and opposed such conflict. She was a unionist, opposed to Irish independence, even as her family were leaving the country of their birth. She made her opinions very clear in the Newnham Political Society debate. The unionists celebrated when the motion condemning home rule for Ireland was carried by a majority of 37.

Outside the debating chamber, Edith took advantage of the ample opportunities for recreational activity. Hockey was the most important team game played in the college. Being small and fast, Edith was a useful hockey player and became a member of the recently formed Newnham hockey team in her second year at Cambridge (Fig. 3.3). The big match each year was for the Elliott Cup between Girton and Newnham teams, but at other times, Edith travelled with the hockey team to play matches against the major girls' schools in the country, including Roedean School on the South Coast. She was also a particularly useful tennis player. Remarkably, in the May Term of 1893, at the same time as she was dealing with her Part 1 Tripos examinations, she won the tennis doubles cup against Girton, three

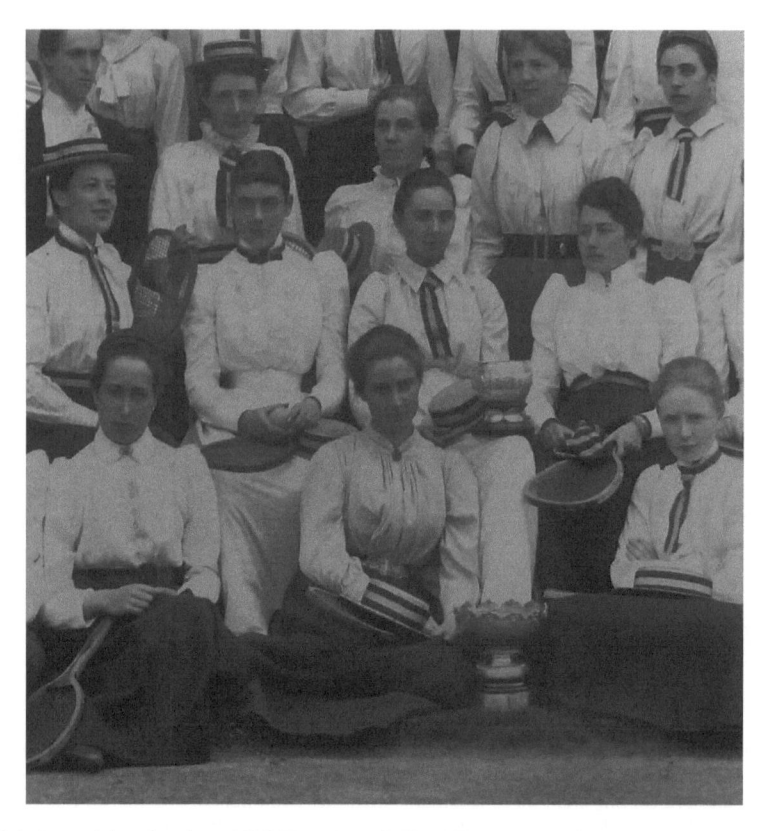

Fig. 3.4 Part of the victorious 1893 Newnham College Tennis team. From the left: Back row: D Jowitt, FJ Davies, EA Stoney, EH Lyster: Front row AMJE Johnson, RV Brooke. Amy Johnstone was Edith's outstanding sparring partner in the Maths Tripos (Newnham College, Cambridge)

sets to one. A photograph shows her sitting next to her stern-looking partner, Florence Davies, another privately educated Winkworth Scholar, both wearing ankle-length white skirts, Edith proudly holding the cup in her lap and her boater in her right hand (Fig. 3.4). She also played in the singles tournament in the same year, though Girton won that time. Edith continued to be part of the team the following year, dominating the competition and winning both in the singles and the doubles. The other popular ball game was fives, mentioned by Edith as one of the important recreational facilities. In the comparative privacy of the fives court, where agility and speed were of prime importance, dress conventions could be relaxed and corsets loosened.

Edith and her friends also relaxed by boating on the Cam, especially in the summer mornings and evenings, times when it was not required to be chaperoned. It was short walk past Ridley Hall and down Malting Lane to the Cam and then left to the boathouse by Silver Street Bridge. A morning trip started early, at 6.00 am, rowing to Baits Bite for breakfast, so they could be back for their first lecture at 9.00 am. The gentle trip along the Backs, gliding past Queens' and Clare, King's and

John's, slowly drifting under the bridges, was a delightful relaxation. The chaperone rules were relaxed further for those who stayed in College during the long vacation, and then they could go for longer, meandering trips, taking a hamper with lunch and tea, idling the time in the summer sun before returning for supper.

And they cycled. The easy availability of new, geared safety bicycles with their pneumatic tyres made cycling steadily more popular. When Edith arrived at Cambridge, she found that, whilst some students rode bicycles, the activity was officially frowned upon. By the end of Edith's time in Cambridge, riding a bicycle was an officially sanctioned freedom. One early student described how, after lectures, they would take 'a five-mile bicycle spin through Grantchester and Trumpington or, at the proper season, through the Madingley woods for primroses' [13]. Cycling was a serious component of student life, and it is possible to sense her hand in its controlled acceptance. The 1894 Newnham College regulations laid down that:

> Students may ride the bicycle with certain restrictions. The art may not be acquired at College. Only inveterate proficiency is countenanced. This is tested by a searching examination in corner turning etc before the candidates receive a diploma.

The dress code was no more relaxed, though. A student described 'the cumbrous skirts covering trouserlegs firmly secured to ankles with broad black elastic'. Gloves and a hat were mandatory in town. By 1895, 'bicycling had became a marked phase in Newnham athletics. Competitors cram feverishly before breakfast to prepare for the fatal test (of coasting round the hockey field).' By the time that Newnham hosted the University Extension meeting, the summer after Edith left, a visiting student from Cheltenham Ladies' College was able to house her bicycle in a shed with stands for 30 or 40 machines. She was astonished to discover that Newnham students had invented a cycling event in which wooden hoops were driven with hoop-sticks, speculating that 'a University Kindergarten had been found necessary for some of these advanced women in whom childhood had had no chance of ripening' [14]. Newnham students had surely benefitted from Edith's enthusiastic influence on the acceptance of cycling as an official part of student life [15]. Nowadays, a metal plate, fixed the wall outside Clough Gate, warns; 'Newnham College. No Cycles Beyond this Point Please. Domestic Bursar'. Student cycling remains an activity subject to external control, in spite of Cambridge now topping the list as the most popular city for cycling.

Edith had reached a watershed in her life. Cocooned comfortably within Newnham, she was in no hurry to leave Cambridge after the examinations in the summer of 1894. She had achieved highly and there was plenty of goodwill towards her. Nevertheless, she needed to give some thought to her future. One of her early aspirations was closed. Medicine was no longer an option, however, much she might have wished otherwise. Florence was still a medical student, and the family budget did not stretch to funding another through medical training. Her sister's career now took priority over hers.

But she had, by now, a clearer idea about where her scientific interests and skills lay. Her modest performance in the Mathematics Part II examinations was evidence that her future should not be in pure mathematics. When an opportunity for travel arose to carry out mathematical research, she was very happy that her friend Ada Johnson was given the opportunity to go. Grace Chisholm from Girton College (who later married and collaborated with one of Edith's lecturers, William Young) had arranged to study at Göttingen University in Germany under the mathematician Felix Klein. There was an offer of a second place that could be filled by a Newnham student. Edith had always kept a sisterly eye out for Ada, encouraging her to take part in college affairs, encouraging her to join the hockey team. She had proposed her as her successor as President of the Debating Society. She knew, too, that Ada's commitment to pure mathematics was greater than hers and that she could benefit from the experience of working with Klein on his theories of symmetries and non-Euclidean geometries. Edith was now clear in her mind that she was much happier working in applied science, using her understanding of physics and her mathematical skills to solve real-world technical challenges.

In spite of mathematical talent, Ada's brilliance failed to bear fruit. Edith even tried to help her after her return from Germany. In 1898, when Edith herself left Cheltenham Ladies' College, Ada briefly took her place teaching there. Sadly, all the time that had been invested in Ada's education, all Edith's efforts on her behalf, would fizzle out. Ada returned home to live with her parents until they died. Newnham had done all it could to develop the exceptional talents of this young woman, Edith all she could do to steer her towards a rewarding career, but academic society was not yet ready to accept a brilliant woman from another social strata into its ranks. She was the only daughter, and convention dictated that she became her parents' carer.

In the same year that Edith was so successful in her Part I Mathematics Tripos at Cambridge, another young woman passed her first major physics examination in Paris. In 1893, Marie Sklodovska graduated in first rank as 'licenciée es sciences physiques' at the Sorbonne. She followed this the next year, by achieving second rank as 'licenciée es sciences mathématiques'. Both Edith and Marie managed to stretch their 3-year scholarships for an extra year. In that same year, Pierre Curie had fallen hopelessly in love with Marie, even though she told him that she intended to return to her native Poland to teach. She returned to Paris in the autumn, nominally for further study but also in response to numerous letters that Pierre had written to her, whilst she was away. By the following June, they were engaged to be married.

Edith did not meet her Pierre in Cambridge: or if she did, there is no record of it. She did not go on a cycling holiday for her honeymoon as the Curies did. The romance between Pierre and Marie Curie is the stuff of legend, two people bound by their love of science and of one another. Perhaps it could only have happened in freethinking Paris, the city of Degas, Debussy and the Folies Begère. Late Victorian, chaperoned, Cambridge gave little scope for romance, requiring formal introductions before there was any opportunity for private intercourse. None of Edith's Maths Tripos colleagues married either, so the trajectory of Edith's personal life was largely set by the British social mores of the time. The book of photographs of the babies of past students, compiled by Millicent Fawcett, Philippa's mother, as a rather obvious hint to her daughter, could not disguise the reality that marriage for Newnham students did not emerge naturally from their time there. Indeed, a survey in 1895 showed that of the 1486 women who thus far received a university education, only 208 had subsequently married [16]. The tongue-in-cheek proposal from Charles Darwin's cousin Francis Galton to Henry Sidgwick that a prize be offered to each Newnham graduate on marriage, and again on the birth of each child, clearly expressing the patriarchal sentiments of the time, was never going to be implemented [17]. These women left Cambridge with confidence in their own abilities, tested against the male-dominated establishment, with a shared experience of women's achievement, based on hard work and mutual support. They sought independence, often in environments in which women were in control, for example, in the expanding sector of girls' education, itself driven by the expectations of the middle classes, and in the foothold gained by women in the medical profession. Men were not required there, and together they were creating islands in which women were the primary actors and decision-makers.

Edith did not want to leave Cambridge. Later, she would recall with fondness the 'life-long joy in the memory of the worth and the keenness of work and play at such a residential College as Newnham' when comparing it with the facilities that were just becoming available for women at Trinity College Dublin. 'In Dublin there is no residential hostel for women, no resident staff of women lecturers, no hall for dancing and debates, no hockey ground or fives court, nor any of the rest that goes towards the wonderful formative power for character of resident life to the students' [18].

An anonymous letter from a Newnham student, published at the end of Edith's second year at Cambridge, echoed her enthusiasm for life as a student at Newnham.

> It is, as I know by experience, a belief current among the ignorant that we Newnham or Girton students are terrible bluestockings, incapable of taking interest beneath classics, mathematics, or various ologies and isms. But I must maintain . . . . that nowhere in England is a set of morally and physically healthier girls to be found that at Newnham. . . . . I think it is only fair to add that the spirit of real fun and hearty enjoyment which pervades Newnham is in great measure due to the influence of Miss Gladstone [19].

The words could almost have been written by Edith herself.

Newnham College Astronomer

Edith was having too good a time at Newnham and disliked unnecessary change. However, in an unforgiving academic environment, her less-than-perfect performance in the Part II Tripos examination was insufficient to gain any research scholarship or formal college lectureship. The list of students in Sidgwick Hall includes her name as a solitary 'Senior Student' for the year 1894–1895, not really a student but not staff either.

In this academic no man's land, she did a bit of lecturing. She was also appointed as the resident College Astronomer. Early in Edith's time at Cambridge, Newnham College had been given an astronomical telescope and funds for an observatory to be built in the College grounds. The American-born Mrs. Mary Boreham, the

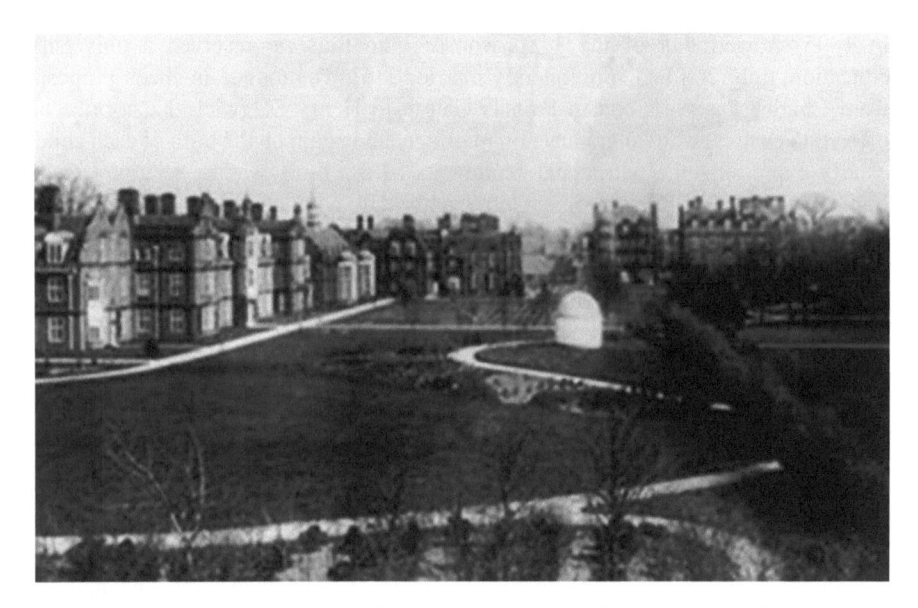

Fig. 3.5 The first Newnham College observatory. Sidgwick Hall is in the centre, Old Hall to the right and Clough Hall on the left (Newnham College, Cambridge)

benefactor, had been recently widowed. After her husband's early death from consumption, she had kept in touch with his well-to-do family from Haverhill, about 20 miles from Cambridge. Her father-in-law, the brewer William Wakeling Boreham, had been an amateur astronomer, and his 6 inch refractor equatorial telescope, with its German achromatic objective lens, had remained unused after he died. Shortly after her husband's death, Mrs. Boreham presented it to Newnham College, with £30 for refurbishment. It was housed within a rotatable copper dome, breached by slit through which observations were made. By the autumn of 1892, this observatory had been erected on a low mound on the old hockey ground to the south of Clough Hall (Fig. 3.5) [20]. The telescope was a high-status and visible statement that Newnham was seriously engaging in science, even though it was much less powerful than the Newall telescope, a 25 inch refractor that had only recently been donated to the Cavendish Laboratory and installed at the University observatory.

The Newnham telescope was mounted on a heavy masonry stand, designed to map the diurnal movements of the heavens (Fig. 3.6). The axis, round which the whole instrument turned, was aligned with the axis of the earth. The telescope was fixed to a circular graduated scale that could turn in its plane and around its centre. Thus the telescope could be set with its optical axis at any known angle to the earth's axis. Vernier scales allowed for very fine adjustment and measurement of angle. A second circular graduated scale was aligned with the equator. Once placed accurately, these two scales measured the ascension and declination of any star. The clockwork drive mounted under the telescope tracked the field of view so as to maintain a star centrally, following the rotation of the heavens.

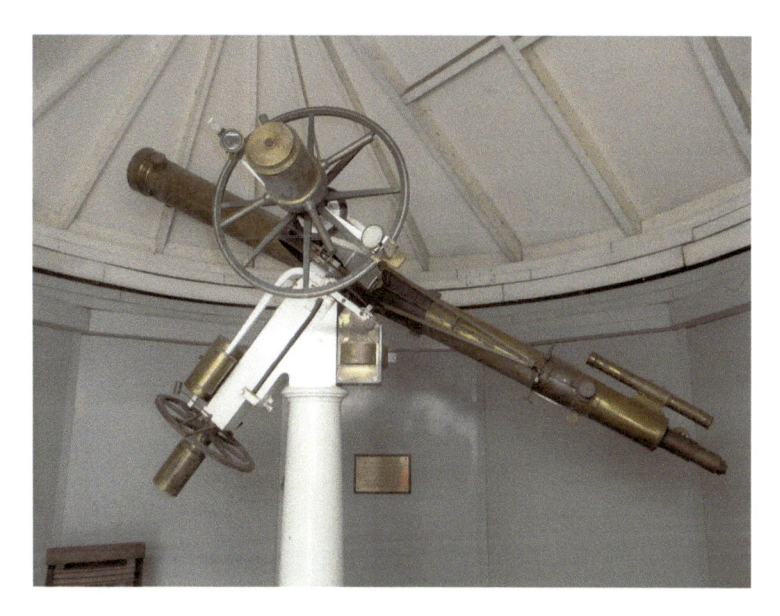

Fig. 3.6 The Newnham College 6 inch refracting equatorial telescope (Francis Duck)

Once Edith had completed her Part II examinations in the summer of 1894, she was given charge and the key of the observatory. This recalls her father's first post with the Leviathan telescope in Birr after he had graduated from Trinity College 50 years earlier. It was reassuring for Eleanor Sidgwick to know that Edith's father was now living in London and might take the occasional trip to Cambridge to see what his daughter was doing, giving them a little astronomical advice on using a telescope that was very similar to the one that he had in Galway [21]. It was one thing installing the instrument, quite another using it for useful astronomical observations and teaching. Edith was a good choice to be its custodian. She had learned the patterns of the constellations in the sky from her father, using his telescope as she grew up. She understood the movement of the planets and the transient appearance of comets. She knew how to sight on a visible celestial object and how to use star maps to locate a minor star or faint galaxy, invisible to the naked eye, by rotating the telescope to a calibrated point in the sky. With the Newnham telescope, she could lock on to the image of an object and track its movement as the earth turned on its axis. Edith supervised students who had no particular knowledge of astronomy and were invited on certain evenings to see, for example, Saturn's rings and Jupiter's moons. Assuming that the old transit telescope that is still in the Newnham Observatory was there in Edith's time, she could have demonstrated how it was used for high-precision star location. She left no evidence of any original astronomical observations, however, and her college role seems to have been limited to ensuring that the telescope was set up, maintained, operated and demonstrated correctly.

Edith's year as the custodian of the Newnham telescope rekindled her father's interest in solving a particular technical challenge in astronomic observation. He had

Fig. 3.7 Johnstone Stoney and the heliostat that he bought from Watson and Sons in 1895. This was Edith's favourite photograph of her father. The instrument is now held by the London Science Museum: item 1936-421

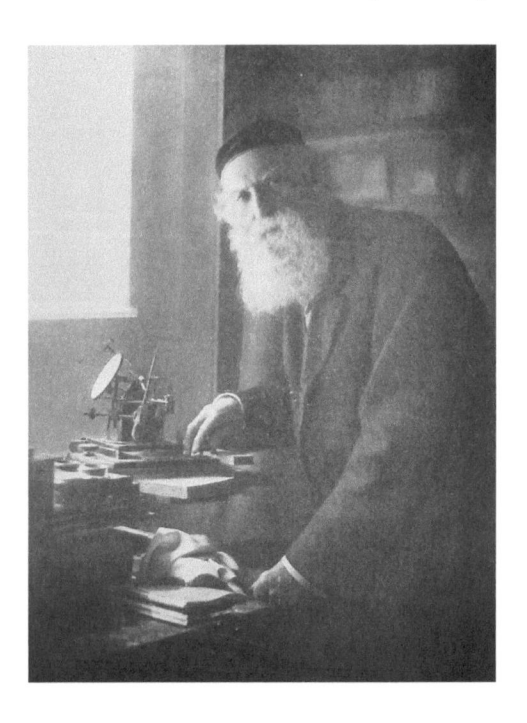

first described his heliostat at the 1869 Exeter meeting of the British Association. This instrument consisted of a mirror turned by drive bands from a clockwork mechanism to compensate for the movement of the sun. It gave a stationary beam of light, aimed towards the North Pole, to be used for optical experiments. With no interest in personal gain, he had not taken out a patent, but arranged for Spencer and Son of Dublin to manufacture his heliostat for sale at five guineas each. His simple design was very popular with amateur astronomers and small institutional physics laboratories, and several other instrument manufacturers offered heliostats using the same principle.

In 1895, her father bought a new heliostat from W. Watson and Sons in Holborn, based on his own design but driven directly from the clockwork mechanism and able to be directed to any azimuth (Fig. 3.7). Whilst this heliostat was quite adequate for general solar studies, he knew that the design was inadequate to act as a 'siderostat', for tracking the image of a small segment of the sky at night. He challenged himself to invent a simple arrangement, capable of greater precision, that would be suitable for use with an equatorial telescope such as Edith's. He presented his design, with Edith in the audience, at the 1895 meeting of the British Association in Ipswich, 'On a movement designed to attain astronomical accuracy in the motion of siderostats' [22]. Edith, resident astronomer at Newnham, needed an accurate siderostat; her father designed one with her in mind.

Edith became a life member of the British Association for the Advancement of Science at this Ipswich meeting. Her father was now a senior statesman of the BAAS establishment, still serving on several committees including the one for electrical standards. He was also helping with another, 'On the uniformity of size of pages of Scientific Societies publications', a thankless task with an unreachable goal. Edith was delighted and honoured as her father proudly introduced his talented daughter to his friends, including Lord Kelvin and Lord Rayleigh and her cousin George FitzGerald's close companion Oliver Lodge.

The Newnham observatory was not unanimously approved, some seeing it as aesthetically displeasing. When the garden was redesigned, these voices were pleased to suggest the addition of some trees to shield the observatory from view from the College windows. The annual report noted, with regret, that these 'do not grow up as fast as might be desired, but perhaps this does not matter so much, as they will inevitably have to be cut down in the interest of science as soon as they do'. After Edith left Cambridge, the observatory was dismantled, and a new one built further from the College buildings, its view towards the horizon unhindered by foliage and where her telescope still resides.

Astronomy was not an unreasonable activity for an aspiring women scientist. Only a few years before, two mathematics students from Girton College, Alice Everett and Annie Russell, had been appointed by the Astronomer Royal, Sir William Christie, as 'computers' to carry out the laborious numerical calculations that underpinned the astronomical observations at the Royal Observatory at Greenwich. The British Astronomical Association made them welcome, and Annie Russell took over the editorship of the Association's journal in 1894. She also married the founder and president, Edward Maunder, in 1895 [23]. Edith knew of these appointments and perhaps saw a possible future for herself in astronomy. Sadly, the salary of a junior 'computer' was only about £4 a month, far less than the £100 or more a year that she might expect to earn as a teacher. Mrs. Sidgwick was clear that exotic careers were for the very few. In 1897, after Edith had left, she was advising that 'women will do excellent work in the subordinate fields of science and learning, will do much laborious work that needs to be done, though it is not very brilliant or striking, and will in particular prove excellent assistants' [24].

Edith, now 26 years old, was coasting. The small amount of lecturing and her role as resident astronomer barely filled her time or her bank account. In spite of the joys and successes of her 5 years at Cambridge, she was left with no tangible benefit, no future career, no degree and no husband. Apart from Helen Gladstone, she was now the longest-standing resident of Sidgwick Hall. In spite of their age difference, the two women had much in common. Both came from liberal backgrounds. Both knew that their time in Cambridge must soon end. Both experienced the inspiration and challenge of being daughters of great men. Both, too, shared a common concern for the future welfare of their fathers, each recently retired. William Gladstone, now well past 80 years old, sight and hearing both failing, finally resigned as prime minister on 3 March 1894, and Helen knew that she must soon leave Cambridge to care for him. At least Edith did not have to worry about her own father for the time being. He was approaching 70, still fit, and Gertrude could keep an eye on him in London. But she could no longer presume on his subsidies to keep her going, especially with Florence's continuing costs for her medical training. Eventually, in the autumn of

1895, Edith finally bowed to the inevitable and opted for the financially secure world of education.

References

1. Stoney EA. Women laboratory assistants. Woman Eng. 1922;1(2):165–7.
2. Stoney GJ. On the cause of double lines and of equidistant satellites in the spectra of gases. Sci Trans Roy Dublin Soc 11th Ser. 1891;4:563.
3. Philips A, editor. A Newnham anthology. Cambridge: Newnham College; 1979. p. 5.
4. Howard JN. Eleanor mildred sidgwick and the rayleighs. Appl Opt. 1964;3:1120–2.
5. Stoney F. OBE, MD. The vote.1932 Oct 28;33:1201.
6. Hamilton E. Quoted in Roy Jenkins. Gladstone. London: Macmillan; 1995. p. 598.
7. Cockburn EO, editor. Catherine Durning Holt. Letters from Newnham College 1889–1892. Cambridge, Newnham College. Edith left no personal record of her experiences in Cambridge.
8. The Melbourne Argus; 1934 Jan 17. p. 15.
9. The higher education of women. The evening telegraph: 1893 Jun 14, and another Woman's year. Morning Post; 1893 Dec 29.
10. Cambridge Independent Press; 1893 Nov 10.
11. Records of Newnham College. Newnham reports 1893 and 1894.
12. Balfour, Letters, p 46. Quoted in Simon Heffer: the age of decadence Britain 1880 to 1914. London: Random House; 2017. p 320.
13. Willcox MA. The sidgwicks in residence. In: Philips A, Newnham A, editors. Anthology. Cambridge: Newnham College; 1979. p. 14.
14. Louch M. The Cambridge meeting. The Cheltenham Ladies' College Magazine. 1896;24 (autumn):304.
15. Quiggin MA. Students may ride the bicycle. In: Philips A, Newnham A, editors. Anthology. Cambridge: Newnham College; 1979. p. 44–6.
16. Searle GR. A new England: peace and war 1886–1918 (The new Oxford history of England). Oxford: Clarendon Press; 2004. p. 69.
17. Francis Galton to Henry Sidgwick. Quoted in Fara P. A lab of one's own. Oxford: OUP; 2018. p. 43.
18. Stoney EA. Collegium sacrosanctæ et individuæ Trinitatis juxta Dublin. Newnham College Letter. 1904:37–43.
19. The beneficent influence of College life on girls. Cambridge Independent Press; 1892 June 29.
20. Newnham College Report; 1892.
21. Ryder AJ. An Irishman of note, George Johnstone Stoney. Privately published; p. 87.
22. Stoney GJ. On the equipment of the astrophysical observatory of the future. With two appendices: appendix I.- on the support of large specula; appendix II.- on making the siderostat an instrument of precision. Mon Not R Astron Soc. 1896;56:452–9.
23. Brück M. Torch-bearing women astronomers. In: Mulvihill M, editor. Lab coats and lace. Dublin: WITS. p. 73–85.
24. Fara P. A lab of one's own. Oxford: OUP; 2018. p. 125.

Chapter 4
Cheltenham

Edith never lost contact with Newnham College, but, for the present, she needed to find paid employment. She had enjoyed what little teaching she had done during the past year and found that she was quite good at it. Bowing to the inevitable, she secured an appointment as assistant mathematical mistress at a provincial English spa town in the west of England. She was becoming part of the English educational establishment, any trace of an Irish accent now lost.[1]

The school, Cheltenham Ladies' College, was far from provincial. Edith knew that she was joining one of the longest-established girls' schools in England and was aware of the reputation that the headmistress Dorothea Beale had established for herself and for the College since its founding 40 years earlier. Miss Beale was one of the outstanding educationalists of the nineteenth century, a pioneer flag bearer for girls' education. She had accepted the post of headmistress at Cheltenham in 1858, only 4 years after the school had been founded, and had been personally responsible for its growth into the school that Edith joined. Edith's first impressions were of a much larger establishment than Newnham College, with 600 full-time pupils. Over half of these were boarders. In the early days, many of the pupils had been daughters of military, civil or church families overseas, boarding in one of several residential houses close to the College. By the time Edith arrived, there was new money in the late Victorian economy. Edith found herself teaching predominantly the daughters of stockbrokers, accountants, civil engineers and factory owners, who now outnumbered those from medical, legal and church parentage.

Unlike Newnham, the College buildings themselves were intended primarily for teaching. They were also intended to impress. Stepping through the main doors, Edith entered a lofty entrance hall, with its broad staircase winding upwards. The stark geometry of the floor, a tessellation of large square black and white tiles known

---

[1] 'She would speak in a clear young voice with perfect enunciation and the purest English'. Hutton IE. With a Woman's Unit in Serbia, Salonika and Sebastopol. London: Williams and Norgate; 1928. p. 26.

as the Milky Way, led towards the vaulted Great Hall, its Gothic windows giving a strongly ecclesiastical feel. Elsewhere she saw graceful chairs, designed and created by local craftsmen in the new Arts and Crafts style. The windows were filled with stained glass, and there were murals on the walls, all similarly crafted. Beautiful wrought iron tracery supported the banisters, and even the simplest stair rails were decorated with a stylised daisy, the emblem of the College Guild.

Mathematics Teacher

Edith taught her Division 2 pupils, up to 16 years old, in the Great Hall. She quickly discovered that it would need all her powers of concentration to do so. It was not the pupils that were the problem: under Miss Beale's 'rule of silence', they did not speak unless spoken to. The difficulty was that several lessons were conducted simultaneously in this large undivided open space. Edith was allocated an open area to the side of the main central aisle, her pupils sitting in their desks with quill pens in hand, gathered round her blackboard. One pupil later recalled 'One of the most valuable lessons I learned within those beloved walls was concentration, and to this day I can work placidly in a babble of noise' [1]. A few yards to Edith's right, a German lesson could be in process, instruction on the Roman empire to the left, whilst immediately behind her back, a fellow teacher was discussing Hamlet with a group of 13-year-olds. Moreover, classes were often taught under the watchful eye of Miss Beale, seated on her large wooden 'throne' against the end wall. Edith had learned how to focus intensively without distraction in Cambridge. She now learned how to focus under much less congenial conditions.

Edith did not give all her lessons under such stressful circumstances. The New Wing had been opened a year before she arrived, with rooms dedicated to teaching the Oxford and Cambridge examination classes. She was pleased to find that some were even preparing for degree-level examinations through the Oxford Extension system or as external candidates at London University. For some years, Bedford College in London was the only other women's college in England where women could prepare for a London degree. Edith taught these Division 1 mathematics pupils in the Cambridge Room, off the corridor on the ground floor, next to the new library. She instructed and guided these most able and senior maths pupils, not overseen by Miss Beale, but instead beneath the watchful portraits of four of Cambridge's greatest minds from the arts and sciences, depicted in stained glass, with the morning sun glowing through the window. Two were poets, Edmund Spenser (Pembroke College) at the top of the window and John Milton (Christ's College) below. The other two were Francis Bacon and Isaac Newton, both from Trinity College, reminding both pupils and teacher of the foundation of the scientific method and of the power of mathematical analysis.

Upstairs was the museum, filled with extraordinary artefacts, including a great brown bear, shot in the Rocky Mountains, an ichthyosaurus whose remains had been found under the playing field during an earlier building phase and some 4000-year-old Babylonian tablets. Several items had been donated by the Natural History Museum, and items continued to arrive during Edith's time at the College. She was entertained to see the arrival, in 1896, of 'two rhinoceroses, a beautiful kangaroo, a fine eland and a handsome anteater' [1, p. 59].

Edith soon found that Miss Beale valued mathematics and science as essential elements of a girl's education. In the year Edith arrived, the College Magazine carried a passionate article by Miss Beale in defence of geometry, which she saw as a cosmic subject leading to 'the heaven which is above the heavens'. In her 1898 address to the College Guild, Miss Beale said 'How can girls be prepared for such work as falls to them as heads of great schools, and hospitals, and settlements, as doctors in foreign lands, if their education was, as I found it, minus mathematics and science?' Dorothea Beale had been the first lady mathematics tutor at Queen's College, London, a girls' school whose foundation predated that of Cheltenham Ladies' College by nearly a decade, and had continued teaching maths throughout her time there as Principal. Edith knew that Miss Beale was taking a special interest in her teaching ability, proudly reporting her outstanding Tripos success in the 1895–1896 College Magazine. Edith soon appreciated that her academic standing was the highest of all the 69 full-time teaching staff. The mathematics department was particularly well staffed, with all three other teachers having completed the Cambridge Maths Tripos examinations in Class I or II. Amongst the other staff, Edith discovered that 16 had degrees from London University, two with MA, eight with BA and six with BSc.

She was well placed to tutor those pupils who were preparing for student life in Cambridge or Oxford, full of advice on what to expect and how to succeed. She did not disappoint. In her last year, one of her pupils, Dorothy Mitchell, was awarded the Winkworth Scholarship, as she herself had been 9 years before. Another, Margaret Pearce, was offered the Clothworkers' Scholarship. Gathered up by Philippa Fawcett, both these young women went on to successfully complete the Mathematics Tripos in 1901.

Edith was surprised by the contrasting view of sports between Newnham and Cheltenham Colleges. Back in Cambridge, several pages of the Newnham Annual Report were devoted to the successes of the students in tennis and hockey matches, both between the halls and against Girton College teams. Edith was looking forward to sharing her enthusiasm and skill in tennis and hockey when she arrived in Cheltenham. She discovered that Dorothea Beale disliked competitive sport. Certainly the pupils could play friendly hockey on some rough ground that had been made available by a local farmer in 1892. In the year that Edith arrived, a further 12 acres of land were purchased for a playground, and 26 new tennis courts were built. Cricket was played in the summer. But Miss Beale's annual reports rarely made mention of sport, and, during her time as Principal, no Cheltenham Ladies' team was ever assembled to play another school. Edith played to win, and she did not really understand the purpose of playing games just for fun.

There were other sports and activities. Calisthenics, movement to music, was very popular. Fencing was introduced in Edith's time, and horse riding was a popular optional extra. Most importantly for Edith was that staff and pupils were free to ride their bicycles where and when they wished. Even Miss Beale, who was initially opposed to such an unladylike activity and was now well over 60 years old, finally gave in. Not wishing to make a fool of herself on two wheels, but wanting to demonstrate that she, too, could move with the times, she acquired a tricycle just before Edith left the College. Around 7.00 am each morning, Miss Beale, whose eyesight and hearing were not what they once were, could be seen cruising erratically down Bayshill, to the alarm of passers-by.

X-Rays and Astronomy

In December 1895, Wilhelm Röntgen, a 50-year-old physics professor from the small German university of Würzburg, made public his discovery of a new radiation that passed through human flesh [2]. The beginning of Edith's second term would have found her involved in lively college discussions, wondering with her colleagues what was her father's opinion of the reports. She was a bit isolated in Cheltenham and had to rely on letters from him and from Florence for the latest news and opinions. A year later Cheltenham General Hospital bought its first X-ray set, which was placed in the care of Dr. Ferguson. Later in 1897, on 8 November at 5 o'clock, the general public in Cheltenham were invited to attend a public demonstration lecture at the Imperial Rooms on 'The Röntgen and Allied Rays' given by Dr. Ferguson. This was the first occasion on which Edith had the opportunity to observe the new radiation in operation, a new science that would play such a significant part in her own life and that of her sister Florence.

Much has been made of the rule of silence at Cheltenham Ladies' College. The pupils were not allowed to talk to one another in the College, in the classrooms, the corridors or the halls. This leaves the impression of quiet calm, encouraging contemplation and careful study. Yet this was not quite Edith's experience. In October 1895, just as she arrived in Cheltenham, the foundation stone was laid for yet another phase of building. During her first 2 years, she was surrounded by the cacophony of a building site, masons cutting Bath and Cleeve Hill stone, bricklayers mixing cement for the bicolour brick walls, scaffolding poles clanking and carpenters sawing and carving the massive roof timbers. A new hall and tower were being built at the southern end of the long corridor, on land previously occupied by the run-down Cheltenham Theatre and pub, procured by Miss Beale a few years earlier (Fig. 4.1).

The hall was sufficiently complete for the Empress Frederick to inspect it during her visit to the College on 29 June 1897. Queen Victoria's eldest daughter was back in England from Germany for her mother's Diamond Jubilee celebrations, and, knowing of her interest in girls' education, Miss Beale had invited her to come down by train from Windsor Castle for the day to inspect the magnificent new building. And magnificent it was. With its two upper galleries, seating 1600 in comfort, it was far larger than the hall in Newnham that Edith remembered using for her Debating Society. The architect, Mr. E R Robson FSA, had used the latest constructional methods to create the space, with structural ironwork clad in carved

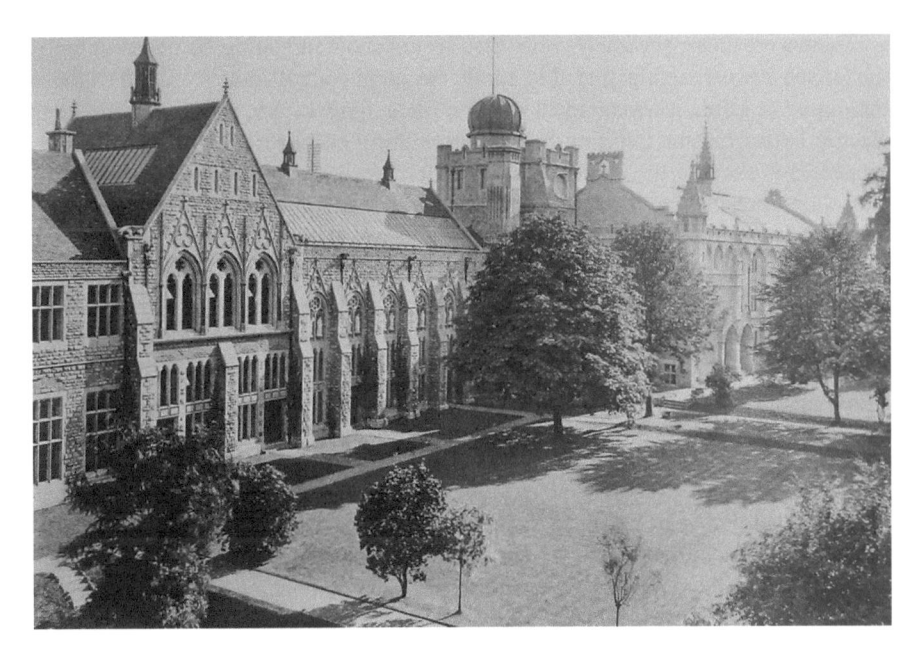

Fig. 4.1 The new hall, tower and observatory, Cheltenham Ladies' College, 1898

pine to support the tie beam roof, 55 feet to the ridge. It was heavily ornamented in the English Gothic design, with many features deliberately included to minimise echoes. The new development was lit with 370 electric lamps, with 5 miles of wires, a move to bring in the changing technology that replaced the old-fashioned, smelly gas lamps that still illuminated the older buildings. Including lighting, the new building cost about £20,000 [3].

When she had arrived at Cheltenham, Edith had been aware that Miss Beale had listened carefully when she spoke of the Newnham Observatory and her role as the College Astronomer. She was interested in how the telescope was mounted and where the observatory was situated. By then, the plans for the new hall and tower had been drawn up, and the building work was starting. Where better to site an observatory like Edith's than on the top of the new tower, giving a much better view of celestial objects close to the horizon than was possible from the Newnham Observatory, on the ground? So, as the building was being completed, the citizens of Cheltenham had been surprised to see appearing a shaped green dome, mounted on top of the 70 foot stone clock tower. This was the new College observatory. A spiral staircase of 85 steps brought Edith to the room housing the clock mechanism, with its two clock faces, one towards the College and the other towards the town. Nineteen more steps up an elegantly curved wooden staircase reached a door, leading directly into the observatory. The view from the platform outside was spectacular, over the town to the Cotswold Hills on the right and the Malvern Hills towards the north.

There were those, she knew, who were unsure about mounting the observatory on top of the tower, feeling that this spoilt the architectural integrity of the Gothic building. For Edith, it was an ideal location for an observatory, above the distracting electric light from the building below and with an excellent view of stars as they dipped low towards the western horizon. It was also a lighthouse for women's education, a visible confirmation that the Ladies' College was fully prepared to be part of the scientific age of the next century. The revolving dome was constructed of steel with an opening shutter, mounted on a circular rack-and-pinion drive that allowed it to follow the movement of the heavens. It was covered with papier maché and canvas, waterproofed with sea green paint. She keenly anticipated the installation of the telescope and other astronomical apparatus. The new buildings commenced use only a few months before Edith departed, and so she had to leave the observatory in the care of other staff when she left [4].

Edith had already made her knowledge of astronomy known to her new colleagues and pupils. After the examinations were over in the summer term of 1896, at the end of her first year, Edith had delivered one of the four end-of-year lectures that were always included at this point in the school calendar. Edith's lecture on astronomy was the only one of scientific interest, the others being on nineteenth-century novelists, Greek myths and modern Italian history.

Not surprisingly, Edith's father continued to support her astronomical activities. In June 1898, just before she left Cheltenham, she arranged for her father to give one of the end-of-year lectures. Edith listened as he developed ideas on the measurement and the knowability of nature, the subject that he had addressed about 10 years earlier before he left Dublin. She was aware that she was amongst the few in the audience in the large new hall of Cheltenham Ladies' College who could grasp the importance of what he was saying. His lecture, 'Survey of that part of the Scale on which Nature works, about which Man has some Information', was considered by some as rather dry, but Edith grasped what he was saying through her previous conversations with him. He wanted to give his audience a sense of the largest and the smallest known distances, ranging from estimates of the spacing of molecules to the distance of the most remote stars. He did not use scientific notation, using powers of 10 to express orders of magnitude on a logarithmic scale, perhaps concerned that this would be too difficult for his audience to understand. Modern prefixes for large numbers, such as giga- and tera- for 10^9 and 10^{12}, and for small numbers such as nano- and pico- (10^{-9} and 10^{-12}) were yet to be established, so he made up his own terminology: he called the series 10, 100, 1000, etc. uno-one, uno-two, uno-three and so on. A metro-ten would be a metre multiplied by the number 1 followed by 10 zeros (10^{10} m). To express fractions of a metre, he added the syllable -et, to form, for example, a tenthet-metre. Using this terminology, he stated that man could only measure from metro-twenty at the largest, the distance of the furthest known star, to about a tenthet-metre at the smallest, the estimated intramolecular distance, that is, a range of 10^{20} m to 10^{-10} m. As far as Johnstone Stoney was concerned, this set the boundaries to man's knowledge of nature. He added 'It is well then that we should recognise Nature as the work of God, and ourselves to be but men'. This is a rare reference to his beliefs, added perhaps because he knew that Miss Beale had experienced a serious crisis of faith in the 1880s and was happy to present a view that matched her renewed belief [5].

His theological position was broadly in line with the consensus accepted by many scientists of the time. He had placed boundaries to the knowledge of nature by carefully defining the part that was beyond man's ability to know, which he had assigned to God. But the world of physics had changed utterly during the previous 10 years, and the world of small things was still getting smaller, encroaching on the terrain that he identified as God's molecular dimensions shrinking towards the atomic and subatomic scale. JJ Thompson, in the Cavendish Laboratory, had found evidence for Stoney's electron in its free state. Numerous physicists were already excitedly measuring the radiations that were being emitted by the element radium, examining the new property called radioactivity that had been discovered for uranium in Paris by Henri Becquerel in 1896 [6]. New radioactive elements, radium and polonium, had been discovered by Marie and Pierre Curie, now husband and wife, challenging the current understanding of the nature of the atom [7, 8]. The physical nature of Röntgen's X-rays was still not accepted. Such matters astonished the world. Edith watched as her father was obliged in due course to extend his 'scale over which man has some information', progressively encroaching on God's allocated sphere. By the time the sisters had reached their 50s, both ends of the range of known sizes had been extended: to 10^{22} m for the most distant star cluster, NGC 7006 and down to the estimated size of the nucleus of the hydrogen atom, 10^{-18}. This represented an increase in the known range of sizes from 10^{30} m to 10^{40} m in about 30 years [9].

Edith's father gave the same lecture that September at the British Association meeting in Bristol. Gerald was already a life member, and Florence eventually also joined at the Dublin meeting in 1908. Edith had become one of a small minority of women British Association members. These were mostly the wives and daughters of male members, about 200 of a total membership of about 5000. But this was still a man's club, her father's space, not hers. It would be another 20 years before Ethel Sargant would become the first woman to be a section chair and a council member. As recently as 1897, a woman had been excluded from a sectional committee on the basis of an earlier council view that 'the time has not yet come when it would be for the advantage for the Association to depart from the established custom'. It was too soon for Edith to gain a foothold in this male territory without help, even if she had wanted to. Instead, from now on, she concentrated her efforts by working in exclusively female organisations.

Visits to the scientific meetings were commonly family affairs. Gertrude sometimes went along, pleased to be part of her father's senior position and to listen to talks from eminent scientists. Much later, following his election to be prime minister in 1924, Gertrude recalled coming across Ramsay Macdonald, whose work in geology and science education had led him into this sphere [10].

Published alongside the text of her father's lecture in the College Magazine was another by the explorer and anthropologist Mary Kingsley about her time with the tribes of West Africa. Edith was fascinated by her achievements and, much later, donated her copy of Kingsley's biography to the library of the British Federation for University Women [11]. Mary was the daughter of Charles Kingsley, the novelist and sympathiser with the women's suffrage movement. At the end of this lecture, Mary Kingsley added the following:

> I may confide to any spinster who is here present and who feels inclined to take up the study of (the African) that she will be perpetually embarrassed by enquiries of Where is your husband? Not Have you one? or anything like that which you could deal with but Where is he? . . . it is advisable to say you are searching for him. . . . . this elicits help and sympathy [12].

Her audience, many unmarried themselves, recognised the same difficulty in social situations closer to home.

Edith had gained a more mature understanding of the place of education in her increasingly female-focussed world, and she took from Cheltenham an inspiration from Miss Beale that teaching was a vocation, a view that would stay with her for her whole life. Teaching was a predominantly female profession, with about 75% of the 230,000 teachers in the 1901 census being female [13]. She also had experienced success, giving strength to her feeling of self-worth. Nevertheless, Edith's life was cyclic. She was now in her late twenties, and, in spite of the evident success of her 3 years in Cheltenham, she felt in need of a rest from the obligations associated with her job. When at work, it was in her nature to focus entirely on the matter in hand, to work at the task with wholehearted dedication. It was not possible to continue to work forever with such intensity, and periodically she would take time off either through illness or just for a break.

So, in the summer of 1898 shortly after her father's lecture, Edith left Cheltenham Ladies' College 'to have a year's rest from teaching' and returned to London and to her father in his house in 8 Hornsey Rise, Islington [14]. At the same time, Florence returned from Hull after her year as surgical house officer at the Children's Hospital there. This was the first time for 8 years that the sisters had lived together, and their interests and experience had diverged somewhat since leaving Ireland. The household that they established in Islington was rather different from the one they left in Dublin nearly a decade before. The financial basis of the household had changed. Their father was now retired, financially secure with his Queen's University pension and investment income.[2] The sisters had both demonstrated that they could earn their own living and could look forward to secure future employment, Florence in medicine and Edith in education.

She did not forget Miss Beale's interest in astronomy. She learned from her father that the Leonid meteors were expected to make another spectacular showing in the autumn of 1898, and Edith passed this information back to Miss Beale, hoping that she would be to be able to view them with her pupils. This posed a slight organisational problem. The show was expected to appear after lights out, which was strictly applied. As reported in the College Magazine:

---

[2]A document in the Queen's University archive at Queen's University Belfast records a negotiation over an additional pension from his employment as Chief Examiner for the Civil Service. On his investments, Charles Parsons recorded that Johnstone Stoney wished to purchase a £10 share in his Marine Turbine Company in 1894.

The Chief Constable, Admiral Christian, kindly instructed the Police where to look for them, and as soon as any appeared to ring up Miss Beale, and she was to pull the alarm bell, on hearing which the girls were to get up. The Fire Brigade was told it would not be necessary to send off engines that night. Alas! the clouds veiled the heavens, and the repose of the sleepers was uninterrupted [15].

New Opportunities

The free time generated by Edith's temporary rest from teaching brought work from a quite unexpected direction. Before Edith had left Cambridge, the Stoney family had travelled north to the village of Corbridge in Northumberland to witness Gerald's wedding to Isabella Lowes on 23 June 1894. The newly-weds called their new home Oakley, in memory of their lost family estate in Ireland. Edith had been interested to hear about his work on turbines and searchlights, and even then they wondered whether her mathematical talents could be brought to bear on the engineering problems that he faced.

Gerald had joined the engineer Charles Parsons, youngest son of William Parsons, the third Earl of Rosse, in 1888. He soon impressed Parsons with his ability, and, in 1893, Parsons promoted Gerald to become manager of the searchlight department of C.A. Parsons & Co at Heaton in Newcastle upon Tyne. At the same time, he was made the engineer in charge of the turbine test house. Parsons had come up with a new method for the construction of a silvered mirror to reflect the searchlight beam, to replace the older heavy silvered glass mirrors [16]. In his new design, a thin sheet of glass was heated and, when sufficiently pliable, formed by vacuum against a cast iron mould. This method allowed him to design and manufacture a wide range of shapes and sizes for the reflecting mirrors, allowing searchlight beams to be tailored to specific uses. In particular, the company created mirrors for the Admiralty searchlights in the Suez Canal that created a flat spreading beam so as to light up the buoys at each side of the canal. This was done by using combined parabolic/hyperbolic or parabolic/ellipsoidal shapes for the mirror surfaces.

The iron moulds were made at first by turning an elliptical section on a lathe and then by finishing off the parabolic shape by hand. It was an empirical approach that relied on skilled hands and judgements. According to Gerald, 'It was about 1898 that the true theory of the parabola ellipse was evolved enabling them to be made accurately from an ellipse template and a series of parabola templates' [17]. It was Edith who developed the fourth-order expressions that enabled her brother to more accurately and consistently engineer the moulds onto which the mirrors were formed. Gerald gave his sister no credit when he recalled this event in his memoir, but neither does he claim it for himself nor for Charles Parsons, and it was only later that it became clear that it was Edith's work. However, no job arose from Edith's contribution to her brother's work in his northern engineering firm. Her future employment may not even have been considered by Parsons and his team.

Florence was occupied, forging her own future in medicine, completing her MD. Gertrude busied herself in her studio, developing an interest in sculpture. Edith's father spent much of his time in his study, returning to his earlier analysis of planetary atmospheres based upon the kinetic theory of gases [18, 19]. Bonded by their common interest in astronomy, Edith listened with interest when he presented to the Royal Society his analysis of the Leonid meteor shower, which had failed Miss Beale in Cheltenham the previous year. Knowing of her previous disappointment, Edith wrote to her again calling attention to her father's analysis and to his letter to *The Times* in which he gave his best prediction of the next times of the shower (15 or 16 November) attributing any uncertainty to perturbations caused by Saturn and Jupiter [20].

Still, Edith needed employment. In the summer of 1899, an opportunity arose that would draw the sisters' careers together again. Several years earlier, in 1892, the General Medical Council (GMC), responsible for the register of medical doctors, had ordained that the study of physics was to form part of the extended course of professional medical study [21]. Then, in 1898, the University of London Act had been passed. Since the London School of Medicine for Women (LSMW) was one of the constituent schools of London University, its activities were now guided and controlled by the provisions of this new statute [22]. The report accompanying the statutes included a commentary on the teaching of the basic sciences, which included physics, in medical education:

> .... the sciences in question are not ...... taught at the present day ..... by men looking forward to the pursuit of a medical career. They are now taught .... by men who propose to devote themselves to a career in the sciences which they teach .... the multiplicity of posts and the smallness of the emoluments lead, more particularly in the smaller Schools, to the undesirable practice of the same teacher attempting to teach two or more branches of knowledge.

Elizabeth Garrett Anderson was still Dean at the LSMW, having seen Florence through her successful time there. Ignoring the gender bias of the wording, she recognised the challenges raised in this commentary as ones that she faced in her own institution. The LSMW was certainly small, graduating only nine students that year. Mrs. McDonald, a London science graduate, had been teaching both physics and biology since physics had been introduced to the syllabus after the GMC statement. Whilst the dean was sure that she was perfectly competent, the arrangement would not stand scrutiny as the LSMW expanded. Some London medical schools were outsourcing their basic science classes to the Royal College of Science in South Kensington. This was not a direction in which she planned to move, diluting the collegiate atmosphere that she wished to cultivate. The teaching laboratories had already been installed in the Pfeiffer Block, opened in July 1898 by the Princess of Wales, containing physics, chemistry, physiology and anatomy laboratories. They now needed appropriate staff and equipment.

Florence was now anatomy demonstrator at the LSMW and heard of the opportunity for her sister to join her as lecturer in physics. When Edith applied for the advertised post in the early summer of 1899, she was one of 12, all of whom had appropriate qualifications. Sufficient women were now graduating in science that half of the applicants were women. There was a final shortlist of two. In competition with Edith was Edward Halford Strange M.Sc., a 25-year-old chemist and Quaker. They met the School Committee at 5.00 pm on 7 June 1899. Edith was delighted to be offered the post, in which she was given sole responsibility for the physics course [23]. She was one of only about 40 Cambridge science women who managed to gain academic appointments during the period before the First World War [24].

References

1. Avery G. Cheltenham ladies. An illustrated history of Cheltenham Ladies college. London: James & James; 2003. p. 55.
2. Röntgen W. Ueber eine neue Art von Strahlen. Vorläufige Mitteilung, Aus den Sitzungsberichten der Würzburger Physik.-medic Gesellschaft Würzburg;1895:137–47.
3. Clarke AK. A history of the Cheltenham Ladies' college 1853–1953. London: Faber and Faber; 1953. p. 80.
4. Hay I. Chronicle. The Cheltenham Ladies' College Magazine. 1898 Spring;37:132–33.
5. Stoney GJ. Survey of that part of the scale upon which nature works, about which man has some information. The Cheltenham Ladies' College Magazine. 1898 Spring;38:259–63.
6. Henri Becquerel announced his work in a series of papers in *Comptes rendus* between 1896 and 1897. The first of these was: Becquerel H. Sur les radiations émises par phosphorescence Comptes rendus de l'Académie des science. 1896 Feb 24;122:420–1.
7. Curie P, Curie M. Sur une substance nouvelle radioactive contenue dans la pechblende. Comptes rendus de l'Académie des science. 1898 Jul 18;127:175–78.
8. Curie P, Curie M, Bémont G. Sur une substance nouvelle fortement radioactive contenue dans la pechblende. Comptes rendus de l'Académie des science. 1898 Dec 26;127:1215–18.
9. Richardson L. Logarithmic scale of distances. J Brit Astron Assoc. 1924;34(8):321–2.
10. Letter from Gertrude Stoney to Archie Stoney. 13 Nov 1924. AS.
11. Gwynn S. The life of Mary Kingsley. London: Macmillan; 1932. Edith's copy is now held in the Martial Rose Library, University of Winchester, part of the BFUW Sybil Campbell Collection.
12. Kingsley M. A lecture on West Africa. The Cheltenham Ladies' College Magazine. 1898 autumn;38:264–70.
13. Heffer S. The age of decadence. Britain 1880 to 1914. London: Random House; 2017. p. 708.
14. The Cheltenham Ladies College Magazine 1898;19(37):325.
15. The Cheltenham Ladies' College Magazine. 1899;20(39):105.
16. Parsons RH. Parsons' work on searchlight reflectors. The steam turbine and other inventions of Sir Charles Parsons OM. London: Longmans Green; 1942. p. 23–5.
17. The development of the Parsons mirror from 1886 to 1930. Gerald Stoney FRS October 23 1933. Science Museum Library: PAR8.
18. Stoney GJ. Of atmospheres upon planets and satellites. Astrophys J. 1898;7:25–55.
19. Stoney GJ. On the escape of gases from planetary atmospheres according to the kinetic theory. Astrophys J. 1900;11:251–8, 357–72
20. Stoney GJ, Downing AMW. Perturbations of the Leonids. Astronomische Nathrichten. 1899;149:33–8.
21. Daniell A. Physics for students of medicine. Preface. London: Macmillan; 1896.
22. University of London. The historical record 1836–1912, being a supplement to the calendar completed to September 1912. London University Press; 1912.
23. Council minutes of the London (Royal Free Hospital) School of Medicine for Women. LMA. H72/SM/A/02.
24. Fara P. A lab of one's own. Oxford: OUP; 2018.

Chapter 5
The London School of Medicine for Women

The London School of Medicine for Women

The London School of Medicine for Women (LSMW) had been founded in 1874, largely thanks to the efforts of Miss Sophia Jex-Blake (1840–1912) and others as part of the movement to admit women into the medical profession [1]. Arthur Norton from St. Mary's Hospital and Francis Astie (1833–1874) from Westminster Hospital had suggested to Jex-Blake that a medical school for women be founded in London, and therefore a meeting was held in Astie's home on 22 August 1874, which included Elizabeth Garrett Anderson (1836–1917). A resolution was made that a 'school be formed in London with a view to educating women in medicine and enabling them to pass such examinations as would place their names on the Medical Register'. Jex-Blake found a suitable house for the new school at Pavilion House, 30 Henrietta Place, Brunswick Square, and so the LSMW opened on 12 October 1874. Prior to the founding of the LSMW, there were only two women on the Medical Register in the United Kingdom, and these were Elizabeth Blackwell (1821–1910) who had qualified in the United States and Elizabeth Garrett Anderson. Elizabeth Garrett Anderson was the dean of the LSMW from 1883 to 1903 and was dean when Florence was at that School [2]. Elizabeth Garrett Anderson was the first woman in Britain to obtain a legal qualification as a physician and surgeon and was the first woman anywhere who was dean of a medical school. Her example was inspiring to the young Florence and also to other young women who aspired to become doctors. During her time as dean, attitudes of the medical profession to medical women were changing rapidly, and at the AGM of the British Medical Association (BMA) held in Nottingham in 1892, it was almost unanimously voted that women be admitted as members.

In 1860 Elizabeth Garrett (as she was at the time) had undertaken a course of private instruction in medicine and had enquired as to the possibility of her being examined at Apothecaries' Hall, and this was a recognised path to qualification as a doctor. As might be imagined, this caused some considerable consternation;

however the Apothecaries' Act of 1815 had indicated that 'all persons' could apply, and this would include women. She therefore took the various parts of the examinations and obtained her medical diploma on 26 September 1865, becoming the first woman doctor in Great Britain. She wrote to her friend Emily Davies, 'I heard a cheering account of the hall examination yesterday. Two of the examiners told Mr. C that it was a mercy they did not put the names in order of merit as in this case they must have put me first. I am very glad, though the exam was too easy to feel elated about'. However the Court of Examiners ensured that no more women would be admitted by changing the regulations so that certificates of attendance at private lectures were no longer to be accepted [3]. In 1870 she obtained a full medical degree in Paris.

In 1869 five women including Sophia Jex-Blake had wanted to become doctors in Edinburgh, with two more joining them making the 'Edinburgh Seven'. The group encountered considerable opposition, including opposition from male students, which culminated on 18 November 1870 when the group arrived at Surgeons' Hall to sit for an anatomy exam. Jex-Blake recorded in her diary 'a disturbance of a very unbecoming nature took place yesterday afternoon', and 'there is no doubt that many of the students look upon the admission of the ladies to the classes with no friendly eye'. This was followed by a serious riot, which resulted in worldwide indignation. Various members of the Faculty of Medicine opposed women graduation, and in 1873 the campaign for women doctors in Edinburgh failed for the time being.

Both men and women opposed women entering the medical profession; however there was a group of supporters for women doctors' inclining the well-known scientists Thomas Henry Huxley and Charles Darwin, and with Elizabeth Garrett Anderson, they secured an Act of Parliament in 1877 that allowed medical examining boards to admit women. London University immediately responded positively, and so the London School of Medicine for Women was founded.

The LSMW became linked to the Royal Free Hospital (RFH) in 1877 although not without some considerable difficulties [4, 5]. The new school nearly failed at the start because no hospital would accept women as students, and by 1877 closure seemed likely with no classes being scheduled for the summer. By a happy coincidence, James Stansfield (1820–1898), the Honorary Treasurer of LSMW, on holiday with his wife in Whitby, met James Hopgood (1811–1897) also on holiday with his wife. Hopgood was a solicitor, and also the Chairman of the Weekly Board of the Gray's Inn Lane Hospital, and the hospital was located close to the new medical school. By March 1877 Hopgood and Stansfield had persuaded the RFH staff to admit women as students with a total payment of £715 as fees and subscriptions. Although there were initially only 16 students, there were to be guaranteed fees to the medical staff of £400 each year for 5 years. Sophia Jex-Blake had expected to become the honorary secretary but, whilst she was away qualifying in Dublin, Isabel Thorne was elected to the position. This was probably engineered by Garrett Anderson, and Jex-Blake subsequently returned to Edinburgh where she subsequently established the Edinburgh School of Medicine for Women [6].

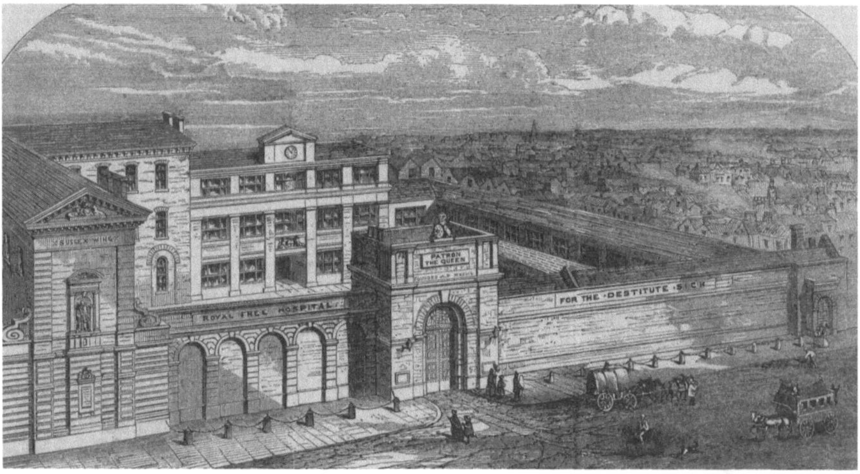

Fig. 5.1 View of the Royal Free Hospital in 1856, in the Gray's Inn Road, showing the new Sussex Wing (from Illustrated Times, 19 April 1856)

In December 1827 William Marsden (1796–1867) had come across a sick girl lying on the steps of St. Andrew's Church in Holborn, and in spite of his efforts, he could find no hospital to accept her for treatment. In order to be admitted to a hospital, she needed a letter from a subscriber, and she had none. Hospitals obtained a significant portion of their funding from their subscribers, and subscribers were entitled to recommend patients for admission. Marsden paid a widow to provide a room; however the girl died 2 days later. Marsden was shocked by the incident and wanted to set up a free hospital. Following a meeting he was determined to set up such a dispensary in 16 Greville Street in Covent Gardens. In 1834 two wards were added, and the name 'Free Hospital, Greville Street' was chosen. There was an attempt to found a medical school, the 'Free Hospital School'; however this proved to be a failure. When Queen Victoria came to the throne in 1837, she agreed to be the patroness, and the name was changed to the 'Royal Free Hospital', and this was so successful that by the 1840s it was obvious that a new hospital building was needed. Traditionally the British State had taken little interest in the provision of health care, and at this time in history, the State was relatively indifferent towards the nation's health. Any new hospital would have to be funded by public and private subscription [7]. The governors found a site in Gray's Inn Lane (later called Gray's Inn Road), and the new hospital opened in January 1843 (Fig. 5.1). The financial position of the RFH was often precarious, being helped however in 1851 by a subscription from the Great Northern Railway to cover railway accidents to those attending the Great Exhibition.

In 1853 the nearby Hunterian School of Medicine in Bedford Square approached the RFH with a proposal to use the wards for clinical teaching. This was expanded into a proposal for a 'Royal Free Hospital Medical School' which ultimately failed.

This turned out for the good, since had it succeeded the RFH would not have been in a position to accept students from the LSMW some 24 years later.

Florence Moves to London

At the time that Florence reached young adulthood, battles had been won, and women were able to study medicine in Scotland and in England; however this was not the case in Ireland. In Dublin University women were not yet admitted to medical degrees. Florence therefore came to England at the age of 21. By the end of the nineteenth century when Florence went to London, there was a degree of parity in education between men and women, and middle-class women had won some battles [8]. In 1878 the University of London had accepted women for non-medical degrees, and the first MD taken by a woman was by Mary Scharlieb (1845–1930) [6]. However by 1894 when Florence was a student, there were still fewer than 180 medical women on the medical register in Great Britain [9]. Mary Scharlieb had started training as a midwife in Madras in 1871 and realising the value of becoming a doctor was one of the first four women students at the Madras Medical College. Scharlieb returned to England and met Elizabeth Garrett Anderson qualifying from the LSMW in 1882. Queen Victoria had a special interest in her Indian subjects and met with Scharlieb in 1883 at Windsor Castle to discuss the suffering of women. The death rate from childbirth in India was high, partly because women were reluctant to consult a male doctor. Scharlieb returned to Madras Medical College in 1883, finally returning to England in 1887 because of ill health. She was appointed as a surgeon at the New Hospital for Women (NHW) where she subsequently succeeded Elizabeth Garrett Anderson in 1892 [2]. Interest in the position of women in India continued at the LSMW, particularly following the setting up of a scholarship by the wife of the viceroy of India, the Earl of Dufferin. The Dufferin Scholarship was awarded from 1885 'to ladies willing to prepare for the practice of medicine in India. (and) awarded at the discretion of the Council to students of LSMW'. A number of medical women went to India, and as a student Florence would have been well aware of the concern. Indeed the most famous Indian doctor of the period Rukhmabai (1864–1955) was a student contemporaneous to Florence, graduating from the LSMW in 1894. Rukhmabai returned to India in 1895 to take up a position as the Chief Medical Officer at the Women's Hospital in Surat. This partly explains Florence's concern for women's obstetric health in India in her later professional life. The concern for woman's suffrage and rights in Great Britain was always part a global movement and was a common cause for women worldwide, although as Carrie Chapman Catt, the US feminist and suffrage campaigner, was to exclaim in 1908, Britain was the 'storm centre' of the women's movement [10].

Florence formally applied to attend the LSMW in October 1891, having matriculated that January based on her own private study. She had taken her preliminary science in London in July 1891, partly studying at the Royal College of Science in Dublin but 'chiefly at home'. The LSMW was located in 30 Handel Street in

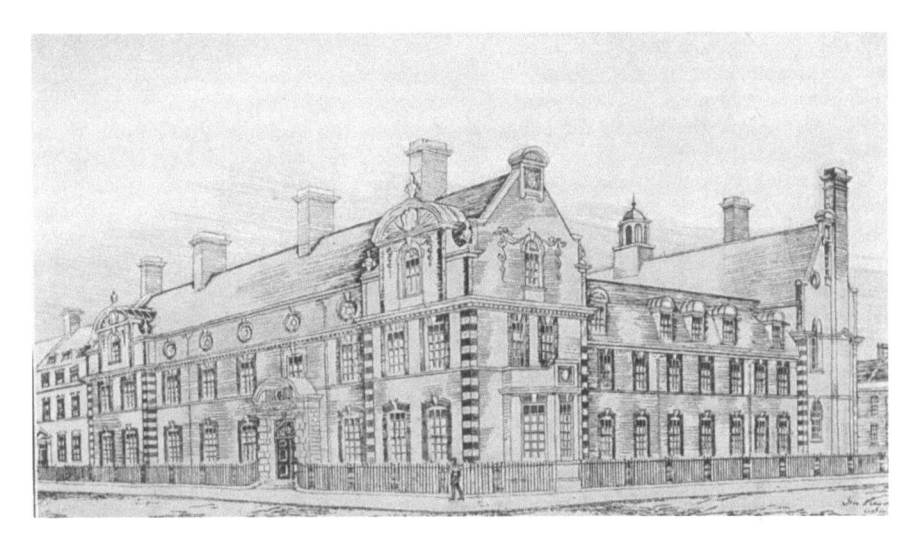

Fig. 5.2 The London School of Medicine for Women, Hunter Street 1899 (from Aesculapia, Women's Work in Medicine in The Lady's Realm, Vol. 61, 1899)

Brunswick Square (Fig. 5.2) and as we have seen was associated with the Royal Free Hospital in Gray's Inn Road. The new buildings of the Royal Free Hospital were opened by the Prince and Princess of Wales on 22 July 1895 (Fig. 5.3). The motto of the LSMW was 'Work is as it is done', and the facilities for students were excellent (Fig. 5.4). Florence's name appears as number 318 on the school's register of students. She entered the LSMW as a compounder, which meant that she paid her fees in a single sum or yearly rather than paying for individual courses.

The testimonial that accompanied her application for admission to the LSMW had been filled in and signed on 24 September 1891 by Robert S. Ball, who gave his address as the Observatory, Co Dublin. This was Sir Robert Stawell Ball FRS (1840–1913), who was a distinguished Irish astronomer. In 1874 Robert Ball had been appointed as Royal Astronomer of Ireland and Andrews Professor of Astronomy at the University of Dublin and based at Dunsink Observatory. In the year after Florence entered the LSMW, Ball was appointed the Lowndean Professor of Astronomy and Geometry at Cambridge University and the director of the Cambridge Observatory. In the testimonial Ball says that he has known Florence for 'ten or more' years. Ball's friendship with Florence's father had started in 1865 when Johnstone Stoney had asked Ball to tutor the three younger sons of the astronomer William Parsons (1800–1867) who was the 3rd Earl of Rosse.

As a medical student Florence initially lived in College Hall, which was located in Byng Place close to the LSMW. The house had been opened in 1882 at 1 Byng Place, in the southwest corner of Gordon Square, with the aim of providing additional accommodation for the increasing numbers of female students who were then attending the University of London. Many students from LSMW lived in College Hall including Louisa Aldrich-Blake (1865–1925), its future dean. The hall proved

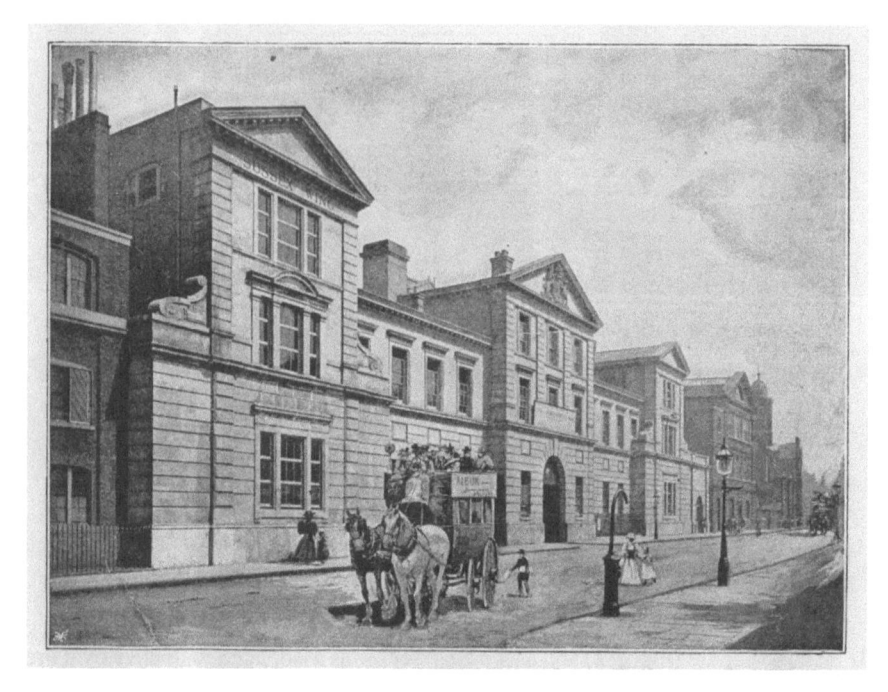

Fig. 5.3 The new buildings of the Royal Free Hospital, Gray's Inn Road, opened by the Prince and Princess of Wales, 22 July 1895 (from The Illustrated London News, 27 July 1895)

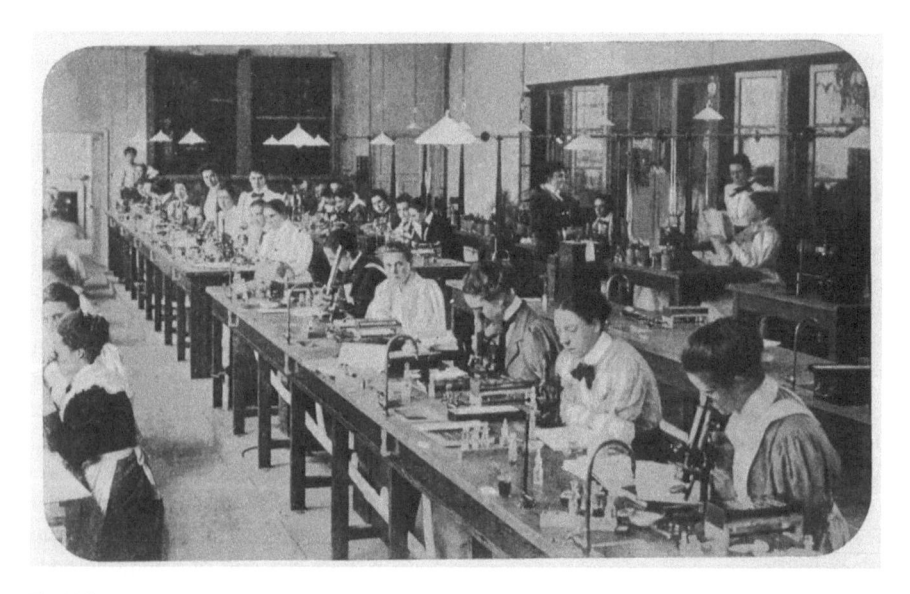

Fig. 5.4 Women students of physiology at work at the LSMW in 1899 (from Aesculapia, Women's Work in Medicine. The Lady's Realm, Vol. 61, 1899)

to be very successful and had been increased in size to occupy two adjacent houses and was affectionately known by the students as 'Byng'. Since it was so successful in the support it was giving to women students, it had been incorporated in 1886 and called 'College Hall London'.

Florence was an able student, and her list of honours was described as impressive by Amy Sheppard in her 1932 obituary in the medical school's magazine [11]. In July 1893 she took the London Intermediate MB examination and received honours in anatomy, physiology and materia medica. Florence was 6th in the 3rd class in anatomy, 1st equal in the 3rd class in physiology and histology and 1st in the 3rd class in materia medica and pharmaceutical chemistry. The LSMW subsequently changed the title materia medica to pharmacology in 1909. Although some men may have felt threatened by women becoming doctors, the *York Herald* [12] noted 'Members of the sterner sex (that is men) who are jealous or afraid of the intellectual attainments of women may, perhaps, find a crumb of comfort in the Class Lists of the Intermediate Examination in medicine of the University of London. In the pass list of the entire examination there are ten candidates in the first division, but not a lady amongst them'. The writer continues 'In the Honours Examinations in the various subjects the men have it so far all their own way, as only one lady—Miss Florence Ada Stoney—is successful in obtaining honours, and she does not rise higher than the third class'. However the writer does acknowledge that the honours were achieved in three subjects.

Florence received class prizes or honour certificates for every subject that she took. Florence was awarded the first Mackay Prize, which was awarded to the head student for the year in general class work, and received the sum of £20. The *Lady's Pictorial* journal for 14 July 1894 recorded the award and printed her portrait, along with a portrait of the second prize winner.

The life of a female medical student of the period is well illustrated in the novel *Mona Maclean, Medical Student* written by Graham Travers [13]. This novel was immensely popular and, having been published in 1894, by 1897 had already passed through 12 editions. The novel deserves wider recognition since it gives valuable insights into medical and social life in the late nineteenth century and particularly since it presents the views of a young woman. Medical fiction was popular then as now, and *The Body Snatcher* by Robert Louis Stevenson had appeared in 1884 and *Round the Red Lamp* by Arthur Conan Doyle in 1894. Graham Travers was the pen name of Dr. Margaret Todd (1859–1918) who was a prolific author and one of the first female medical students at the Edinburgh School of Medicine for Women, which had been founded by Sophia Jex-Blake, where Todd wrote Mona Maclean. Margaret Todd was the associate and romantic partner of Sophia Jex-Blake, and wrote her biography after her death [14]. Following Todd's death, a scholarship was created in her name at the LSMW.

The novel chronicles the life of the young Mona as a female medical student at the LSMW. Mona has just failed her intermediate examinations, and so she takes a break from her studies and goes to stay with her cousin who is a shopkeeper in Scotland. Whilst the medical woman is presented as scientific, she is also shown as feminine, and her friend Lucy tells Mona that '.... the art of dressing one's hair is at least as important as the art of dissecting'. When she was with her cousin, Mona kept her identity as a medical student hidden, and her cousin wrote, 'Nobody here knows anything about your meaning to be a doctor, and what we don't know does us no harm. They would think it queer[1] as you know I do myself, and keep hoping you will find some nice gentleman---------"("Gentleman"!" groaned Mona.)'. Throughout the book there is a theme of the 'genus Medical Woman' not being understood. Mona's aunt spoke of 'Mingled pride, affection, disgust and fear. Disgust for the life-work she had chosen, fear of her supposed 'cleverness.' Lady Munro despised learned women'. For Lady Munro a woman was not to appear too intelligent in society. Mona's uncle was, if anything, even less comprehending about the nature of the medical woman. ' "The fact is," he broke out impulsively at last, "I am torn asunder on this subject of women doctors—torn asunder. There is a terrible necessity for them—terrible—and yet what a sacrifice!"' And so, in the view of her uncle Sir Douglas, a medical woman becomes hardened and loses something central to womanhood. He exclaimed 'It is bad for a man, but a man has some virtues which remain untouched by it. A woman loses everything that makes womanhood fair and attractive. You must be becoming hard and blunted?' Mona replied that she was not becoming hardened.

Mona's uncle raised the question of dissection and likened it to human butchery. Mona realises the gulf in viewpoints between herself and her uncle. 'How could she talk of that ever-new field for observation, corroboration and discovery; the unlimited scope for the keen eye, the skilful hand, the thinking brain, the mature judgment?' She continued '"To be a true anatomist," she thought with glowing face, "one would need to be a mechanician[2] and a scientist, an artist and a philosopher."' So a woman was perhaps particularly suited for the study of anatomy and for dissection, and so the comparison could be made to Florence with her love of anatomy and her work as an anatomy demonstrator at the LSMW.

However whilst Mona might have a strong belief in the ability of woman to enter the world of medicine with the challenges of dissection and clinical medicine, other work was viewed as far less congenial. In her letter to Mona inviting her to stay, her cousin wrote '.... although you will have plenty of time to yourself, you will be of the greatest use to me. Both in the house and in the shop----'. Mona greeted this letter with horror, '"Good God!" said Mona; and letting the letter fall, she buried her face in her hands'. And so for a well-brought-up young lady from a privileged background, becoming a doctor and entering a high-status profession was a goal to be desired, whereas working in a shop was something entirely different, even if it was only on a temporary basis.

At the opening of the winter session of the LSMW for 1894, the formal address to the 'lady students' was given by Mary 'Maida' Darby Sturge MB (1865–1925), who was a recent graduate. This must have been of considerable public interest since it was reported in *The Daily News*, *The Times* and the *Daily Chronicle*. Sturge

---

[1] Queer as meaning strange or odd.
[2] Mechanician means a mechanic.

emphasised to the students the need for having a scientific outlook and a reverence for the laws of nature. However in order to have a right understanding of others, a deep knowledge of culture was important, and with what sounds like a very contemporary outlook, Sturge stressed the individualisation of treatment. Sturge spoke on the wisdom of 'learning something of the nature and vitality of normal children', and indeed without this, the needs of children when sick can scarcely be understood. This latter topic was to become important to Florence once she had graduated. The lecture also indicated that in the future doctors would be surprised that in the nineteenth century 'the sick were largely tended in wards instead of carrying them into fresh air and sunshine outside our cities'. This is perhaps a lesson that we still need to learn. The lecture finished with an observation on the rewards they would find as doctors since 'every morning brought with it new horizons, every night new stars'.

In 1893, Florence's father had packed up the house in Dublin where she had been raised, offered it for rent and moved to London. He took a lease on 8 Hornsey Rise, Islington, which was a six-bedroom, semi-detached house in the Northern Suburbs, easily large enough to also accommodate Florence. The motive for this move has been explained by a major biographer as being to give his daughters the opportunity of a university education in England, a view that has been sustained in later accounts of his life [15]. This interpretation must be viewed with some caution. John Joly's biography for the Royal Society, informed by Edith's letter to him, makes no such claim nor does another contemporary account of his life by their family friend Robert Ball [16]. Neither is the explanation supported by the chronology. Edith had already completed her first 3 years in Cambridge, and Florence was well established as a medical student in London. In truth, Johnstone Stoney was now approaching 70, and Gertrude was the only one of his children left in Dublin. Gerald was in Newcastle, and Robert was permanently settled in Australia. The pendulum of family dependency was swinging, and his motivation was as likely to be to assure his old age as to give support to his increasingly independent daughters. Her father immediately took a direct interest in her work, as he had done with young Gerald's bicycles in Dublin and more recently with Edith's astronomical work in Cambridge. Florence had brought her Leitz microscope to London, making good use of it in her anatomical investigations. Her father set about a detailed analysis of the physical optics of the microscope and proposed ways in which the resolution could be improved [17].

Florence graduated MB in November 1895 and BS in December 1898, both from the University of London and both in the second division. At this time the MB and BS degrees were taken separately and were classified into first and second divisions. She also qualified for the Prideaux prize, which was awarded for the writing of an original essay within 2 years of taking the MB examination.

Florence was active in the life of the school. A school magazine was started in 1895. It was a great success and gave many details relating to the professional, sporting and social aspects of the LSMW and the RFH. When the original committee stood down in early 1897, a new committee was elected, and Florence became the editor. The original name of the magazine was *Magazine of LSMW and RFH*, and this was changed to *Magazine of RFHSMW*.

The New Hospital for Women

Following her graduation as a doctor, Florence held a series of medical appointments before she was able to obtain a residential appointment in Hull. When she qualified as a doctor, she was automatically registered for independent medical practice with no restrictions, and the current probationary preregistration year was not introduced until considerably later. In this period it was commonplace for doctors to have multiple appointments concurrently, unlike the present time when having a single appointment is more common, and certainly when a junior. For several periods of 6 months duration, Florence worked as a clinical assistant to the New Hospital for Women. Clinical assistants worked under a departmental head, and the position may or may not progress to a more senior appointment.

The NHW had been founded by Elizabeth Garrett Anderson in 1866 as the St. Mary's Dispensary for Women and was then located in Seymour Place in London. It was the first dedicated hospital for women and run by women. It was renamed the New Hospital for Women in 1872, moving in 1874 to 222–224 Marylebone Road. The hospital moved to a new purpose-built building in 1890 on the site of Somers Place West in Euston Road, and this is where Florence worked (Fig. 5.5). Most London hospitals received no state support, and were often built in poorer areas where the need was greatest. Their difficult position was described by Charles Booth who wrote 'But their (hospitals) annual expenditure far outruns this settled income (benefactions and legacies), and to supplement the funds obtained from regular and annual subscribers, the general public is appealed to every year to enable the management to perfect and extend their work' [18].

The NHW building is of red and white brick and was described by ACS in an article in *The Illustrated London News* of 10 February 1892 as having a somewhat unprofessional air. One of the patients described the NHW as 'more like a gentleman's house than a hospital'. The internal decoration was the design and work of Agnes Garrett, the sister of Elizabeth Garrett Anderson, with the aim of providing a beautiful and restful environment, as can be seen in the design of the common room (Fig. 5.6). In 1874 Agnes Garrett with Millicent Fawcett had started the first all-woman interior decorating business A&R Garrett House Decorators [8]. The four wards were decorated with Italian bas-reliefs, including casts from work by Luca della Robbia and Donatello (Fig. 5.7). For the poor women who attended the hospital, it must have seemed like a palace. Many women who were not prepared to attend the general hospitals were very willing to attend the NHW and found the women staff more sympathetic to both their bodily and mental needs. The building is now the headquarters of Unison and houses a museum dedicated to the hospital, which may be visited. This new hospital also contained the Women's Medical Institute, which was located on the ground floor. This contained a library and reading room. Following the death of Elizabeth Garrett Anderson on 17 December 1917, the NHW was named the Elizabeth Garrett Anderson Hospital, joining the National Health Service. The name continues today as the Elizabeth

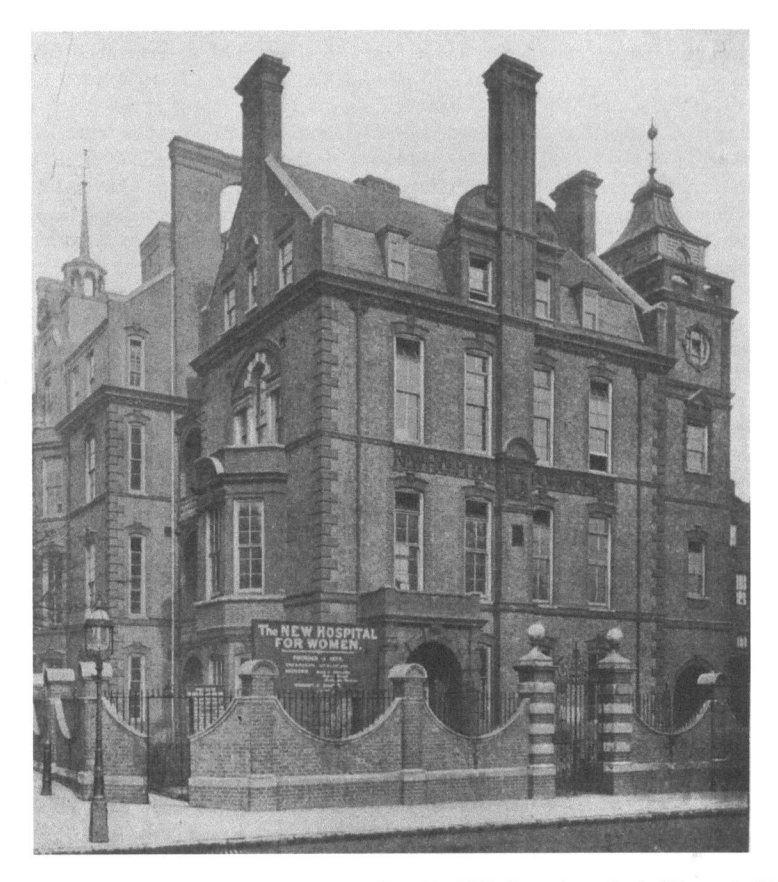

Fig. 5.5 The New Hospital for Women, Euston Road in 1899 (from Aesculapia, Women's Work in Medicine, The Lady's Realm, Vol. 61, 1899)

Garrett Anderson Wing of the nearby University College Hospital and is providing gynaecology, maternity and neonatal care.

Following qualification Florence was also appointed as clinical assistant to the Southwark Eye Hospital (Fig. 5.8). The Royal Eye Hospital was located in Southwark as the successor to the South London Ophthalmic Hospital. The hospital was at St George's Circus and was a modern hospital with 40 beds, having opened in 1892 and finally closed as late as 1980. Florence will have given treatments for common eye conditions; however at this time the treatments available were quite limited, and many conditions were untreatable. In the latter part of the nineteenth century, it might be imagined that the general public greeted each new hospital with some enthusiasm. In fact this was often not the case. In a perceptive article about the new Eye Hospital in Southwark, FHL wrote in *The Illustrated London News* of 17 December 1892 that the public usually greeted a new hospital with complete disapproval and distrust. FHL has the public saying 'Have we not too many hospitals already; are not many of them grossly ill-managed, hopelessly in debt, and designed

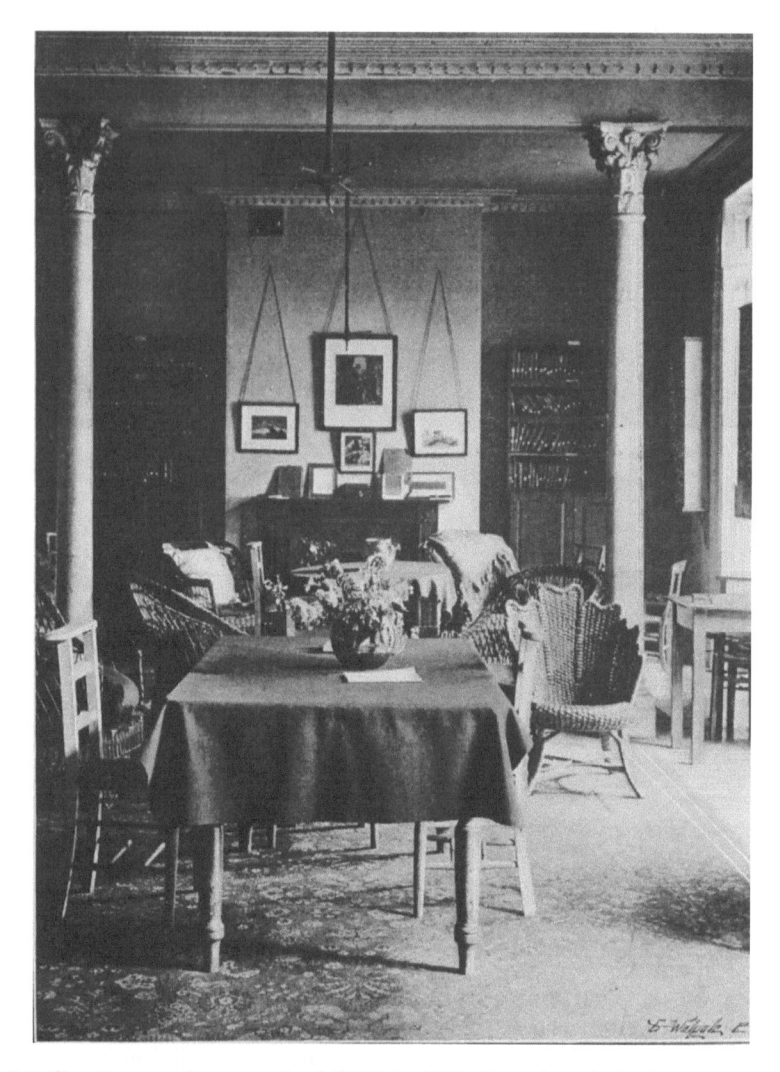

Fig. 5.6 The Common Room at the LSMW in 1899 (from Aesculapia, Women's Work in Medicine, The Lady's Realm, Vol. 61, 1899)

to further the interests of the medical staff rather than those of sick humanity?' However the article was favourable to the new hospital and emphasised its value to the surrounding working or destitute poor. The hospital had been designed with the latest antiseptic principles and for the best care of the blind. In these days before antibiotics there was a significant risk from infection, and the article drew attention to the 'frightful mortality from blood-poisoning to which nurses fall victims in such large numbers'. This risk applied as much to the doctors as to the nurses. The hospital was described as the most perfectly equipped eye hospital in the kingdom. The outpatients department with its waiting area where Florence worked was

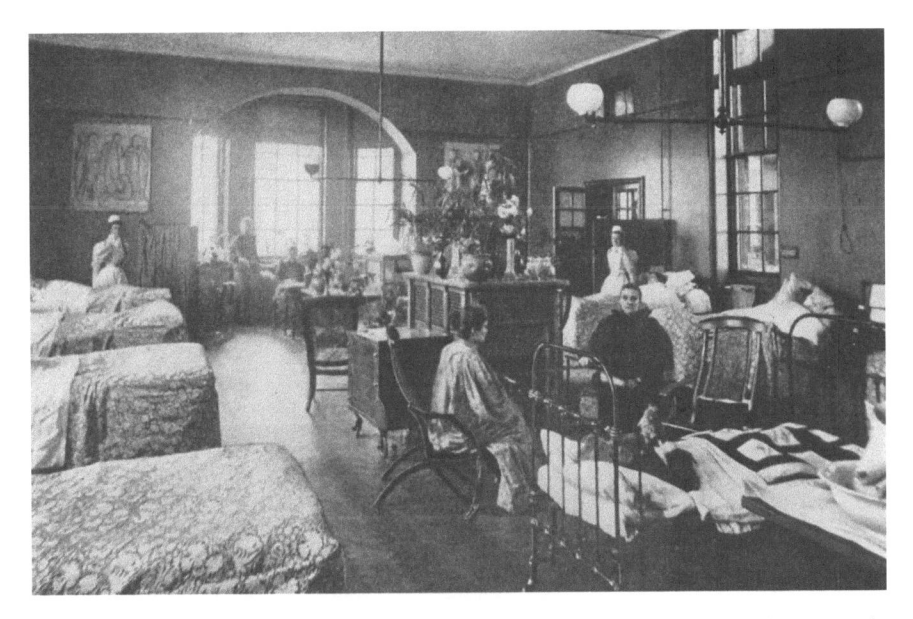

Fig. 5.7 A Ward in the New Hospital for Women in 1899. An Italian bas-relief can be seen on the wall on the left of the photograph. (from Aesculapia, Women's Work in Medicine, The Lady's Realm, Vol. 61, 1899)

commended as being big, well warmed and electrically lit, with refreshment stall and dispensary (Fig. 5.9).

Other appointments that Florence undertook included that of assistant anaesthetist to the RFH to which she was appointed in 1896. Louisa Aldrich-Blake had been appointed anaesthetist to the RFH in 1894 and was the first woman to hold the post. The anaesthetic apparatus of the period was relatively simple and employed a face mask holding a piece of gauze. The volatile anaesthetic agent, either ether or chloroform, was dripped onto the gauze and thereby inhaled. In addition for 3 years Florence was an assistant to the Throat and Ear Department, also at the RFH.

The Victoria Hospital for Sick Children, Hull

In 1897 Florence left London and travelled to Hull where she was appointed house surgeon at the Victoria Hospital for Sick Children (VHSC), replacing Miss Mabel Jones MD (Lond) (c1865–1923) who had resigned to move to Brighton. The appointment was noted in the Eastern Morning News of Saturday 29 May 1897. Mabel Jones was a LSMW graduate and was later become well known for her support and medical care of suffragettes who became ill or were injured whilst in prison.

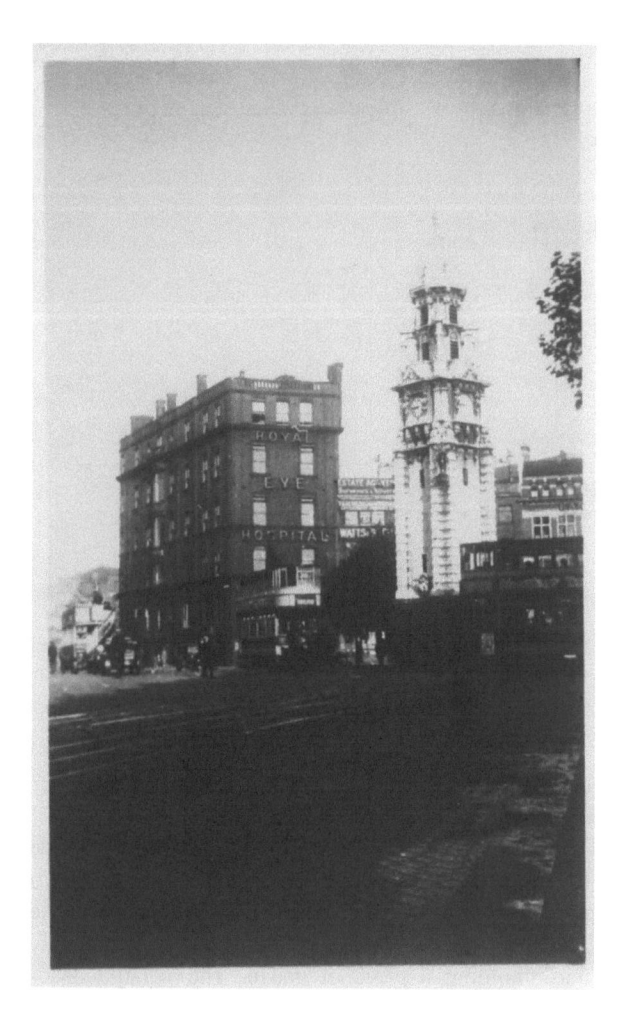

Fig. 5.8 The Royal Eye Hospital in 1929 (from an old postcard, unidentified publisher)

Mabel Jones had been appointed junior assistant in anaesthetics to Louisa Aldrich-Blake in 1894, and Aldrich-Blake was appointed the next year as surgical registrar. These events were seen as encouraging, since, as Neil Macintyre exclaimed, 'It was galling to those qualifying at LSMW that they could not get jobs at their own hospital' [6]. It would seem for the Board of the RFH that being associated with an all-woman medical school with the associated financial advantages was one thing, but actually appointing women to your medical staff was a little different. In order to progress to appointments in other hospitals, it was necessary to obtain experience as a resident at the RFH. Many prestigious children's hospitals, such as the Hospital for Sick Children in Great Ormond Street, where LSMW graduates wanted to work, would not even consider an application unless a previous residential appointment had been held. In 1898 a petition was made to the RFH by 51 LSMW students and 32 graduates that its residential posts be opened to women.

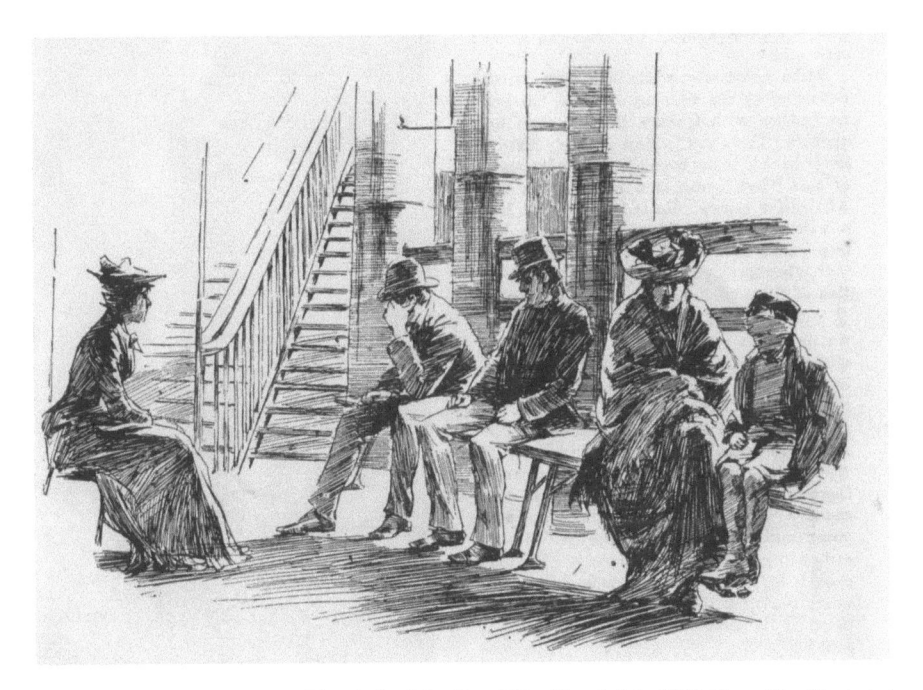

Fig. 5.9 Outpatients in the waiting hall of the Royal Eye Hospital in 1892 (from The Illustrated London News, 17 December 1892)

There were prolonged discussions; however it was not until April 1901 that two female residents were appointed, Louisa Garrett Anderson as house surgeon and Louisa Woodcock as house physician. It was an important public statement that these names were included in the annual report for the year-ending 31 December 1901. Florence would not have obtained a residential post at the RFH in 1897 but was able to do so at Hull, partly because of the work there done by Mary Murdoch.

Florence held this post for 14 months. The VHSC had been founded in 1873 with 30 beds to serve the poor of Hull and was initially opened in a house in Story Street. An outpatients' department was opened for the young patients to be seen and treated. In 1876 a working men's collection was mentioned, and a Working Men's Committee was established in 1890 shortly before Florence arrived. This Working Men's Committee was necessary since the VHSC was part of the Voluntary Hospital Movement [19], and fundraising was an important source of its income. Indeed if the finances were not forthcoming, the service stopped, such as in 1914 when the Babies' Ward was forced to close temporarily. There was no state funding for these hospitals. In 1891 a new hospital, now with 44 beds and designed by S. Musgrave, was opened in Park Street, and it was in this new building that the young Florence worked (Fig. 5.10). The *Hull Daily Mail* of 23 June 1898 described the sad case of a young lad who died of his injuries after a stone had been 'hurled at his head'. The deceased was a 10-year-old boy who had been struck over his right eye and cut. Although the cut had not seemed serious initially, the wound was contaminated, and

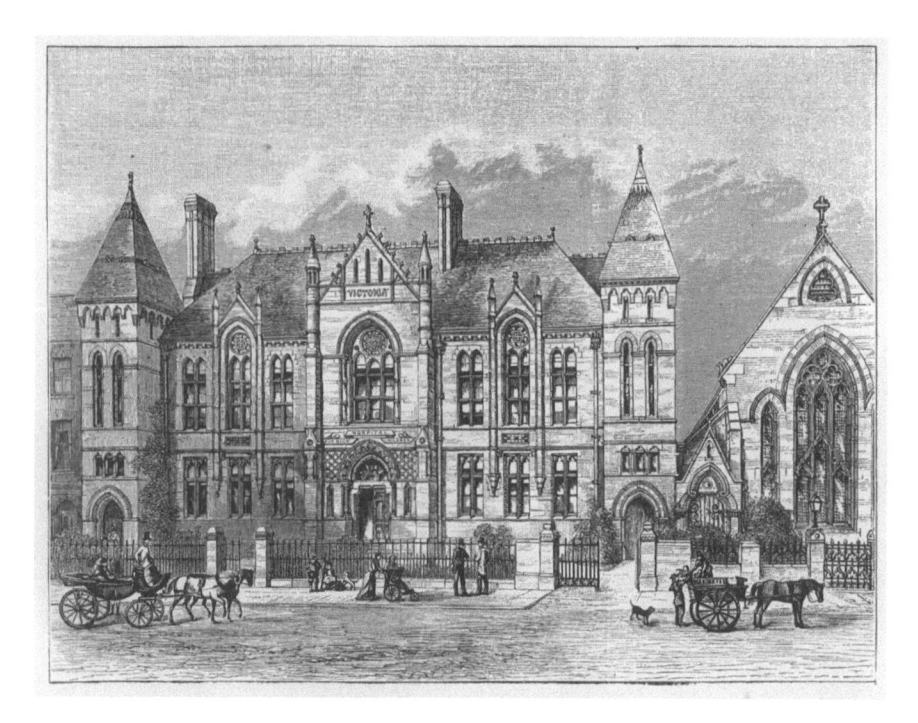

Fig. 5.10 The Victoria Hospital for Sick Children, Hull in 1891 (from the Graphic 25 July 1891)

the boy died of 'blood poisoning'. This illustrates the seriousness of even apparently trivial injuries that became infected in the era before antibiotics. Florence, as house surgeon, was quoted at the inquest saying 'that when the deceased was admitted it was almost a hopeless case' [20].

There were connections between the LSMW and Hull. Dr. Mary Murdoch (1864–1916) had graduated from the LSMW in 1893, and her first post was as house surgeon at the VHSC where she remained until 1895 [21]. After returning to London for a year, she went back to Hull where she was appointed honorary assistant physician, becoming honorary senior physician in 1910. In 1900, Mary appointed Dr. Louisa Martindale (1872–1966) as her assistant. Martindale had graduated from the LSMW in 1899 [22]. Martindale subsequently worked as a surgeon in Brighton, and during the Great War her practice was increasingly busy since many of the male doctors were leaving for the front. She therefore decided to use her holiday allowance to work as a locum for one of the women surgeons working in France. As a result on 6 August 1915, she left for the SWH in the Royaumont Abbey. In Paris she stayed in the Lyceum Club and was able to visit the famous French radiologist Antoine Beclère (1856–1939) and to observe his X-ray treatments of fibroids and non-malignant uterine haemorrhage. At Royaumont she observed all the work that was being done, including the X-ray work. The work was very busy, and she described over 300 patients being admitted in 3 days. Frances Ivens and her staff had to work for 22 h in the day, and were unable to take off their clothes for days at a time, and were lucky if they could have 3 h sleep at a time. Martindale was tremendously impressed by Frances Ivens the CMO for her endurance, courage and surgical skill and for the 'wonderful work that women were doing'. In 1931 Martindale was President of the Medical Women's Federation. As a gynaecological surgeon in Brighton, Martindale shared with Florence an interest in the use of radiotherapy for benign and malignant pelvic disease, and she develop an effective service and made major contributions.

Mary Murdoch was a remarkable person being particularly concerned with public health and the education of mothers and was Hull's first female general practitioner. In 1904 Murdoch founded the Hull Women's Suffrage Society but left when it became militant. Murdoch shared an interest in motoring with Edith and was one of the first car owners in Hull. Whilst it now seems obvious to most that women should be able to drive the motor car, there was considerable early opposition. The pioneer New Zealand doctor Agnes Bennett (1872–1960) noted that 'it was looked on as madness for a woman to drive a car and I had great difficulty in getting a man to teach me to drive' [23].[3] After Murdoch was appointed to the VHSC, only female house physicians and house surgeons were appointed, and these were preferentially from the LSMW, which will be why Florence went to Hull. Murdoch expected a high standard from the house staff expecting self-confidence and independence but working in a supportive environment. Murdoch 'believed in men and women working together in harmony for a common end, but she never compromised or pandered to prejudice. She treated men with a fine directness and fearless self-confidence, and when she knew herself to be in the right she never allowed herself to be overborne'. These words could as easily been spoken about Florence.

Florence obtained her University of London MD in 1899 from the RFH. Unfortunately current London University records give no further information on the topic of her MD; however Florence must have been working on her thesis, whilst she was a house surgeon at Hull.

The Anatomy Demonstrator

Florence had always been interested in anatomy, and for 5 years, from 1898 to 1903, she was demonstrator in anatomy at the LSMW, whilst at the same time setting up her general medical practice in London. The role of the anatomy demonstrator was important, although relatively junior. The role of the anatomy demonstrator has often been performed by junior surgeons whilst training for examinations in surgery as a part-time post. The demonstrator performed dissections to demonstrate specific anatomical regions of importance, supervised dissections by medical students and helped surgeons in training. Helen Chambers (1879–1935), who became the

---

[3]Edith worked with Agnes Bennett during WW1 in Serbia, helping her to set up the radiology equipment at Ostrovo in 1916, where Dr. Bennett was the first CMO.

pathologist at the LSMW, testified to the good teaching that Florence gave to both herself and to other students. By the 1890s anatomy teaching was well developed, and the older days of 'body snatching' were long passed. The Anatomy Act of 1832 had given a licence to medical students, anatomy teachers and doctors to dissect donated bodies, and this Act had been passed in response to public concerns over the illegal trade in stolen corpses. Florence used to say that her time as an anatomy demonstrator had been of the greatest help in her later work as a radiologist, so that in a case of an injury she could always describe to a surgeon exactly what had happened. Florence was able to indicate which muscle was likely to be lying between any bony fragments, and was able to give the exact level of a nerve injury, and indicate the best way to remove a foreign body.

The practice of dissection was also considerably more pleasant than that experienced by previous generations. Historically the bodies had not been preserved, and physical decomposition was a problem particularly in the summer months. Preserving agents were gradually introduced, and until the 1890s methylated spirit was used as both a fixative and preservative agent, at which point formalin became the preferred agent. In the late 1890s, when Florence was an anatomy demonstrator, formalin was superseded by Kaiserling's fixative. Johann Carl Kaiserling (1869–1942) had come up with a technique for preserving histologic and pathologic specimens without changing their natural colour. Kaiserling's fixative was an aqueous solution made from formalin, potassium nitrate and potassium acetate.

On 17 November 1899, the Anatomical Society of Great Britain and Ireland held its annual meeting at the LSMW. The ASGBI (now called the Anatomical Society) was a relatively new society having been founded in 1887 following a suggestion of Charles Barrett Lockwood, who was a surgeon and anatomist at St. Bartholomew's Hospital in London. The aim of the ASGBI was to 'promote, develop and advance research and education in all aspects of anatomical science', and the first annual meeting was held on November 1887 at University College London. In May 1894 two ladies, Mrs. Percy Flemming and Miss Annie Frances Piercy from the LSMW, were admitted to the ASGBI, and so it is perhaps not surprising that the annual meeting was held there in 1899. The main business of the 1899 meeting was to confirm Professor Alfred Young of Owens College in Manchester as president. There were many interesting papers presented at that meeting, and particularly noteworthy was that by Charles Lockwood who presented a paper on the 'Lymphatic system of the Appendix'. Florence demonstrated a dissection of an oesophagus with 'well-marked diverticula'. She said 'I have here a specimen of an oesophagus showing the unusual occurrence of two diverticula' and there was a full description of the specimen and accompanying was a carefully drawn line diagram. The meeting was written up in the Magazine of RFHSMW.

In 1901 Florence attended the 69th Annual Meeting of the British Medical Association, which that year was held in Cheltenham from 30 July to 2 August. At this time the BMA meetings were of major scientific significance and leading doctors and scientists presented their researches, and Florence was to be active in the Association throughout her career.

Florence resigned her post as anatomy demonstrator in September 1903 for a number of reasons. It was partly because on an increasing amount of time that she had to give to her private medical practice; however Helen Chambers said that part of the reason was that Florence realised that there was no possibility at that time of a woman being appointed to the lectureship, and so Florence began to specialise in the new field of X-rays.

Madame Bergman Österberg's Physical Training College and Women's Health and Education

Florence lectured in anatomy to the physical education students at Madame Bergman Österberg's Physical Training College, which was then located at Kingsfield in Dartford Heath in Kent (Fig. 5.11). In the 1903 prospectus, Florence is recorded as being a visiting teacher of anatomy. Florence lectured the Österberg students in their first year, and the students also visited the LSMW to watch Florence's dissections. Watching dissections and viewing specimens would be helpful for the students since teaching at the college in anatomy and physiology was by lecture and not practical. One can only wonder at how observing dissections affected non-medical students. An illustration in the 1903 college prospectus shows Florence giving an anatomy tutorial at the Training College. The subject being taught is the anatomy of the brain as shown on the blackboard (Fig. 5.12). The student sitting third from the right is Emma Silvia Cowles (1881–1975). Silvia Cowles subsequently joined Florence's team as a masseuse in Belgium in 1914.

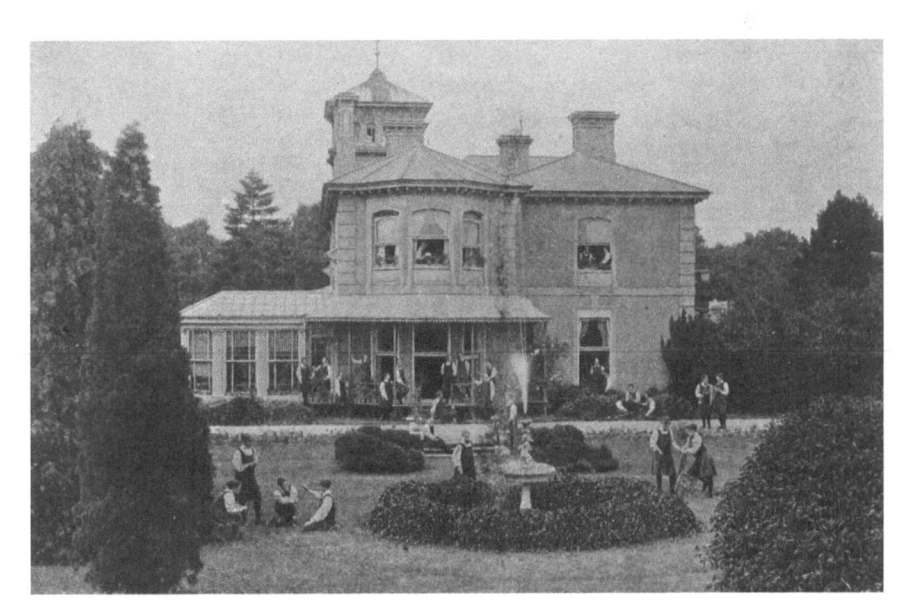

Fig. 5.11 Madame Bergman Österberg's Physical Training College at Dartford (from Stevens, C L McC. A Unique School. The Windsor Magazine 1897, 589–593)

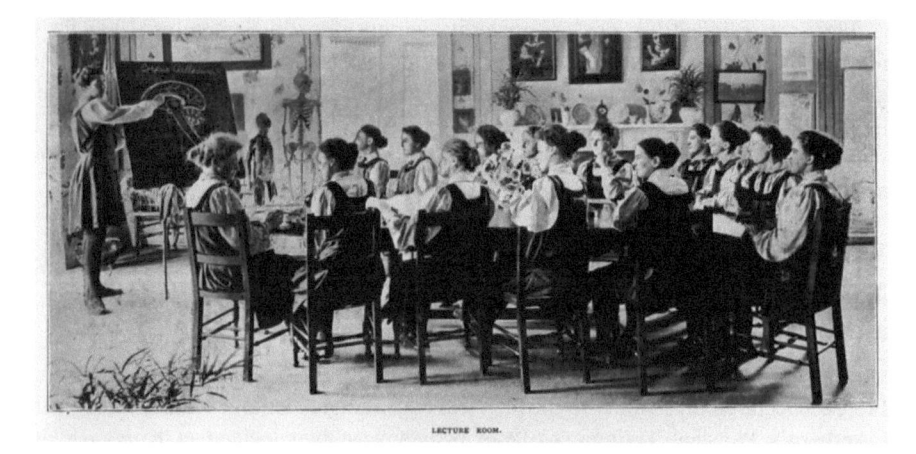

Fig. 5.12 Florence giving an anatomy tutorial at the Training College in 1903. Florence is seated on the left. The student sitting third from the right is Emma Silvia Cowles (from Madam Bergman Österberg Physical Training College 1903 Prospectus. Courtesy of Jane Clayton)

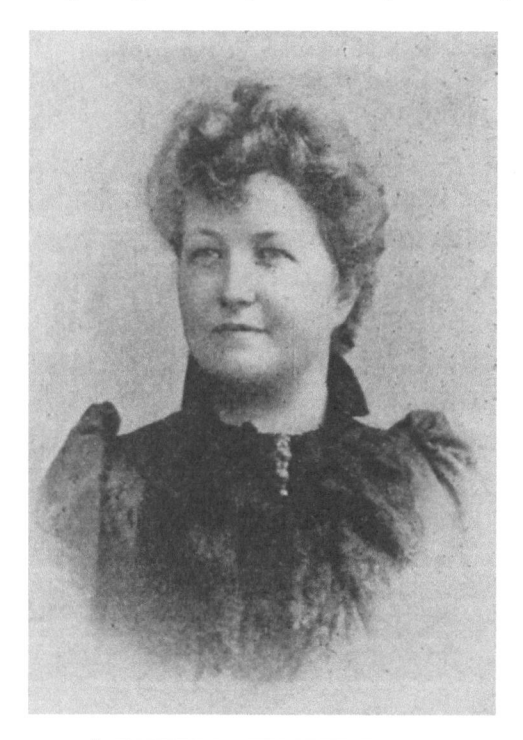

Fig. 5.13 Martina Bergman Österberg (1849–1915) (from Stevens, C L McC. A Unique School. The Windsor Magazine 1897, 589–593)

Martina Bergman Österberg (1849–1915) was a remarkable woman, described as being a 'handsome, well-built, imperious woman' [24] (Fig. 5.13). She was born in Sweden and subsequently moved to England. She trained at the Royal Central

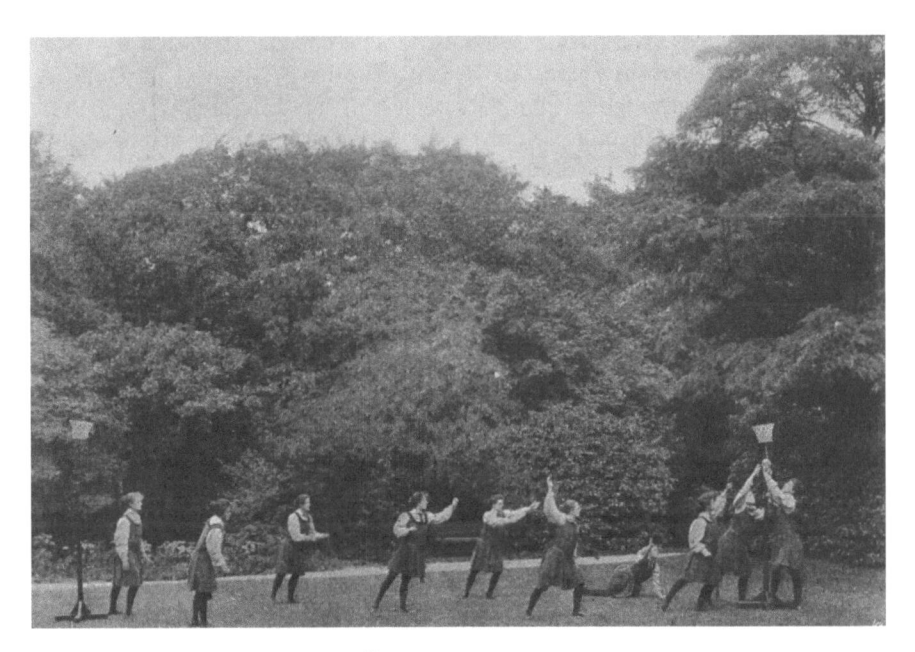

Fig. 5.14 Playing basketball at the Österberg's Physical Training College. The girls are seen wearing their gymslips. (from Stevens, C L McC. A Unique School. The Windsor Magazine 1897, 589–593)

Gymnastic Institute in Stockholm and developed the ideas of Pehr Henrik Ling (1776–1839) on health and exercise. Ling saw the value of anatomy and physiology for health, the knowledge of both of which was developing. After Madame Österberg came to England, in 1881 she was appointed to the London School Board and was instrumental in developing physical education as a core part of the school curriculum [25]. By 1909 the Ling system was standard in British schools. Her Physical Training College, which was for women's physical education and instructor training, was located initially in Hampstead. When the Hampstead site became too small, the college moved to Dartford Heath where it continues today as part of the North Kent College [26]. The college was instrumental in the importing of basketball from America (Fig. 5.14), lacrosse from Canada, the invention of netball and the wearing of gymslips in place of older heavier garments that young women were obliged to use for exercise. The girls also played cricket, many years before the formation of the Women's Cricket Federation. It is noteworthy that women were so much involved in the development of British gymnastics. Florence must have been very sympathetic to the aims of Madame Österberg with the latter's emphasis on physical health and education and also her commitment to women's progress, and Österberg donated money to organisations related to women's emancipation in her native Sweden. Österberg was convinced that the key to the emancipation of women was in economic independence and justified her high fees since her graduates were assured of employment as teachers of women's physical education. Florence's anatomical knowledge was put to very good use at the college. The Österberg system emphasised that every gymnastic movement must have a distinct physiological objective and would progress from the simplest of movements advancing to the most complex. Knowledge of anatomy was therefore essential for optimisation of exercise and in the avoidance of injury.

Many of the principles that Madame Österberg valued were emphasised by Florence in a lecture that she gave to the Bristol Centre of the Parent's National Educational Union at the Kensington School of Art in Berkley Square and reported in the *Western Daily Press* of 18 November 1904. The lecture was entitled 'Children's Health', and some of her points sound surprisingly contemporary. She emphasised the importance of preventing disease and in the need for good air and healthy breathing. Gymnastics and the use of light, loose and warm clothing were all recommended. Florence supported to regular medical examination of schoolchildren with an emphasis on the chest and spine. Florence took her own advice and between 1906 and 1908 was the Medical Advisor to two girls' schools in London, which were Blackheath High School and South Hampstead High School.

In due course Florence became involved with the Chelsea College of Physical Education, which was founded in 1898 in 'order to give a sound education in Physical Training' [27]. There was to be a broadly based curriculum, and students would be taught the fundamental principles of physiology which underpinned the various systems of gymnastics that were then in vogue in different countries. A scientific approach was seen as being essential 'for all whose task in after life[4] will be to teach others and to design and to adapt exercises and games for children and adults under different conditions of physique and environment'. The aims of the College were similar to those of Madame Bergman Österberg, and indeed there were connections between the two colleges. The importance of physical education to the women's movement should not be underemphasised. Agnes Bennett [23] pointed out that playgrounds in girls' schools in Wellington had been looked upon as superfluous, with only three quarters of an acre being allowed for girls and some 50 acres for boys. When Bennett complained, the Chairman of the College described her views as 'windy piffle'. This incident is another example of the stereotype of active boys and passive girls.

Students for the professional course were to be between the ages of 18 and 25, and their height should not be less than 5 ft. 3 in. All of the candidates for admission to the College were to have a medical examination and must either 'be examined by the College Medical Adviser (Florence A. Stoney, M.D., 4, Nottingham Place W. Hours 11-1), for which a fee of 5s. is charged', or alternatively the medical entrance forms could be filled in by the candidates' own doctor. In the 1912–1913 report, it is recorded that 'Dr. Stoner (that is Stoney) - writing pamphlet - treatment with X-Rays of Exopthalmic goitre', and Florence indeed presented that paper at the Annual Meeting of the BMA that year.

---

[4]After life refers to the work that the students would undertake after qualification.

Florence was now financially independent, and, around 1903, she bought a house in West London at 30 Chepstow Crescent, Ledbury Road, Notting Hill (now demolished), on a large corner plot at the junction with Chepstow Villas. She moved in with Edith, her father and their domestic help. The telephone line (1473 Western) made it easy to contact friends, colleagues and patients. Being the owner, Florence was the family member with a vote in the local elections, not her father [28]. Edith, on the other hand, had to wait until the sisters bought a house together after their father died before she could vote locally [29]. Their cook and domestic help, Mary Kennedy, came with them, and they employed a parlour maid, Catherine Gaffney. They lost the view over the park that they had enjoyed in Islington, but the new house had advantages. It afforded much easier access to the LSMW and the various hospitals and colleges in London where she worked, using the newly opened Central Line from Notting Hill Station. They no longer had to use the awkward Victorian network of railway lines that had served their previous house in the Northern Suburbs.

References

1. Todd M (Graham Travers). The life of Sophia Jex-Blake. London: Macmillan; 1918.
2. Manton J. Elizabeth Garrett Anderson. London: Methuen; 1965.
3. Hunting P. A history of the society of apothecaries: The Society of Apothecaries; 1998.
4. Lord R. Dame Louisa Aldrich-Blake. London: Hodder & Stoughton; c1930.
5. Crawford E. Enterprising women: the Garretts and their circle. London: Francis Boutle; 2002.
6. McIntyre N. How British women became doctors: the story of the Royal Free Hospital and its medical school. London: Wenrowave Press; 2014.
7. Evans AD, Howard LGR. The romance of the British voluntary hospital movement. London: Hutchinson; n.d.. undated c1930
8. Ashton R. Victorian Bloomsbury. New Haven\London: Yale University Press; 2012.
9. Gleadle K. British women in the nineteenth century (Social history in perspective). Basingstoke: Palgrave Macmillan; 2001.
10. Mukerjee S. Sisters in arms. History Today. 2018;68:72–83.
11. Sheppard A. Obituary. Dr. Florence Stoney, OBE. The Magazine of the London (Royal Free Hospital) School of Medicine for Women. 1932;27:128–13.
12. Higher Education of Women. York Herald, Friday 11 August 1893.
13. Travers, Graham (Margaret Georgina Todd). Mona Maclean, medical student. A novel. 12th ed. Edinburgh: William Blackwood; 1897 (first published 1894).
14. Todd M (Graham Travers). The life of Sophia Jex-Blake. London: Macmillan; 1918.
15. Owen WB. Stoney, George Johnstone (1826–1911) Dictionary of National Biography (12) 922.
16. Ball RS. Dr G. Johnstone Stoney, F.R.S. Observatory. 1911;34:187–290.
17. Stoney G J. Microscopic vision. London Edinburgh and Dublin Philosophical Magazine Ser 5. 1896;42:332–49, 423–42.
18. Booth C. Life and labour of the people in London. London: Macmillan; 1903. p. 150–1.
19. Evans AD, Howard LGR. The romance of the British Voluntary Hospital movement. London: Hutchinson, undated.
20. Hull Daily Mail, 23 June 1898.
21. Malleson H. A woman doctor. Mary Murdoch of Hull. London: Sidgwick & Hackson; 1919.
22. Martindale L. A woman surgeon. London: Victor Gollancz; 1950.
23. Bennett A. Epilogue. In: Manson C&C. Doctor Agnes Bennett. London: Michael Joseph; 1960.

24. May J. Madame Bergman-Österberg. London: George Harrap; 1969.
25. Inglis S. Played in London. English Heritage: Populus; 2014.
26. Stevens C L McC. A unique school. The Windsor Magazine 1897;589–93.
27. Webb IM. The history of Chelsea College of Physical Education with special reference to curriculum development, 1893-1973. PhD thesis, University of Leicester; 1977.
28. Parliamentary Borough of Kensington (North Division), No 3 (Pembridge) Polling District. Division three – county and parochial electors. Elector 11956; 1902.
29. Childs Hill Ward of the Urban Parish of Hendon. Occupational electors. Division three county electors and parochial electors. Electors 5694 and 5605, 20 Reynold's-close; 1915

Chapter 6
Florence and X-rays

Pioneer Radiology

Florence became interested in the new subject of radiology at time when the apparatus and facilities were still in a primitive stage, and there was very little awareness of either radiological protection or the basic tenets of radiobiology [1]. The X-rays had been discovered by Wilhelm Conrad Röntgen on 8 November 1895, which was the year that Florence had qualified as a doctor. The discovery caused an international sensation, and the general public had to be reassured that the discovery was actually true and that it had been made by a serious German scientist. A series of reports were made by Sidney Rowland and had appeared in the *British Medical Journal* in 1896 and were read with interest. It was not long before the medical potential of the new discovery was appreciated and the apparatus was acquired by hospital electrical departments. The articles in the *BMJ* showed the potential of the new discovery, and as a member of the BMA, Florence would have followed the dramatic developments of the new subject. For example, in the *British Medical Journal* in 1896, there is a description of a subaltern[1] who fell off his horse whilst riding in Hyde Park. He had an elbow injury, and the radiograph revealed a simple dislocation with no fracture, and this was reduced with confidence. This alerted doctors to the diagnostic possibilities of what was being called 'the new photography'. Sidney Rowland went on to found the first ever radiology journal the *Archives of Skiagraphy*, and as a radiologist Florence went on to make many contributions to this journal and its successors.

The early apparatus was of low power and was difficult to use for many reasons. The electricity was provided by either batteries or by static electrical machines such as that devised by Wimshurst. A Ruhmkorff induction coil was used to make the high electrical tension required to operate the X-ray tube. The X-ray tube was

---

[1]A subaltern is an officer, and especially a second lieutenant, in the British army below the rank of captain.

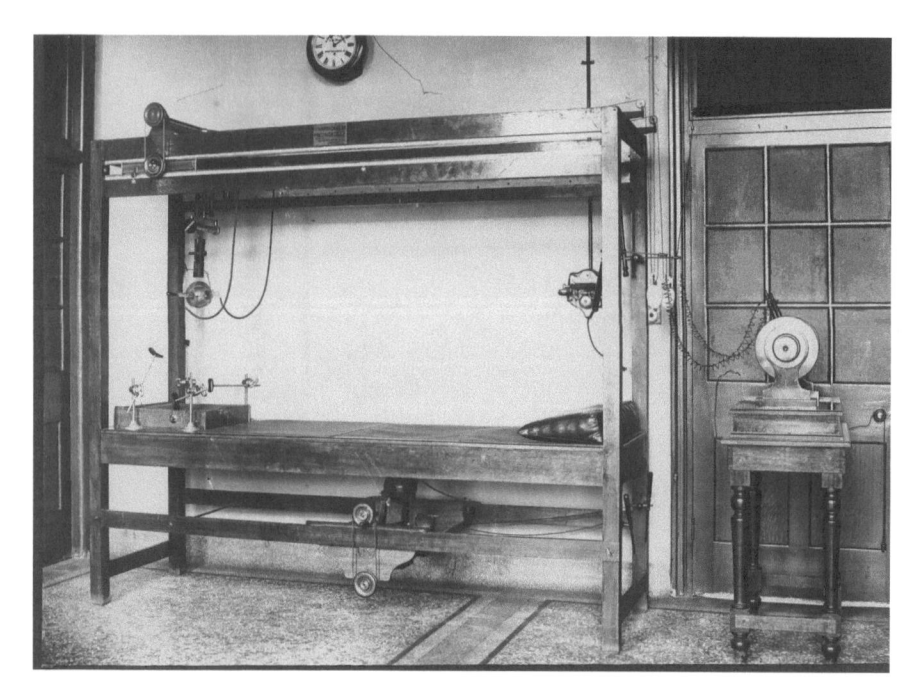

Fig. 6.1 An X-ray couch from 1910, The London Hospital (original photograph in author's collection)

attached to the high tension by wires, and the tube resembled a light bulb with no surrounding protection. Although the apparatus in use prior to the Great War may look primitive to modern eyes, at the time it was cutting edge technology (Fig. 6.1). There were dangers from several directions. The operators were at risk from electrocution, and this was a major concern for the pioneers. Shockproof apparatus was not to be introduced until the 1930s. Radiation was emitted in all directions, and protection was not common until after 1900 when the tube was either encased in a lead lined box or a lead glass cover. Unfortunately many of the pioneers suffered from radiation injuries. The injuries started as a dermatitis, which was painful and debilitating, and persistent exposure would result in the development of malignancy and fatalities. Amy Shepherd (d1936), who became the ophthalmic surgeon to the EGAH, noted about Florence that 'Much of her work, like that of many early radiologists, was done under adverse, and even dangerous conditions. Always ready to help and always resourceful, she gave too freely of a generous spirit in a not over-robust frame, and enlivened even the common task with her flashes of wit and wisdom' [2]. There was a certain bravado about radiation displayed by the pioneers, and the editor to the BJR obituary comments that 'she (Florence) never hesitated to risks in localisation work on the operating table, and since the war had suffered from dermatitis of the left hand'. The final source of harm for the operators was chemical irritation from the wet processing of the glass plates.

Radiology and Anatomy

Florence's anatomical interest and knowledge were to serve her in good stead when she worked as a radiologist. This was an interesting period for the study of anatomy, and Röntgen's discovery of X-rays in 1895 was transforming the understanding of both our anatomy and of ourselves. The discovery of the X-rays created a popular sensation, with both the general public and the medical profession being fascinated. So as an example, Charles Thurstan Holland (1863–1941), a general practitioner in Liverpool, saw some of the early X-ray work of Sir Oliver Lodge, which he was making at University College Liverpool in February 1896. Lodge had taken a radiograph of a boy who had shot himself in the hand. A successful radiograph was obtained, and Holland described the excitement they both felt when the plate was brought out into the daylight and the shadow of the bullet was seen. By the end of May in 1896, Holland had acquired an X-ray kit, and as he later recalled, 'There were no X-ray departments in any of the hospitals. There were no experts. There was no literature. No one knew anything about radiographs of the normal, to say nothing of the abnormal' [3].

On 17 September 1896, Holland examined the hand of a child at the age of 1 year and was fascinated to see the ossifications in the skeleton [4]. The bones were seen with a clarity never before possible. Holland noted the absence of ossification of the epiphyses, and Holland immediately realised the role that X-rays could have for anatomical studies and in observing skeletal growth. He started collecting radiographs at different ages of development, and later that year he showed them at the annual meeting of the British Medical Association in Liverpool.

More local to Florence, and also in London, John Poland (1855–1937) of the Miller Hospital in Greenwich had a particular interest in epiphyseal anatomy and trauma. Considerable effort was made in the late nineteenth century and early twentieth century in understanding the anatomy of the developing epiphyses and radiographic anatomy [5]. Eugene Corson (1855–1946), from Savannah, GA, wrote to John Poland on 21 November 1900, admiring his book on the *Traumatic Separation of the Epiphyses* and enclosing some reprints. In the November 1900 *Annals of Surgery* article 'A Skiagraphic Study of the Normal Membral Epiphyses at the Thirteenth Year,' Corson had written 'The X-ray will prove to be a valuable aid in the study of many points of normal anatomy' and that 'The bone relationships in joints, the various joint movements, and the different steps in bone development can all be studied in a striking way by the X-ray'. It was the clarity of radiography that impressed Colson, who commented that 'the discovery of Röntgen, a discovery which makes possible and easy and an absolutely correct diagnosis where previously uncertainty and error outweighed definite knowledge'. Poland had shown his series of films at the first conversazione of the Röntgen Society in 1897, and the anatomical possibilities of the new technique would have appealed to Florence.

The Royal Free Hospital Röntgen Ray Department

On 4 December 1901, the weekly board meeting of the Royal Free Hospital opened a fund 'to defray the cost (about £100) of a Röntgen Ray apparatus' [6]. Within a few weeks, it was clear that the target would be soon met, and the opinion of the surgical staff was sought on further actions. They declared that the apparatus 'had to be obtained from Miller and Co' and that Edmund Roughton, the ENT surgeon, and Wilmott Evans, the skin surgeon, would supervise the order. Having sorted out the purchase, two more practical matters were put in hand, which were staffing and how the equipment would be looked after. In other hospitals, new X-ray equipment was often placed in a department for medical electricity, but as no such department had been established at the Royal Free Hospital, everything had to be set up from scratch.

Several major London hospitals had installed the Röntgen ray apparatus in 1896, and there was a general positive response from the various boards of managements to requests from the medical staff. The first department set up in London was at the Miller Hospital in Greenwich. Others followed rapidly, including the London Hospital and St. Bartholomew's Hospital. The first practical demonstration of radiography in London had been on 13 February 1896 when Stanley Kent made a presentation at St. Thomas's Hospital. Those interested in 'the new photography' as it was called had founded a society, the *Röntgen Society* [7][2], which Florence was to join in January 1903. By the time that the Royal Free Hospital set up its new department in 1902, radiology was well-established, and even smaller hospitals such as Beckenham Cottage Hospital were acquiring apparatus.

On 1 January 1902, Mr. Evans reported that he had arranged with the LSMW for the 'maintenance and care of the appliances' and that it was proposed to appoint a special officer to work the apparatus. Although Wilmott Evans did not know it, with these two actions, he had set in train a sequence of events that would create Florence's career and reputation and eventually lead to both sisters' major contributions to radiology during the Great War. Applications were invited for the post on 19 February, although the post was not advertised [8], and only those with a medical qualification were considered. Florence was appointed as the medical electrician on 19 March at a salary of 20 guineas per annum.

Florence was known to Edmund Roughton through her work as a Clinical Assistant in the Nose and Throat Department at the RFH. She had not, as far as it is recorded, gained any prior experience with X-rays, although she would have been fully aware of the new discovery. Florence would have known about the use of electricity in treatment, as in electrotherapy. Remarkably, several sets of surgeons' case notes remain, and from these a particular patient treated in Florence's time can be used as an example [8]. Mr. Evans was recorded as using electrolysis to treat a naevus. Under anaesthetic, a direct current of 10 mA from a large battery was passed between a pair of needle electrodes on the skin placed at several places over the

---

[2]The Röntgen Society continues today as the British Institute of Radiology and is the oldest radiological society in the world.

disfiguring naevus, a treatment that was repeated once a week for 6 weeks. The notes recorded that the 'result is probably not immediate', and indeed there appeared to be no benefit at all. Such experimental uses of electricity were not uncommon at the time but gave promise of future developments. There was little real understanding of the changes that were taking place in the body with various forms of treatment, and as a result such treatments were made on a pragmatic basis.

Roughton and Evans would have been aware that Edith, who was now in her second year as physics lecturer in the School of Medicine, would be able to provide the technical and scientific backup that would be needed when this new technology was introduced into the hospital. Electrical equipment was delicate and needed to be used carefully. For example, at the beginning of 1900, the students had damaged the batteries that were used in electrotherapy, and it was part of Edith's role to ensure that this did not happen again.

It should also be noted that the RFH was coming under increasing pressure to demonstrate its commitment to women doctors beyond that of allowing women LSMW students to gain their clinical practice on the hospital wards. This followed the March 1898 petition presented by 83 past and current students and so it did no harm to include a woman in the new post of Medical Electrician.[3]

Mr. Evans could anticipate treating his patients' skin conditions with X-rays, adding to the light therapy and electrotherapy that he already used. Florence had now secured her first senior hospital post, and Edith and Johnstone could be justifiably proud of her achievements. And, finally, the arrangement meant that the sisters could officially work together, sharing the challenge of setting up and operating a new department of radiology. Working together would be of mutual benefit. Florence learned from Edith about the physics and technology of X-ray equipment, and Edith gained a knowledge of practical anatomy and pathology from Florence's clinical work. This would be essential in their work in the Great War.

The much needed electrical department at the Royal Free Hospital was opened in April 1902. The Magazine of the RFHSMW in May 1902 stated, 'an advance has been made . . . .by the organisation of an electrical department. An X-ray apparatus is now fitted up in Elizabeth Ward . . . .Miss Stoney is appointed as electrician [with] two students as assistants, who will be initiated into the mysteries . . . .Miss Stoney attends on Wednesdays at 12.30 p.m. and on Fridays at 9 a.m.' [7].

The department had taken some time to get into good working order. In the RFHSMW Magazine for January 1903, Florence was to write, 'but now the X-rays are available twice a week, ...and . . . .patients are treated by electricity with the constant or interrupted current as required'.

The rooms were badly ventilated, and there was no separate room for the X-ray work. The apparatus could only be used when the room was not needed for other purposes. The X-ray apparatus was initially left open for all to use, including for casualty work by the house surgeons, but it had to be locked after the equipment was damaged within a week of opening. Florence noted that with 'a delicate electrical

---

[3]The 1901 annual report was not printed until after Florence had been appointed in March 1902.

instrument connected with an electric main with over 200 volts it does not do to blindly do to turn one handle after another and observer results'. The electrical power was obtained from the nearby St Pancras main supply. The apparatus although appearing primitive and simple to our modern eyes was in reality complex and needed considerably practical skills in order to obtain good results. It was only following the development of the Coolidge vacuum tube that the exposure parameters could be predictable and standardised. Florence wrote describing the need for experience in judging the timing of exposures. The factors that the radiographer needed to consider included the body part to be examined, the strength of the current passing through the tube, the distance from the object radiographed to the photographic plate and whether the tube has a high or low vacuum. With the early ion tubes, the intensity of vacuum changed depending on the use of the tube. With use the vacuum increased and the tube 'hardened', and therefore choosing exposure factors was difficult compared to today, when the radiographic apparatus has automatic control of exposure factors. The radiographer therefore needed to know how the tube had been used, and tubes were selected depending on the part of the body that was to be examined. The process of development was time consuming, and many glass photographic plates needed over half an hour processing to reveal the image. Florence commented that the photographic work was tedious. The photographic process was also complex and required the making of developing, fixing, intensifying and reducing solutions. The processing parameters had also to be varied to suit the needs of a particular plate and to optimise the image. A knowledge of paper printing was essential since it was common to include a paper print of the negative with the written report. She often took the plates home and developed them in her bathroom in the evenings.

At that time, the radiologist, commonly called radiographer, was not a member of the hospital medical staff, and Florence was not a member of the committee that discussed the work of her department. An appeal for improved conditions resulted in the purchase of second-hand apparatus; however there had not even been an enquiry about its suitability for use with the other equipment! This must have irked both Florence and Edith who were knowledgeable about the technology and knew about how to purchase and assemble the equipment.

The work that she undertook was varied. The examinations were particularly helpful for foreign bodies, and she describes a needle in the knee of a patient referred to her by a former student. Florence was particularly pleased in locating a round tin whistle that could not be felt, but could be easily seen radiographically lodged at the level of the suprasternal notch at the base of the neck. At this time the apparatus was still of low power, and abdominal foreign bodies were not visible. She examined a bullet wound in a man, who was employed by the Society for the Protection of Cruelty to Animals and was injured when a horse he was holding was shot. His radius was fractured; however the retained bullet was easily seen and removed. Other cases included medical conditions such as phthisis (tuberculosis), bony deformities such as coxa vara and pes cavus, a sarcomatous tumour of the humerus, finger clubbing and a dislocated elbow (Fig. 6.2). When Florence started to use the screen (fluoroscope) for examinations, she emphasised the need for a history and a

Fig. 6.2 A dislocated elbow from 1903 (from Magazine of the RFHLSMW 1903)

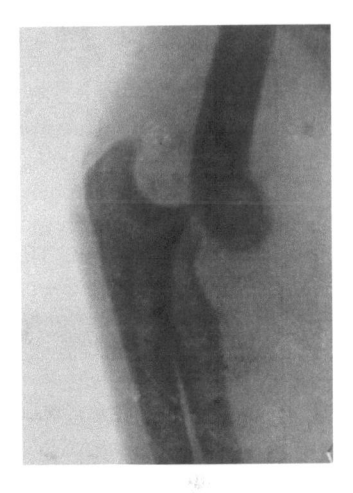

physical examination before starting and particularly before performing an opaque meal examination, performed in those time with oral bismuth before it was replaced by barium.

Her first X-ray treatment was of a man who had had a rodent ulcer for 20 years. Florence gave 23 exposures over a month. The tube was placed at 8–9 inches from the patient, and initial exposures of 5 min were gradually increased to 20 min. Florence was pleased with the results. Throughout her career, it was said that she was a 'firm adherent of the school of big dosage, often alarming her colleagues'. In therapy with X-rays, there is a balance, and giving too small a dose will avoid complications but risk under treatment, whereas giving too high a dose may well cure the clinical problem but at the risk of causing unnecessary complications. It was said that 'she seemed to know instinctively which patients would stand intensive treatment' and that 'many malignant cases are alive to-day as the result of what some would have termed her temerity, and many others had their lives prolonged to an unsuspected extent'.

It cannot be overstated how unusual Florence's department was. It was the first ever radiology department to be fully staffed by women. Florence herself may have been the first women radiologist. The two student assistants from the LSMW were both women. And, uniquely, the care of the equipment was in the hands of a woman physicist.

Florence's main interest was in anatomy, so it is unsurprising that she spent the first months using the X-ray equipment to take radiographs, rather than using it for therapy. Perhaps it was never going to be possible to serve both the physicians and the surgeons to their full satisfaction. Expectations were high on both sides, but Florence could only fit so much into the 2 days for which she was paid. She had to explain to the physicians that it took a long time to develop the radiographic films that showed the surgeons exactly where to find an embedded needle. She had to explain to Dr. Evans that it took a long time to treat the rodent ulcer with X-rays and that many days were needed.

Before the end of 1902, the perceived unsatisfactory operation of Florence's department was being discussed at the Medical Committee. An initial scheme for its reorganisation was referred back from the Board to the Medical Committee in December, where a subcommittee consisting of Buzzard, Evans and another surgeon Mr. Legg was set up to 'consider the question of Electrical (Röntgen Ray) Department and to make recommendations for the more efficient working of that Department' [9]. Buzzard and Evans, physician and surgeon, proposed that the department should be split into two. The surgical registrar should take charge of the X-ray equipment under the advice of Mr. Evans. The medical registrar should take charge of the 'electrical testing and the batteries' with the advice of Dr. Buzzard. Each person should gain an allowance of £15 for the additional work. Each would attend daily, but at different times.

The new arrangements were accepted by the Board in April, and, on 1 June 1903, there was no mention of a 'medical electrician'. Florence, who had set up the equipment and had successfully run the department for not much more than a year, lost her position.

There was a surprising corollary to these events. During that year, two new women took over as registrars and hence took roles in the electrical and Röntgen departments. Florence Willey (later Lady Baxter) took over as surgical registrar and so took charge of the X-ray equipment. She went on to be appointed as Assistant Physician for Diseases of Women at the Royal Free in 1908 and Lecturer in Midwifery at the LSMW in 1913. After the war she was one of the women doctors who established the Marie Curie Hospital for radium treatment of uterine cancer. Willey was replaced as radiographer in 1904 by Frances Ivens, a remarkable doctor with whom Edith would work in France during the war. On the medical side, the electrical equipment was taken on first by Christine Murrell and then by Adeline Roberts. In 1933, Murrell was the first woman to be elected to the General Medical Council, although she sadly died before she could take up her seat. Thus, although Florence herself did not continue at the Royal Free, her position was filled by four eminent women doctors during the next few years. As each gained experience with X-rays, they too would know that Edith was close at hand to give technical advice if it was needed. The split operation of the department did not survive. When the two posts were recombined in 1906, a man, G. Harrison Orton, was appointed as the 'Radiographer and Medical Electrician'. However dividing X-ray departments was not uncommon, and at Guy's Hospital there were medical and surgical departments for many years.

Radiology at the New Hospital for Women

In 1902 Florence started the X-ray department at the New Hospital for Women located in Euston Road and was appointed as the 'rayologist'. The New Hospital for Women was only a short walk from the Royal Free Hospital in Gray's Inn Road.

Using her experience from the Royal Free Hospital, she was able to propose several changes, altering a pre-existing order for a rheostat and using the money to provide a motor for £16, a significant expenditure at that time. She arranged that the X-ray department was enlarged 'by removing the linen cupboards and altering the tea-room' [10]. At first Florence saw very few patients, and this was only on one or two mornings a week. The entry from the Röntgen Ray Department for the 1905 Annual Report shows only 59 diagnostic cases and 22 cases for treatment for the whole year. These data were not recorded before Florence took over and show that she was concerned to publicise the importance of the work of her department.

The largest single therapy group comprised ulcers (4/22 in 1905, 10/29 in 1906 and 8/37 in 1909), although by 1909 she had also treated 9 cases of ringworm. The largest single group of diagnostic cases was for renal calculi (13/59 in 1905 and 11/45 in 1906, 36/96 in 1909). Otherwise, both lists include very small numbers of cases in any single category. For therapy these include single cases of migraine, lupus, lumbago, tuberculosis of the vulva, and acne, for example, with a handful of diagnostic cases for rheumatoid arthritis, foreign bodies, fractures, and general examinations of chest and abdomen. Whilst Florence's experience would have been extended in her own private practice, these are still very small numbers on which to create any firm therapeutic conclusions, or strong diagnostic confidence, during these early years. During the next years, however, the department steadily expanded under Florence's guidance and enthusiasm [11]. By the 1906 report, Florence was included as one of the medical staff, in charge of the electrical department. The financial challenge to the hospital of equipping an effective and modern X-ray department was beginning to become clearer, and a special fund for the X-ray department of £154-9s-6d was reported. The following year, Florence contributed some of her own money.

By 1910 the X-ray department was promised a new room within the existing hospital, since it was 'almost dangerous in its old quarters'. Pressing her advantage, Florence was able to get an agreement in 1911 for £123-3-6 for X-ray equipment for her new room, and this was the single most expensive item purchased by the Hospital Guild that year.

Up to this point, the X-ray department had no formal representation in the committee structure of the hospital. However, in March 1911, the Pathology Committee expanded its remit to become the *Pathology, X-ray and Mechanical Therapy Committee* [12]. This formal representation, her new room and her new equipment allowed Florence to present an argument that X-rays should be available during 2 full days a week, rather than only two mornings as previously stated. By 1914, the diagnostic workload had doubled from that reported a few years before, suggesting that this extension was granted. Florence also suggests appropriate charges: two shillings and sixpence for a diagnostic X-ray and seven shillings and sixpence for a month's radiation treatment. These charges would be for outpatients. She argued against cross charging for in-patients, considering that this should be covered by the overall hospital costs. At the same time, she pressed for the appointment of a darkroom technician to carry out all the photographic development, which she had previously done herself. A Miss Wortham was appointed who had previously worked as an assistant at the Royal Free Hospital.

Florence suggested that a nurse should be appointed to the X-ray department at an enhanced nurse's salary. Perhaps not unsurprisingly, the response suggested that there were no spare nurses. However managing and caring for patients without nursing support, particularly if therapy was undertaken, would have been very difficult. When the department at the Glasgow Royal Infirmary had opened in 1897, there was a staff of nurses at its inception, as well as two medical officers and an unqualified assistant. More costly requests followed. The management committee meeting on 2 December 1913 discussed a request from Miss Stoney for a new coil for which the cost would be more that £42. Management seems to have become concerned about the escalating cost of running an effective X-ray department by now, and the decision was referred back to the Medical Council to 'go thoroughly into the matter with Miss Stoney'. More financial requests followed on 30 January 1914 for £300 for X-ray tubes (they were stated to last about 3 months of therapeutic use and 6 months of diagnostic use). By 11 June that year, there was 'an urgent need to enlarge the X-ray department', a request which was rejected at the management committee meeting in July because 'Enlarging the X-Ray accommodation would amount to approximately £250' so nothing could be done in the present state of finances.

When war broke out in August 1914, and Florence started to work for the war effort, she was at first given leave of absence and then replaced. The X-ray work was taken on by Miss Christine Bernard LMSSA, who was also working from Florence's consulting rooms at 4 Nottingham Place. Although the service did not grow further under Miss Bernard, Florence had left a robust and respected service, which the hospital continued to support.

Graves' Disease

Florence Stoney continued with her X-ray work including the treatment of exophthalmic goitre (Graves' disease or Graves-Basedow disease), which became a major interest. In 1912 she presented a paper on the treatment of thyrotoxicosis using radiation to the annual meeting of the British Medical Association held in Liverpool from 19 to 26 July. The Section on Electro-Therapeutics and Radiology was chaired by Charles Thurstan Holland, and the first paper was by G. Fedor Haenisch (1874–1952) who spoke on radiation treatment of uterine fibroids. Florence described her experience of treating exophthalmic goitre, or Graves' disease, with X-rays [13, 14]. This was a well-established treatment for this condition, and whilst external radiation is no longer used, today radiation treatment continues with the use of radioiodine introduced following the Second World War. Florence thought 'It is to me rather terrible to see these patients subject to operation, where the risks are considerable, and shock in their nervous systems very severe and sometimes fatal'. Her patients were often very sick, and described as 'a weak, twitching, emaciated, anxious object—become day by day more placid, and happy, and fat, till they attain a sense of well-being and are again able to enjoy life'. The oral antithyroid drugs that are used today were not yet developed, and, for example, propylthiouracil only came into medical use in the 1940s and methimazole was introduced into use as late as 1954. Florence started to treat Graves' disease in April 1908, which was slightly earlier than Haenisch, and by 1912 had seen 48: 10 in private practice and 38 seen at the NHW. Of her 41 completed treatments, she had 14 complete cures, and 22 had great improvement and returned to ordinary life. Only one case did not do well. This was a patient with acute disease who left Florence's care and returned to Edinburgh and died following surgery. In Florence's series described in full in the paper, 87.8% of women resumed their normal lives.

X-ray Notes from the United States

Florence paid a visit to the United States just prior to the outbreak of the Great War, specifically to observe up-to-date American practices in radiology, which were widely reported in the British radiological literature. Florence published a most interesting account of the trip in the *Archives of the Roentgen Ray* (the forerunner of the *British Journal of Radiology*) in October 1914 [15]. This was at a time of rapid technical development in radiology, and it must have been hard to keep up with the many developments.

She took passage in the SS Baltic, departing from Liverpool on the 26 March and arriving in New York on the 5 April 1914. Travelling at this time was time consuming. Florence stayed in America for a month and returned to Plymouth on 3 May 1914 having taken passage on the SS Lapland, which was operated by the Red Star Line. She visited several Eastern towns and also made a special visit to Schenectady in New York. She found the doctors to be very helpful and made the interesting observation that 'I found the doctors in America, both in the hospitals and in private, very ready to allow me to see the work in their departments—medical women not being kept out of everything so much as in England'.

In the early decades of radiology, considerable problems resulted from the relatively low power and unpredictable output of the early gas or ion X-ray tubes. These problems were resolved by the inventions of William Coolidge (1873–1975) [16, 17] who was an engineer working for General Electric Company at Schenectady in New York. In the ion tubes, the cathode was a simple cup, and the anode was set at an angle, hence the name of focus tubes. The working of these X-ray tubes depended on the ionisation of the gas inside the glass bulb, and their function was unpredictable. Coolidge designed an entirely new type of tube with a hot spiral cathode and a high vacuum. This new tube was stable with a predictable radiation output. The new tube was first demonstrated at a dinner in a New York hotel on 27 December 1913. The new tube was enclosed in an open-topped lead glass bowl for radiation protection. This tube was revolutionary, and all modern tubes are variants of this design. During the First World War, Coolidge became involved in producing a dependable portable radiographic unit for military use by the US Army [18]. Significantly Florence brought back a new Coolidge X-ray tube, which was only the second to arrive in England. These Coolidge tubes only slowly replaced the older ionic gas tubes. This was partly related to their higher cost, but also because if you were experienced in the use of the ion X-ray tubes, excellent results could be obtained.

In America she found that there was a major concern for radiation protection. The radiologists and technicians were perfectly correct to be concerned, and by this period there had been many radiation martyrs who suffered greatly from the harmful effects of radiation. Although knowledge of radiobiology and radiation protection at this time was poor, there were some basic principles that had been established. For example, Florence observed that nowhere was the operator left exposed to radiation apart from when performing fluoroscopic examinations. The X-ray control unit was always placed behind a metal screen, which was usually lined with lead, and the X-ray tube could be activated with the operator safely behind the switchboard as is done today. The apparatus was also not shock proof, and, although the wires were simply insulated, touching the tube or cable would result in fatal electrocution. The cables supplying the tubes were run across the ceilings and were attach to the ends of the tube using a rheopore, and Florence described this as being both elaborate and excellent. She felt that the wires were quite well insulated and would not be constantly leaking current and sparking.

In most hospitals there was only plain film radiography performed with no fluoroscopy at all. This was because of the dangers of fluoroscopy and a justified caution about exposing the operators to radiation. In one office she observed that the fluorescent screen was viewed via a mirror, and the operator stayed behind a lead screen, even for setting the photographic place in position. She thought this was elaborate but very efficient, and the aperture could be narrowed down to include only the actual region that was being observed and obtaining an improvement in detail and dose reduction.

Florence visited Boston, New York, Washington, Baltimore and Philadelphia and reported on the very highest standard of radiography that she encountered. At Massachusetts General Hospital, Florence observed gastrointestinal work using bismuth, prior to the more universal use of barium sulphate, and fluoroscopy was assisted by the use of a palpation spoon designed by Guido Holzknecht of Vienna. Florence noted that the standard of gastrointestinal examinations was far in advance of the work that was being done at that time in London. Bismuth was used as a suspension, and from 6 to 40 radiographs were taken to diagnose gastric or duodenal ulcers. These contrast examinations either as an opaque meal (OM) or opaque enema (OE) were the mainstay of diagnosis in the gastrointestinal tract and only passed away with the development of modern endoscopy. It was a common practice to include a reduced-sized print of the abnormality with the written report. The newly invented Coolidge X-ray tube was seen by Florence to be in frequent use, and she was most impressed with its performance.

The practice that she observed in some larger hospitals was for one assistant to radiograph extremities and for another to radiograph the chest and abdomen. This was because in these days, before the universal use of the Coolidge tube, certain ion tubes were better suited for some examinations than for others.

Florence spent some considerable time describing the use of transformers in the United States. She found that most places used a transformer, rather than the older induction coil, with an output of between 2 and 4 kW which was adequate for most radiological uses. Occasionally 10 kW transformers were used. She gives the advantages of the transformer as:

1. Allowing rapid radiographic exposures of 1/10 of a second and 100 mA giving instant radiography of a chest and abdomen. This gave good views of moving organs such as stomach and colon for contrast studies using bismuth, with instantaneous radiography.
2. The transformers were much easier to use and keep in good order than were the induction coils.
3. The transformer could work on either alternating (AC) or direct current (DC). In the 1880s there had been considerable controversy in the United States about the relative value of AC and DC. By 1913 the use of AC was prevailing mainly due to its lower cost of power distribution; however some DC systems persisted.

However it was found that transformers were noisy and resulted in an increased wastage of X-ray tubes. The Wimshurst static electricity machines that were so common in the initial period of radiology were still being used. Florence described a splendid large one designed especially for Dr. Williams at the Boston City Hospital, which could provide enough current for the entire X-ray department.

Florence noted that most of the hospitals did not practise treatment with radiation and that even the cancer hospital in Boston performed only radiography. However she was able to observe some treatments with radiation. This was mainly carried out using radium emanation also known as radon, which was usually contained in small metal needles that were inserted directly into the tumour. She visited Philadelphia and observed radiotherapy with X-rays. She was impressed by the treatment of a 36-year-old woman with breast cancer who was treated directly after surgery and noted that they used heavy doses, heavily filtered and frequently repeated. The surface was carefully marked out and exposed in turn with a crossfire being directed on the tumour from as many points as possible.

She observed cases of cancer of the cervix that had been treated and also case of abdominal cancer. She described patients with inoperable cancer who had reduction in size of the tumour followed by treatment with radiation and also patients with advanced malignancy with a fixed mass that became mobile following radiation and could then be treated with surgery. She was interested to observe the use of radium for various uterine conditions and also radiation treatments of Graves' disease, as both were her major clinical interests.

Professional Life

In 1906 Florence took up consulting rooms at 46 Harley Street. Harley Street was the premier location in London for doctors engaged in private medical practice. In 1910 Florence also moved her professional address from Harley Street to rooms in 4 Nottingham Place. Nottingham Place was close to the medical streets of Devonshire Place and Harley Street and was also in walking distance of the RSM in Wimpole Street with its meeting and library facilities and the NHW. There were a number of medical women who had rooms in Nottingham Place, and Florence may have moved so they could be close together for professional support and for further opinions (Table 6.1). The group of medical women were distinguished and included two deans of the LSMW.

In 1914 Florence moved from Bayswater back to North London to 20 Reynolds Close in Golders Green. As a residential area Golders Green grew significantly in the early twentieth century, following the opening of a tube train line on the London Underground and the opening of the adjacent Golders Green Hippodrome. Golders Green station has frequent trains to Euston Station, which was in easy walking distance of the NHW or Nottingham Place. Florence took an active part in local affairs and in May 1914 took part in a public meeting celebrating the anniversary of the Garden Suburb Mothers' Rest Home where she was on the platform [19]. The Garden Suburb Mothers' Rest Home supported nursing mothers who were in difficulties. Florence maintained her interest in gardening and at the end of June 1914 took part in the Hampstead Garden Suburb Horticultural Society's gardening show. In the novice's section, Florence was awarded second prize for cut roses and was highly commended for outdoor grown flowers [20].

Table 6.1 Consulting rooms of medical women along the east side of Nottingham Place, London (post office directory)

House number	Occupant
4	Miss Florence Ada Stony, Physician and Surgeon
4	Miss Christian Constance Bernard, Physician
14	Miss Helen Webb MB, Physician and Surgeon
14	Miss Connie Surge MD, Physician and Surgeon
14	Miss Jessie Crossfield, Physician
15	Miss Julia Cock MD, Physician (Dean LSMW 1903–1914)
17	Miss L Aldrich-Blake, Physician (Dean LSMW 1914–1918, 1918–1925)
18	Mrs Louisa Atkins MD

The Association of Registered Medical Women

Florence actively participated in the Association of Registered Medical Women (ARMW) and attended, chaired and presented at its meetings. The ARMW had been founded in London in 1879 with the intention that it would 'speak on behalf of all medical women and represent their interests' [21]. The ARMW developed into the Medical Women's Federation, which was founded in 1917 and continues today. A stimulus for founding the MWF was the British government's dismissive attitude towards the women doctors who had wished to serve in the Great War.

The ARMW was not afraid to express its views on 'The Suffrage Issue', and in 1913 an entire page of the *Daily Herald* was given over to the subject [22]. It was signed by President Constance Long, and other signatures included Louise Aldrich-Blake, Mary Murdoch, Agnes Savill and Florence Stoney. The letter comments on the incongruity of a Bill before Parliament that would extend the franchise to all adult men, whilst at the same time excluding women who were working in the same areas as men, and with the same duties and responsibilities. Medical women were working in prisons, schools and in public health. Women were also serving on County and Borough Councils, Boards of Guardians (of Workhouses) and Education and Insurance Companies. The Bill was not therefore a just extension of representative government.

In an interesting meeting of the ARMW on 2 December 1913 [23], and chaired by Mary Scharlieb, there was a discussion for a proposed 'Indian medical service for women' as described by Sir Charles Lukis in his inaugural address to the LSMW on 1 October 1913 [24]. Lukis saw medical woman as the key to improving the health of India because of their influence on the women of India. Whilst there were strong long-term links between British medical women and India, the reaction of the meeting to Lukis was mixed. The overall conclusion was that 'no first-rate medical women will consent to work under such conditions'. Particularly objectionable was the significant gender pay gap compared to men. The men could receive £1400 per year but the women only received £400. Women were also subordinate to a local lay committee with powers of suspension, and this was not acceptable.

Most of the patients shown by Florence at meetings of the ARMW were ones that she had treated personally (Table 6.2). Her presentation of 6 February 1906 is of particular interest where she presented six women with varicose leg ulceration and one with tertiary specific (syphilitic) ulceration, and she wrote it up fully showing its importance to her [25]. Florence described the need for multiple treatments for varicose veins, and if there were varicose ulceration or specific (syphilitic) ulceration, then treatment would be longer. Florence gave two treatments lasting half an hour, and 'a high–frequency brush is played over the offending part, just avoiding large sparks'. This was followed by massage and rubbing at home, and the patient could then attend to daily activities. Florence believed 'that electricity. . . . causes the muscular walls of the veins to contract. . . . (and) the ozone from the high-frequency brush also stimulates the ulcerated surface'. The healing could be slow but ulcers would eventually be healed. The patients were all treated at the NHW, and some

Table 6.2 Florence's contributions to the London meetings of the ARMW

Date of ARMW meeting	Florence's contribution to the ARMW meeting
6 December 1904	1. The first was a 62-year-old woman with a rodent ulcer of the face present for 3 years. Florence gave seven X-ray treatments each of 2 min, and there was healing with minimal scarring 2. A 28-year-old woman with rectal prolapse present since birth cured by ten treatments with Faradism and high frequency. Florence noted that 'High frequency proved most successful where there was lack of tone and flabbiness of tissues of not too long duration; such cases may be local, as in varicose veins, piles, prolapse, or general, as sleeplessness, overwork, and loss of tone after influenza' 3. A 50-year-old woman with chronic abdominal eczema for 5 years cured by 12 X-ray treatments. A recurrence was cured by further four treatments 4. A 65-year-old woman with chronic psoriasis cured by six exposures 5. A 69-year-old woman with multiple trunk papillomata cured without scarring after a month's treatment 6. A 60-year-old woman with rheumatoid arthritis of the wrists showed increased movements and loss of subjective symptoms after 14 high-frequency treatments. Florence noted that only the fibrous and inflammatory thickening could be influenced and that the bone elements were unaffected. Two or three month's treatments were needed 7. Three cases of breast cancer were shown, all too advanced for surgical treatment. The X-ray treatments did not heal the tumours, although the pain was improved. Florence commented that 'X-ray treatment of mammary carcinoma would be most satisfactory when applied to the neighbourhood of the scar immediately after removal of the new growth by operation, and such treatment had been found to reduce the frequency of recurrence'. Essentially Florence was advocating lumpectomy followed by immediate radiotherapy
6 February 1906	Florence presented five patients with congestion and venous ulceration of the legs [15]
6 February 1912	1. A patient with lupus vulgaris of the face being treated with X-rays 2. Enlargement of the shoulder joint presented on behalf of Maud Chadburn (who had been senior to Florence at LSMW). The differential diagnosis was between syphilis of the shoulder, sarcoma and rheumatoid arthritis 3. A forearm skin lesion in a 20-year-old woman presented on behalf of Louisa Garrett Anderson. In the discussion Florence expressed the view that it was self-inflicted, even though it had been present since the age of 2
4 February 1913	A 59-year-old patient with scirrhous carcinoma of the left breast and considered inoperable. Florence had seen the patient 17 months earlier, and the patient had received fortnightly treatments. The disease had remained stationary, and the ulcerated area had healed. In the last 2 months, further nodules had appeared, and the patient had lost weight
8 January 1914	Florence took the chair for the meeting, but showed no cases herself
3 February 1914	1. The first patient shown was a case of scirrhous carcinoma of the breast sent to her as incurable and successfully treated with X-rays for 2 1/2 years 2. The second patient was one with uterine fibroids treated with X-rays and induction of premature menopause. The uterus shrank considerably in size under her treatment

patients had travelled a considerable distance. The patients were working-class women and were suffering significant long-term distress and disability. Florence's care for women and for common medical conditions is seen when she says 'I am afraid these cases are dull, but, still, we cannot all hope to do major operations, and there is room for good treatment of minor ailments as well, which, though not dangerous, may yet make life a misery unless attended to'. It is all too commonplace for doctors to become interested in the rare and exotic and neglect the common.

All of Florence's busy private and public medical work in England was brought to an abrupt end when the Great War, or First World War, started on 28 July 1914. Whilst hostilities had started in Europe, the conflict was to spread throughout the world, and the impact on individuals and society would be incalculable and irreversible.

References

1. Thomas AMK. Florence Stoney and Early British military radiology. In: Nushida H, Vogel H, Püschel K, Heinmann A, editors. Der durchsichtige Tote – Post mortem CT und forensische Radiologie. Hamburg: Verlag Dr. Kovač; 2010. p. 103–13.
2. Sheppard A. Obituary. Dr. Florence Stoney, OBE. The magazine of the London (royal free hospital) school of medicine for women, vol. 27; 1932. p. 128–13.
3. Holland CT. X-rays in 1896. Liverpool Medico Chirugical J. 1937;65:61.
4. Holland CT. X-Rays in 1896. Br J Radiol. 1938;11:1–24.
5. Thomas Vesalius AMK. Röntgen and the origins of Modern Anatomy. Vesalius. 2016;22(1):79–91.
6. Minutes of the Weekly Board meeting of the Royal Free Hospital between December 1901 and April 1902. LMA H71/RF/A/02/01/006.
7. Neil McIntyre How British women became doctors. Wenrowave Press. 2014.
8. Evans' case notes. 1897–1903. LMA. H71/RF/B/02/14/001.
9. Royal Free Hospital Committee minutes. LMA. H71/RF/A/06.
10. Minutes of the Management Committee of the New Hospital for Women, March 3rd and June 2nd 1904. LMA. H13/EGA.
11. Annual reports of the New Hospital for Women from 1905 to 1919. London Metropolitan Archives H13/EGA/06,07,08.
12. Reports of the Pathology, X-ray and Mechanical Therapy Committee of the New Hospital for Women. LMA. H13/EGA/064.
13. Stoney FA. On the results of treating exophthalmic goitre with x-rays. Br Med J. 1912;ii:476–80.
14. Stoney F. On the results of treating exophthalmic goitre with x-rays. Arch Roentgen Ray. 1913;17(8):317–22.
15. Stoney FA. X-ray notes from the United States. Arch Roentgen Ray. 1914;19:181–4.
16. Liebhafsky HA. William David Coolidge, a centenarian and his work. New York: Wiley; 1974.
17. Miller JA. Yankee Scientist, William David Coolidge. Schenectady: Mohawk Development Service; 1963.
18. X-ray Studies. Schenectady: General Electric Company, 1919.
19. Garden Suburb Mothers' Rest Home. Hendon & Finchley Times – Friday 22 May 1914.
20. Hendon & Finchley Times – Friday 03 July 1914.
21. http://www.medialwomensfederation.org.uk/about-us/our-history. Accessed 16 Nov 2018.
22. The Suffrage Issue (What Women Doctor's Say). Daily Herald – Thursday 23 January 1913.

23. The association of registered medical women. Br Med J. 1914;i:30.
24. Lukis CP. The medical needs of India. Br Med J. 1913;ii:837–9.
25. Stoney FA. Chronic congestion treated by electricity. Arch Roentgen Ray. 1906;10(12):325–9.

Chapter 7
Teaching Physics

Having explored Florence's developing career as a doctor, we will return to 1899 and consider what her sister was doing meanwhile.

Edith was now employed full-time as a lecturer at the London School of Medicine for Women. Her academic status was proudly declared in the Annual Report: 'Physics Lecturer: Miss E. A. Stoney, Cambridge Mathematical Tripos Pt. I. and Pt. II. Associate of Newnham College Cambridge'. These qualifications were very important as the London School of Medicine for Women strove to establish its status and credentials. At this time, medical students at Guy's were taught physics by Professor Arnold Reinold from the Royal Naval College at Greenwich and at University College by Professor (later Sir) William Ramsay. The professors who gave lectures in physics in the medical schools outside London were even more impressive: Oliver Lodge in Liverpool, Arthur Schuster in Manchester, John Henry Poynting in Birmingham and JJ Thomson in Cambridge. Edith's cousin George FitzGerald was teaching physics to the medical students at Trinity College. It was a time when a sound grounding in physics was considered to be an essential part of medical training [1].

Edith was initially offered a salary of £78-15s per annum, but negotiated an increase to £100 per annum, possibly based on her salary at Cheltenham. This was further increased to £140 in 1903. The same year that Edith was appointed, Florence was taken on as a part-time demonstrator in the anatomy laboratory, so the two sisters were back together again, both working in the new Pfeiffer Block. They were delighted to let their father know of their first academic appointments in a university department.

As soon as her appointment was agreed, Edith received a request for an estimate of the cost to equip the new physics laboratory. On 26 June she wrote from her home at eight Upper Hornsey Rise: 'When you hand in my request for a grant of £210 for the fittings of the Physical Laboratory, may I ask you to mention ... that I was only able to get a preliminary estimate the evening before I understood that I must send in my request for the grant—and that, owing to the pressure of time, many details of my total estimate must, I fear, be somewhat inaccurate'. This reaction is only too familiar

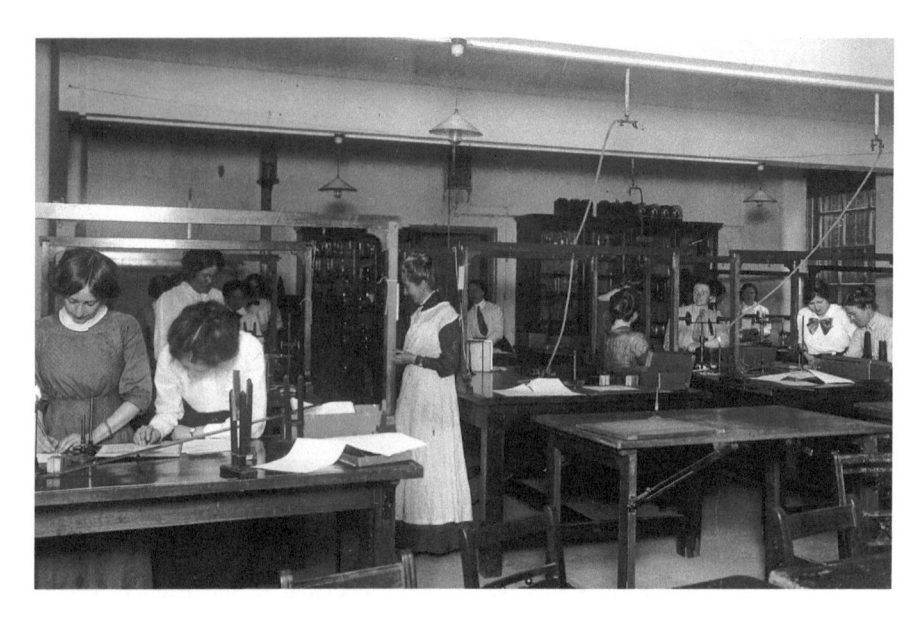

Fig. 7.1 Edith Stoney and her physics laboratory. London School of Medicine for Women c. 1910. (Women's Library, London School of Economics)

to anyone who has ever been asked to provide a complex estimate at the drop a hat. The laboratory, planned for a maximum of 20 students, turned out well in spite of her concerns and is shown in Fig. 7.1.

Having sorted out the laboratory accommodation, Edith was faced with the challenge of designing an appropriate course in physics, now a requirement for medical students in their first year. Her only reference points were the published examination requirements of the Universities of London and Durham, of the Scottish Colleges and of the Society of Apothecaries. There was no need to concern herself yet with requirements of the London College of Physicians or the College of Surgeons, because they had yet to open their doors to women. The LSMW had approached both colleges in 1895 to accept women to their examinations, but both declined.

In order to deal with the various requirements, Edith meticulously separated her course into three parts: Class A for those wishing to prepare for the examinations of the Society of Apothecaries, Classes A and B for Durham and Classes B and C for London. During her first year, 5 of her 11 students were studying for the membership examinations of the Society of Apothecaries or for the University of Durham examinations. The content throughout was pure physics, as required by the examination syllabi: mechanics, magnetism, electricity, optics, sound, heat and energy. It contains only one medical application, the correction of short and long sight by optical lenses.

Building on her experience in Cheltenham, she developed an effective style of teaching, with a sympathetic rapport with her students. The challenge was to link her teaching of the rather dry physics syllabus to the medical motivations of her students. An ex-student later wrote, 'Her lectures on physics mostly developed into informal talks, during which Miss Stoney, usually in a blue pinafore, scratched on a blackboard with coloured chalks, turning anxiously at intervals to ask "Have you taken my point?". She was perhaps too good a mathematician ... readily to understand the difficulties of the average medical student, but experience had taught her how distressing these could be' [2]. It was in her nature and education to present physics mathematically and, viewing the course as being at degree level, set an academic standard that some of her medical students were unable to reach.

Edith had joined the growing sector of higher education for women. By 1900, about 16% of full-time students in British universities were women, most studying arts subjects. This grew to about 20% by 1910 [3]. During her first few years at the LSMW, the small student numbers allowed Edith to use a personal, tutorial approach to her teaching, which suited her, opting for analogies to explain difficult concepts. By the spring of her second year, she was provisionally recognised as a Teacher of London University, an important formality in establishing her position and credentials as a university lecturer. This was a notable achievement. There were only 26 women in the list of recognised teachers in 1901, about 5% of the total. Six were from the LSMW, the others being Julia Cock (medicine), Mary Dowson (medical jurisprudence), Charlotte Ellaby (ophthalmology), Clare Evans (chemistry) and Mary Schlieb (midwifery). Edith joined the 21 registered male physics lecturers and professors to become the first woman ever registered to teach physics at London University [4].

Retaining her interest in secondary education, she was appointed examiner for mathematics for the Intermediate Board Examinations for Schools in Ireland in 1902, a position she maintained until 1906.

She now had committed to her future career in science education. She was comfortably settled back with her family in London where they could attend any of the many public events on offer. On 20 June 1900, they went along to Carlton House Terrace for 'Ladies Day' at the Royal Society. Women had been permitted to attend one of the Conversazioni in the Royal Society yearly programme, by invitation, since 1876. After the pleasant parochialism of Cheltenham, Edith enjoyed having access to the intellectual buzz of the Metropolis. She knew that Miss Beale would be pleased to share her new experiences, so she wrote her a short report about what had been presented that day [5]. It was an eclectic mix of science, lectures and exhibits, under the presidential care of Joseph (Lord) Lister. She was delighted that all the drawings and photographs from an expedition to view a recent solar eclipse in Algiers had been prepared by women. Her report is notable for the frequency with which she remarks on new techniques, delighting in the many emerging applications of new technologies. Edith was taken by a radio-controlled clock mechanism and an invention adopted by Lloyds' Bank to remotely obtain signatures to various documents. Professor Hadden showed moving, cinematographic photographs of native dances from the Torres Strait; Professor Fleming demonstrated experiments with radio waves. Taking a pedagogical view, Edith noted how useful this last demonstration could be in showing the analogy between radio and light waves to a class of students.

But women attended the Royal Society as guests, not in their own right. This was the same year that Marian Farquharson, the first female Fellow of the Royal Microscopical Society, petitioned the Council of the Royal Society that 'duly qualified women should have the advantage of full fellowship'. The Council chose to interpret its Royal Charter so as to deny this possibility. This was still her father's world, into which women could be invited, or rejected, depending on the prevailing male consensus.

Florence and Edith were pleased to have successfully completed their first year in the teaching laboratories of the Pfeiffer Block. They planned an adventurous summer walking holiday together in the Harz region of Germany, where they explored the magnificent wooded mountainous terrain, dominated by the Brocken with its panoramic views from the summit. They were particularly interested in the 'beautiful, great, deep Rübeland Caves', with their stalactites and numerous bones of prehistoric cave bears [6]. Both had been trained to observe and interpret. They noticed the patterns of vegetation that had grown near the old oil lamps deep within the caves, in comparison with that close to the brighter electric lamps, installed in 1892 on the command of the Kaiser. From the patterns of growth, they concluded that it was not the warmth or infrared radiation of the lamp that had enabled the growth, but instead it was the shorter wavelengths of the light that was needed to energise the growth. The other puzzle was how the spores had managed to reach such depths within the cave, an observation to be stored away and commented on later.

Edith received an important request during January 1902. She had been a lecturer at the LSMW for just over a year, and already the value of having someone with her specialist knowledge of physics had been recognised. The Medical Committee of the Royal Free Hospital were planning to install their first X-ray equipment and recognised the need of an expert to look after it. They looked no further than the School of Medicine, delighted to find there an expert physicist who could take responsibility for the care of the X-ray equipment. It was doubly satisfying for Edith when Florence was appointed to take clinical charge of the Rontgen Department in March. Working closely together, sometimes developing the exposed X-ray plates at home, Edith began to learn at first-hand the potential of radiological diagnoses.

Florence and Edith spent other holidays together, their trips sometimes having a scientific theme. In August 1905 they joined a cruise to view the total eclipse of the sun in Spain. It was with huge excitement that they boarded the Royal Mail steamship Ortona in London on 25 August. The ship went to Plymouth the following day to pick up some more passengers and then proceeded across the Bay of Biscay, past Porto and Cadiz to Gibraltar. They left there at 11.00 a.m. on 30 August to be in place off the Spanish Coast at Alcalà de Xivert, where the main body of the world's astronomers were assembled under the track of the total eclipse, in time for the moon's shadow to darken the day. Florence later wrote of her own recollections of seeing 'one of the grandest spectacles in nature. We saw the corona splendidly and the great flames of incandescent hydrogen' [7]. They were delighted to listen on board to Sir Oliver Lodge's descriptive lectures and to socialise with the other passengers, who included Sir Arthur Rucker, Physicist and Principal of the University of London; the Irish Physicist Professor Joseph Larmor, who had been teaching mathematics at Cambridge during Edith's time there and had previously lectured in natural philosophy at Queen's College Galway; Sir Alfred Hopkinson, the Vice Chancellor of Manchester University; and Professor William Tilden, Dean of the Royal College of Science. Continuing via Marseille, they left the Ortona at Naples on 3 September. They knew that their father would have deeply enjoyed the trip and delighted in recounting their adventures to him on their return. He continued his interest in astronomy well beyond his eightieth birthday the following year. His last scientific paper, on 'Telescopic vision', was published in 1908, in which he discussed, amongst other matters, the possibility of seeing very small markings on the surface of Mars with the telescopes that were available at that time.

The Stability of Marine Turbines

Their brother Gerald brought another challenge to tease Edith's mathematical skills. By this time he was deeply involved with the design and development of Charles Parsons' marine turbine engines, an innovation that revolutionised ocean transport. They had started testing the *Turbinia* in 1894, 100 feet long with a displacement of 44 tons, the first ship to be powered by a turbine engine. Gerald had taken part in all its sea trials. They had reached a maximum speed of 34 knots, at a time when the fastest destroyers could hardly reach 27 knots [8]. Parsons, with Gerald Stoney aboard, demonstrated the *Turbinia*'s speed at the Great Naval Review to celebrate Queen Victoria's Diamond Jubilee. As a result, two further vessels, HMS Viper and HMS Cobra, were commissioned. Tragically, both vessels were lost within a short while of one another, Viper when she ran ashore in fog on 3 August 1901, and Cobra when she broke her back in a storm in the North Sea 7 weeks later. By then, the first commercial vessels had been commissioned for service on the River Clyde. Whilst Gerald and Charles Parsons were convinced that the losses could not be attributed to the design of the turbine engine, inevitably questions were raised about the stability of this new engine design when buffeted by high seas. They needed to produce evidence to convince others that the underlying engineering design was safe.

Gerald approached Edith for her help. The particular concern was whether the bearings supporting HMS Cobra's drive shaft might have failed from the gyroscopic forces exerted during vessel movement at sea, so being the cause of its loss in the North Sea. He could give her the details of the size and mass of the engine and vessel, the speeds of travel and shaft rotation and the expected greatest movements of the vessel. Could she work out the associated forces on the bearings? She did so to Charles Parsons complete satisfaction. He could confidently report, in 1903, that 'the actual gyroscopic forces on the bearings of Cobra's engines, when making 1100 revolutions at 34 knots, and in the heaviest and shortest sea, could not exceed one-half of the normal weight on the bearings, and at a speed of 18 knots, which was never exceeded during her ill-fated voyage, the gyroscopic forces on the hull could not exceed those produced by one person walking about on the deck' [9].

Edith's father was sufficiently proud of his daughter's achievements to write to Charles Parsons to ask him to confirm her contributions to the work of his firm. Most likely he also felt that she had had insufficient recognition for the work that she had done for them. On 2 June 1903, Parsons replied. His letter is couched rather formally as a testimonial that could support any future application for a research or other scientific post should Edith wish to follow such a path. He starts by saying 'I have much pleasure in bearing testimony to your daughter's great and original ability for applied mathematics'. Reading between the lines, there is a suggestion that he had not been aware, until her father and brother had pointed it out to him, that Edith had made any earlier contributions. He simply confirms that he is aware of her calculations made on behalf of his firm, Messrs C.A. Parsons and Co.

First he referred back to the calculations that she had made for Gerald for the shape function of his searchlight mirrors:

> The problems she has attacked and solved have been in relation to the special curvature of our mirrors for obtaining beams of light of particular shapes. These investigations involved difficult and intricate original calculations, so much so that I must confess they were quite beyond my powers now, and probably would have been so also when I was at Cambridge and graduated 11th Wrangler in 1876.

He considered that the calculations were correct in every detail and gave valuable and satisfactory results. He then confirmed the work she had done more recently on the stability of his marine turbines:

> Your daughter also made calculations in regard to the gyrostatic forces brought on to the bearings of marine steam turbines through the pitching of the vessel (steam turbines being those of the "Turbinia"), and showed that such forces were not sufficiently large to cause trouble in practice.

It was a substantial endorsement of her ability as a mathematical physicist and must have given a considerable boost to her self-confidence. Perhaps this was all she wanted and needed, because there is no evidence that she then set about using this testimonial to seek alternative employment [10].

Meanwhile, their other brother, Robert, was getting settled into his life as a doctor in Australia. He was married to Louisa McComas in 1893, and they started a family: Archibald, Margaret (Madge), Gerald and finally William in 1899. At last there were grandchildren to maintain the Stoney name, even though they were on the other side of the world. Robert practiced medicine in several towns on the south coast of New South Wales, moving every few years, finally settling in Nowra in 1898. Very sadly, his wife Louisa found her life very stressful and, following William's birth, suffered a severe mental breakdown from which she never recovered. Postnatal depression was not sufficiently understood at that time, and mental illness was not treated with any understanding, especially in relatively unsophisticated rural Australia. Louisa never left mental hospital and died, still a patient, in 1952.

Letters between Islington and New South Wales kept them in touch with the difficulties afflicting Robert and his family. Finally, in May 1901, Gertrude volunteered to go out to Australia to help him with his four children. She stayed as his housekeeper for about 9 years, as her nieces and nephews grew up, much as her aunt had done after her own mother's death. She returned to Dublin once Madge, the only daughter, was 13 and was considered old enough to look after the family [11].

Other sad news had arrived from their family back in Dublin earlier that year. Their brilliant and much-loved cousin, George FitzGerald, had died on 22 February, shortly after an abdominal operation on a perforated ulcer. He was not yet 50 and had been suffering from abdominal problems for a number of years. His death was a huge loss to the family and to science.

Edith herself was not immune to sickness. At the beginning of the 1902–1903 academic year, she was allowed sick leave for two terms. Her role was covered by a talented physics demonstrator from Guy's Hospital Medical School, John Ryffel. He was a First Class Cambridge Natural Science graduate who eventually gained a B. Chir degree and went on to become Reader in Biochemistry and lecturer in forensic medicine at Guy's and analyst to the Home Office.

Graduation at Last

Edith moved with her father and sister to their new house in Chepstow Crescent Notting Hill at about this time. Florence, a London graduate, could now announce herself as 'Dr. Florence A Stoney B.S., M.B., M.D.'. It was slightly galling for Edith to have to content herself with just 'Miss Stoney', after all her earlier Cambridge examination successes. Some of her fellow Tripos students had chosen to sit for the London University examination as external candidates, open to women applicants, so enabling them to formally demonstrate their academic credentials with letters after their names. When, in 1904, another means to rectify this deficiency appeared, which did not require sitting further examinations, Edith grasped it enthusiastically. Her father had been in Dublin in the summer of 1902 when, on 1 July, he was awarded an honorary Doctor of Science degree from his *Alma Mater*, Trinity College Dublin. His interest in Irish higher education remained undiminished, and he listened carefully when he heard of plans that Trinity might be considering conferring degrees on women. Back in London, they watched developments in Dublin with great interest.

The rumours were correct. On 13 March 1903, the Board of Trinity College agreed to put forward a scheme for the admission of women, and by 9 June the Senate accepted the resolution 'that it is desirable that degrees in the University of Dublin shall be opened to women'. It was passed by 74 votes to 11. On 8 December, a letter from King Edward VIII instructed the Senate to interpret the College statutes in such manner that women may obtain degrees. From 1904, the University of Dublin opened all its lectures, examinations and degrees in arts to women. In addition, women could also be admitted to the medical school, with the provision that classes in dissection were to be taken separately.

None of this would have had any direct bearing on Edith's academic position if it had not been for the action of Edith Badham, an earlier student at Newnham (History Tripos, 1888). She had made contact with the Trinity College Board, and, at its meeting on 16 April 1904, it was agreed to inform her that 'a Grace will be proposed by the Board to the Senate on Thursday next, to give the degree of B.A. to women who have obtained the certificate for that degree at the Cambridge Tripos Examination'. By this time she was headmistress of St Margaret's Hall, Dublin, and was therefore known to the Board members, giving strength to her case. During the next few weekly meetings of the Board, a form of words was developed that was finally agreed at the meeting on 21 May, and the Senior Lecturer was instructed to effect the final corrections and arrange for their publication. It was Clause 7 that was of particular importance to Edith: 'Those educated in Oxford and Cambridge will be treated (subject to the above time limitation) as if they had been admitted to the academic status in these Universities corresponding to their educational exercises'. This arrangement, by which Dublin degrees could be awarded to Oxbridge *women ad eundem gradum*, was to remain in force for a period of 3 years [12].

The summer degree ceremonies, the Commencements, were to take place at the end of May. If Edith was to graduate that year, as the new regulation now allowed, she had no option but to travel to Dublin in order to complete all the formalities as quickly as possible. She was one of only six women who succeeded in submitting their applications in time, all ex-students from Cambridge. The two Ediths, Stoney and Badham, were from Newnham, and the other four had been to Girton: Leota Bennett, Agnes Brooke, Helen Bartum and Sophie Nichols. These six were awarded B.A. degrees at the ceremony on 30 May 1904 [13].

On arriving for the Commencements, they realised that they were the centre of considerable attention. The event had caused great public interest, and the hall was packed half an hour before the ceremony was due to start, largely with women. The press delighted in reporting on the appearance of the new graduates: 'The ladies sported their brightest summer garments', with their academic caps and gowns adding to the rich colour of the occasion.

The formal agreement by the Senate to accept the arrangement was not made until 11 June, 2 weeks after the commencement ceremony [14]. The process of registration of students was even slower, and Edith's name was not entered as being registered until 30 June, a month after her degree had been awarded.

Edith spotted a further possibility. Gaining a master's degree from Cambridge did not need any further examination, only that a sufficient passage of time had passed since her successful completion of the Tripos. This qualified her to be admitted for both the B.A. and M.A. degrees from Dublin. As a result, on 30 June 1904, Edith became the first woman ever to be granted the M.A. degree from Trinity College Dublin. The alphabetical list of 27 new Master of Arts graduates includes Edith Anne Stoney after Rev James M'Ivor Stevens and before Rev Cecil Brook Welland, the only woman in the list. Edith did not attend on this occasion, having been granted the right to receive the award *in absentia*, to save her a second journey from London to Dublin.

Edith wished to inform her fellow Newnham students and to share the exact details of the process. She wrote an article for the Newnham College Letter giving careful instructions to any other young woman who had completed the Cambridge examinations on how to gain a Dublin degree [15]. Applications should be made to the Senior Lecturer at least a couple of days before the Commencement and should be accompanied by the Tripos certificate and a formal character reference. The fee for the B.A., payable to the Junior Bursar, was £10 3s in total. Application for M.A. should be made to the Senior Proctor, for which the fee was £9 16s. 6d with an additional charge for a testimonial. Caps and gowns for the ceremony could be hired from one of the college porters for £3 12s. 6d. At the same time, in Oxford, the Somerville Students' Association Report estimated that the whole package, including the fare and accommodation, could be had for £27. Edith did not included information on hotels: she was lucky enough to have relatives in Dublin, so had somewhere to stay.

Edith added that any prejudice about gaining a degree from an Irish university was misplaced, tracing the history of Trinity College, Dublin, from its earliest foundation by Queen Elizabeth in 1562 to the present, proudly pointing out that with 1000 students it was now much larger than Trinity College, Cambridge. The historical links with Cambridge were close, she wrote, and 'some of the first Provosts were Puritans who found Cambridge rather too hot for them' noting Trinity's tolerant tradition of accepting students of all creeds. She was particularly pleased to report the opening of the medical school to women, with its extra accommodation for the women medical students, 'setting an example of open-mindedness to the hitherto so very jealously guarded great and wealthy medical schools of London, Cambridge or Oxford... This opening of the Medical School is no mere figure head, but a real reform for which I fancy we may long whistle at Cambridge'. She even had a go at Newnham, suggesting that her College had no particular enthusiasm to introduce medicine for women at Cambridge.

In retrospect, all this might seem to have been a rather silly exercise in playing with the regulations. Certainly some Cambridge women remained content with their certificate of completion of the Tripos examination. However, the Trinity Registrar was soon to discover that there were a very large number who did not and wanted to have the academic endorsement of B.A. or M.A., after their names. Thanks to Edith's publicity in Cambridge, together with that circulated in Somerville College in Oxford, a further 40 or 50 Oxbridge women received B.A. or M.A. degrees on 20 December that year. By the end of the 3 years set by the Trinity, over 700 women had graduated in this way. Such was the visibility of the scheme, these graduates became known as the 'Steamboat Ladies' from their need to use an Irish ferry line to achieve their objective. There were those who said that the University Senate were not averse to the commercial side of the arrangement: the income would have reached more than £7000 in 3 years. In the University's defence, this unexpected windfall was used to pay for the new accommodation for women medical students.

One of the notable Newnham mathematicians who took Edith's advice and obtained the Dublin M.A. was Hilda P Hudson OBE. She completed the Mathematics Tripos in 1903 with a mark equal to the 7th Wrangler and had followed in Edith's footsteps as Custodian of the Newnham Observatory. During the war she worked for the War Ministry as an aeronautical engineer and was one of the very few women of her time to serve on the council of the London Mathematical Society.

Becoming an Educationalist

Edith had already visited Germany and Spain with Florence for recreation and scientific interest. She now planned a visit to America in support of her continuing commitment to education. In March 1907 she joined a group of teachers who crossed the Atlantic to learn about the American approach to education [16]. The visit was a direct outcome of the Mosely Education Commission visit in 1903. British politicians and industrialists had become aware that industrial innovation and output in the United States was, by then, considerably greater than in Britain, and this was attributed to the American investment in training and education [17]. Similarly, Britain was lagging behind Germany too, worker productivity and efficiency remaining stubbornly low. On 6 June 1906, Mr. Alfred Mosely announced in the press that he had arranged a £5 return fare for those teachers who wished to visit educational institutions in the United States. The scheme was heavily oversubscribed, but Edith was fortunate to secure one of the 500 places. These were roughly equally distributed between the sexes. Sadly there remains no record of the educational institutions that she visited, but the event emphasises her own professional interest and commitment to teaching and to vocational education, stimulated no doubt by her father's deep educational principles. Her outbound week-long Atlantic crossing to New York from Liverpool was on the Cunard line RMS Etruria, and, after about a month of visits, she arrived back in Britain from New York on the White Star Line RMS Oceanic on 1 May.

Her main impression was of the numerous educational and career opportunities open to women in America in comparison with Britain. In the words of another Mosely visitor, she learned that 'at the age of 18 or 19, the majority of girls enter one or other of the numerous colleges dotted all over the United States' [18]. These were largely all-women's colleges in the Eastern States, whilst the colleges on the west coast were mostly co-educational. One of the colleges that Edith could well have visited was Simmons Female College in Boston, founded in 1899. Here, the women could follow courses in vocational subjects, leading to a B.Sc. in horticulture, social work, secretarial studies, library science or household economics. They were definitely not 'bluestockings'.

Edith found greater difficulty in finding inspiration from her visit for her own challenge of placing physics into medical education. Not much had changed in the medical colleges of the United States since a reviewer of John Draper's textbook on medical physics (1885) had written, 'Thus far our colleges may, with but few exceptions, be said to have thrown physics to the dogs' [19]. Draper died shortly after his book was published, so there was no second edition, and Fred Brockway's *Essentials of Physics Arranged in the Form of Questions and Answers Prepared Especially for Students of Medicine* was no more than another physics textbook written by a doctor, omitting any reference to the applications of physics to medicine. Even in the second edition, published in 1902 over 6 years after Röntgen's discovery of X-rays and their widespread introduction into medicine, there were no references to either radiology or radioactivity [20]. It remains surprising that Edith herself did not develop her own lecture notes into a textbook of physics for medical students.

Florence and Edith socialised, met their friends and relaxed at the Lyceum Club, where they were members. Constance Smedley had established this all-women's club in 1903 to serve as a forum for intellectually and artistically minded women [21]. Entry was limited to those 'who had published any original work in Literature, Journalism, Science, Art or Music' or who possessed a university-level qualification, for a joining fee of one guinea and an annual subscription of three guineas. When its new home at 128 Piccadilly was opened on 20 June 1904 by the Chair, Lady Frances Balfour, the wife of the prime minister, she described the club as 'A house built by women, lived in by women, run by women. It is to be a place for rest and relaxation for everyone who comes here; a place where ideals became reality'. Not that this was the only all-women's club to have been established at that time, but this was the one where Florence and Edith chose to be members. The accommodation, which *The Times* described as excellent, included lounges, reception rooms, a rest room, billiard room, library, dining room, bedrooms, etc. Notably it had an international reach: 'It will afford an opportunity for the women-workers from every country to meet on common ground, for the club premises will provide a house in London for each member from the Colonies, America, and foreign countries, in which she may obtain introductions to her English *confrères*' [22]. A second club was soon established in Berlin, followed by one in Paris, the national clubs eventually coalescing to form the International Association of Lyceum Clubs. In their future travels, during and after the war, Edith and Florence knew there would always be a home wherever they roamed. By contrast, the University Women's Club, formerly the University Club for Ladies, founded by Gertrude Jackson of Girton College, remained firmly British.

The Lyceum Club was a meeting place, and the members did not necessarily live in London. Amongst the doctors in its membership was Dr. Louisa Martindale, who trained at the LSWM and who settled in Brighton where she became a leading figure there in women's medicine. Martindale briefly acted as a locum surgeon in the Scottish Women's Hospital in Royaumont in its early days in 1915: this was where Edith would work towards the end of the war [23]. After the war Louisa Martindale was a leading force in the introduction of gynaecological radiation therapy using radium and X-rays. There were several writers, including Rosaline Masson and the Irish author Violet Martin. The educationalist Henrietta White, who became Principal of Alexandra College Dublin from 1890, was a member, as was Crystal MacMillan B.Sc. M.A., who, in April 1896, had become the first female science graduate from Edinburgh University after it had opened its doors to women in 1892. These women and many others of similar standing to Florence and Edith had the opportunity to meet at the Lyceum Club. And every one of the women identified had another characteristic in common: they were all vocal and public participants in women's suffrage and as such had their names included in the 1913 Suffrage Annual and Women's Who's Who.

References

1. Annual reviews of medical training. The Lancet. From 1890–1900.
2. Obituary. Edith Stoney, M.A. The Lancet. 1938 July 9;108.
3. Dyhouse C. The British Federation of University Women and the status of women in universities, 1907–1939. Women's Hist Rev. 1995;4:465–85.
4. University of London. Recognised Teachers. 1901 Jul 11.
5. Stoney E. Royal society conversazione. Cheltenham Ladies' Coll Mag. 1900;42:230–2.
6. Stoney EA. The carrying power of spores and plant-life in deep caves. Nature. 1920;105 (2650):740–1.
7. Letter from Florence Stoney to Archie Stoney. Christmas. 1921. AS.
8. Parsons RH. The steam turbine and other inventions of Sir Charles Parsons, O.M. London: The British Council/Longmans Green; 1942.
9. Parsons CA. The steam engine and its application to the propulsion of vessels. Institute of Naval Architects 1903. Science Museum Library. PAR 23.
10. Letter from Charles A Parsons to Johnstone Stoney. 1903 Jun 2. Newcastle University Archives MSA-2-22.
11. Personal correspondence from Edith McInnon.
12. Trinity College Board minutes. Trinity College Dublin archives MUN/V/5/18, from 16 April to 4 June, 1904.
13. Parkes SM. The 'Steamboat Ladies' the first world war and after. In Parkes SM, editor. A Danger to men? A History of Women in Trinity College Dublin 1904–2004. Ch 4. Dublin: Lilliput; 2004. p. 87–90.
14. Mackenzie AM, editor. The Englishwoman's Review of Social and Industrial Questions No 37. 1904 Jul 15.
15. Stoney EA. Collegium sacrosanctae et individuae Trinitatis juxta Dublin. Newnham College Letter; 1904. p. 37–43.
16. London School of Medicine for Women School Committee. 1906 Sept 26. LMA. H72/SM/A/04.
17. Lupton MC. The Mosely Education Commission to the United States, 1903. Vocat Asp Second Furth Educ. 1964;16:36–49.
18. Women's education in America. Pall Mall Gazette. 1907 Mar 4.
19. Book review: a text-book of medical physics. J Am Med Assoc. 186(7):83–4.
20. Brockway FJ. Essentials of physics, arranged in the form of questions and answers prepared especially for students of medicine. Saunders Question-Compends No 22. 2nd ed. Philadelphia: Saunders; 1902.
21. Lyceum Club. Wemding: Association Internationale des Lyceum Clubs. 1986.
22. The Lyceum Club. The Times. 1904 Jun.
23. Martindale diary, Wellcome Library, London. MS3472.

Chapter 8
Challenge and Loss

Edith had finally earned her position as a respected member of the academic staff at the LSMW. In February 1909, 10 years since her original appointment, she was elected to serve on the School Committee, recognition both of her academic standing and, Edith believed, in the importance of basic sciences in medical training. This gave her a stronger platform from which to argue on behalf of physics, always a Cinderella science in medical training in comparison with its established sister disciplines, chemistry and biology.

As the numbers of women students recruited increased, it became more difficult for Edith to manage all the teaching and practical work on her own, and some expansion of the physics staffing became necessary. Her position on the Council enabled her to argue for the extra staff she needed. Anyone who has been faced with the need to expand a small department within a large bureaucracy will recognise the difficulty she faced. The ideal solution would have been to appoint a full-time demonstrator to assist with lectures and practical classes. Other departments, too, were under pressure and needed extra staff, and the basic sciences were not deemed by some to be as relevant to medical training as, for example, anatomy or pathology.

In September 1909, Edith put in a request for further leave of absence due to ill health. The cause is not known. Even though she was small, she was not physically weak, having been excellent at sports and showing considerable stamina, later, during the war. On this occasion, she offered to resign, an offer that was not accepted at once. Instead, she was given the option to return in 12 months' time on the presentation of a health certificate from her doctor. After a false start to find a locum, a new advertisement for a deputy lecturer gave rise to a short list of three good candidates. Mr. James H. Brinkworth, physics demonstrator at St. Thomas's Hospital Medical School, was appointed. He had impressive academic credentials, a national scholar who had gained a first in physics from the Royal College of Science in 1906. The other two shortlisted were Helen G. Thompson B.Sc., Silvanus P. Thompson's daughter and biographer, who was Demonstrator in Physics at Bedford College, and Mr. F. Lloyd Hopwood, who later became Professor of

Medical Physics at St. Bartholomew's Hospital Medical School, where he carried out pioneering work on the biological effects of ultrasound.

Edith used her time away from the LSMW well. She was free to read academic journals that were delivered to their house and, on two occasions, commented by letter on what she had read. To *Nature* she added her own explanation of the anomalously low speed of fall of lycopodium spores, previously reported in the journal. Edith's ideas were based on her own microscopic observations of minute hairs on the spores that would, she predicted, create eddies and so greater resistance to movement. She had her father's love of analogy and pointed out that this was 'much as the speed of a ship is lessened when its bottom is foul' [1]. In a letter to the *Mathematical Gazette*, she revealed her continuing commitment to science education. Using a published example of a question about thermal expansion, she recommended that pupils be taught to distinguish between algebraic approximations arising during calculations and approximations arising from physical definitions [2].

Visitors to Chepstow Crescent

Johnstone Stoney, at home in Chepstow Crescent, continued to write. He remained irritated about the influence that, in his view, the Catholic Church retained over education in Ireland [3, 4]. He was pleased to be asked by the Irish physicist Edmund Fornier d'Albe to prepare a preface for his book *The Electron Theory* [5]. They shared outside interests other than physics. Fornier d'Albe, an originator of pan-Celticism, had a deep interest in Celtic music, which could now be heard at home using their father's 'most enormous gramophone'. They had both developed an interest in the international language Esperanto: Fournier d'Albe is credited with making the first translation from Irish into Esperanto. This interest was less linguistic than political. They understood the central place that language played in creating national identity and were exploring a view that Esperanto could be a diluting force against growing Irish Nationalism.

The frontispiece photograph of Fornier d'Albe's book on the electron shows Johnstone Stoney, not the author, portrayed as an eminent sage with balding head and long flowing white beard. Another lovely photograph, almost certainly taken during the same sitting, shows him seated with Edith and Florence, wearing the same suit and watch chain (Fig. 8.1).

They were pleased when other friends and relatives visited their house in Kensington. One who came was Ethel Sara Turing (née Stoney), the distant cousin who had attended Cheltenham Ladies' College. Ethel wrote of their father 'He was one of the great who nevertheless retained into old age a childlike simplicity'. Edith could be forgiven for not knowing Ethel in spite of the family connection: their common Stoney ancestor was born in the seventeenth century. Ethel had been born in India and had been sent home to England for her education. She had come over to England from Alexandra College, Dublin, to complete her education and matriculated from Cheltenham in the summer of 1899 in Division 1. In 1907 she married

Fig. 8.1 Edith Stoney, Florence Stoney and G. Johnstone Stoney c.1907. Photograph probably taken by Elliott and Fry, Baker St., London. (Newnham College, Cambridge)

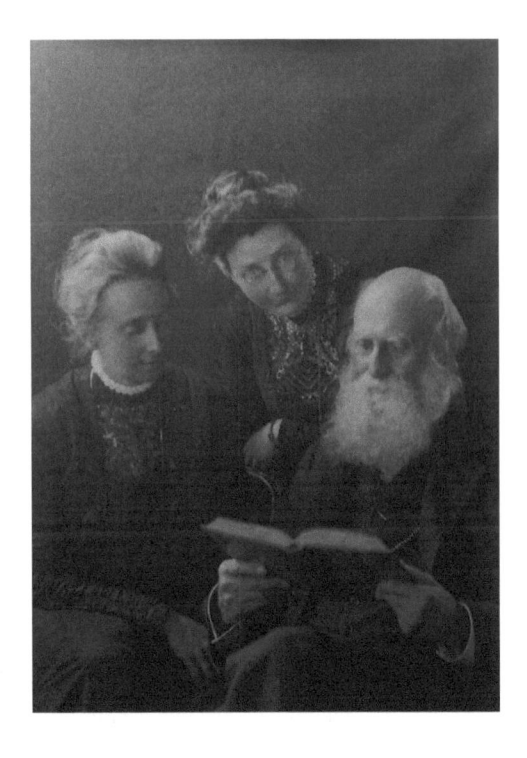

Julius Turing, a civil servant working in India, in Dublin, a union that produced two sons, John and Alan. Alan Turing's career as a mathematician and cryptanalyst sets him amongst the highest mathematical minds of the twentieth century. The brief association between his mother and Edith Stoney in Cheltenham makes a genetic and mathematical link between these two remarkable individuals [6].

Another visitor was their old friend, the Irish astronomer Robert Stawell Ball. In his obituary of their father, he gave a delightful account of Johnstone at home during these final years, which is worth quoting at length:

> His health is no longer strong. His life is confined to a single floor of his house in the west of London. He greets his visitor with the kindness and courtesy that were characteristic of him throughout his life. "I am now verging on 80," he remarks, "so there is not much more time left for working"; and then at once plunges into scientific matters. His room is filled with books and papers and scientific instruments, often with great additional interest that the instruments have been homemade. He will first ask his visitor to sit down at a remarkable arrangement of screens and lenses with ingenious makeshifts by which he is studying abstruse problems in the theory of telescopic vision. Then we are bidden to look through the spectroscope, where he has been investigating some delicate point about the new mercury light. Then a fine microscope will be opened, and Stoney will demonstrate how inadequate are the ordinary geometrical optics to the explanation of the microscope ... Then he will summon a domestic to blow the air-blast and give a performance from Sir Charles

Parsons' latest gramophone.[1] Then he will sit down again, and with pen and paper explain some profound point in the Fourier analysis of waves. We cannot leave until we have heard his views, always broad and far-seeing, on the latest phase of the University question [7].

This had recalled a visit in about 1906, when their father was still quite active. By the autumn of 1910, he was very ill, suffering from heart failure and jaundice. When his old friend John Joly was awarded the Royal Medal for researches in geology and physics that year, Johnstone was too weak to raise himself in bed to write, dictating to Edith his letter of congratulation. In her covering letter, Edith was careful to add 'May my sister and I also say how glad we were to see that you have one of the Royal Medals this year' [8]. Perhaps reminded of their father's support for women entering medicine and of Florence's radiological work, in 1914, Joly was instrumental in setting up a Radium Institute in the Royal Dublin Society. 200 mg of radium bromide was purchased and given to local surgeons for use in emanotherapy, a technique that used the emitted radon gas for therapy [9].

During Edith's period of sick leave, she had been able to give some help with her father's care. She considered resigning her post in order to look after him as Helen Gladstone had done for her elderly father, but decided it was more sensible to return to work, which she did in October 1910, employing two domiciliary nurses to care for him during the final months of his life. As his end drew near, Gerald and Gertrude both spent time close by, staying with a friend.[2]

In the letter that she wrote to John Joly on 1 April 1911 (see Chap. 2), Edith expressed her feelings as her father approached his final days.

> My father is—we fear—sinking—he may however last a few days—but he might collapse at any moment. He is in no active pain, but so fearfully weak and thin that no nursing can hope to keep him for much longer in reasonable comfort—and those of us that love him must be content the end is so near.

Not knowing how to express herself correctly, she added 'It seems morbid to write of such while we still have the, to us, inexpressible blessing of having him'.

Edith was uncertain to whom to leave the task of ensuring that her father's legacy was correctly recorded. Her letter to John Joly was triggered by a visit the day before from a mutual friend, James Reynolds FRS, who was now living in London having left Dublin in 1903 where he had been Professor of Chemistry at Trinity College. Edith had shown him her notes on her father's life, and he planned to write also to Joly with a summary of these. She let Professor Joly know that she was also writing to Professor Edward Culverwell, even though Reynolds had suggested Joly to be

---

[1] He is referring the Parsons' 'auxetophone', a device for sound amplification which did not cause the harmonic distortion associated with a purely mechanical gramophone. Sound was produced by controlling the flow of compressed air through a valve. The design was superseded once amplification was possible by electronic means.

[2] At the 1911 census on 2 April 1911, Gertrude and Gerald were staying with Florence Gladstone at 19 Chepstow Villa, very close to their father's house in Chepstow Terrace.

more knowledgeable about Johnstone's science and contributions to the Royal Dublin Society.[3]

They were in that uncertain time when a death is inevitable, but the timing is unknown, wanting action where none is possible. In fact Edith was wrong in her estimate that her father would die in the next few days. His frail old body clung to life throughout April, into May and then June. Time stopped, while the family was left in emotional limbo for these interminable weeks. Gerald was torn between his feelings for his father and his responsibilities to his employer, with whom his relationship was becoming increasingly fractious.[4]

The Death of Johnstone Stoney

Johnstone Stoney finally died, at home, in the morning of Wednesday 5 July 1911. A small service was held at Golders Green Crematorium. They had made plans to carry the ashes back to Ireland and to inter them in the family grave in Dundrum, but the industrial unrest that characterised this period threatened to derail the rest of their funeral arrangements. There had been an arson attack on a White Star Line vessel berthed in Liverpool, part of the protests of the seamen's strike there. In Dublin, 'the traffic of several of the principal shipping companies remains in a disorganized condition' with 16 vessels tied up on the River Liffey. It was with great relief that they read, on 10 July, that the strike had been settled, for the moment, and that the dockworkers and seamen were returning to work. Trouble erupted again in August, but they were back in London by then.

So, on 13 July, they interred their father's ashes alongside the remains of their grandmother, mother and aunt, in the churchyard of tiny St. Nahi's Church at Dundrum [10]. It was a quiet, modest final resting-place for such an extraordinary man. The funeral used the same route from Bindon's house in Elgin Road that their grandmother's funeral had followed almost 30 years before: past the end of Palmerston Park, down the hill and over the River Dodder by the narrow, cobbled Classon's Bridge and then, rising again, left at the entrance to Weston House, along Churchtown Road to the church. He was the last to die of the children of George Stoney of Oakley Park. His younger brother Bindon had died 2 years earlier. Bindon's widow Frances and her three daughters paid their respects.[5] The service was conducted by their uncle, their mother's brother, Canon Robert Stoney. They were joined as chief mourners by their cousin Maurice FitzGerald, who had travelled

---

[3]Edward Parnell Culverwell (1855–1931) married Edith Fitzgerald, second daughter of Johnstone Stoney's elder sister Anne. He was a mathematician and Professor of Education at Trinity College, Dublin, who endorsed the child-centred Montessori approach to education.

[4]Gerald Stoney resigned from C.A. Parsons and Co. on 30 June 1912.

[5]Bindon's only son George died a few months before him, from tuberculosis, aged 28, on a visit to Robert in Australia.

down from Belfast where he had just retired as Professor of Engineering at Queen's University. They arranged for a headstone to be erected, deciding how best he should be remembered in the inscribed epitaphs. He had a public life: this was honoured by a phrase from the Old Testament, *Righteousness Exalteth a Nation* (Proverbs 14:34). A more personal epitaph recalled his scientific persona: *Felix qui potuit rerum cognoscere causas.* (Fortunate is he who is able to know the causes of things) [11].

It was not only a private family funeral. The chief mourners, including Edith and Florence, welcomed numerous eminent men who had been associated with him during his life, from the worlds of astronomy and medicine. Sir Howard Grubb was there, head of Grubb Telescope Co., which had supplied the 28-inch refractor to the Greenwich Observatory in 1893. Edmund T. Whittaker, FRS, Royal Astronomer for Ireland, came to pay his respects, representing the Royal Society alongside John Joly, FRS. The Irish mathematician, Professor William Snow Burnside was amongst the mourners. Several representatives from the Royal Dublin Society attended. Sir Charles Bent Ball, representing their father's interest in medical education, was able to hear about Florence's career as a doctor. He was the Irish surgeon who had introduced antiseptic surgery to Dublin in 1898. Three doctors from the family attended. Their uncle Dr. Hugh Stoney from Birr and his son Dr. George Bindon Stoney, on leave from South Africa, were there, together with Hugh's nephew, the Canon's son Dr. R. Atkinson Stoney [12].

More personally, one wreath was inscribed 'from his maids, Mary and Kate'. A second, from Mrs. Ayrton, indicates the close relationship between Edith and the engineer Hertha Ayrton, through their respective senior positions in the British Federation of University Women.

This was a sad and emotional time for Edith. She was closer to her father, in interests and in character, than Florence, and probably felt his death more deeply than her siblings. Five years later, she would still recall that 'all our life centred round him—he came long before either of us to the other. As we made no newer ties—our lives are now in the past' [13]. Edith and Florence were executors of his will, and not his eldest son Gerald as might have been expected. His estate was valued at about £6000.

Returning to her lecturing post in October 1910 gave Edith a means to refocus her grief about the slow dying of her father. She considered the deficiencies of her physics course, and how the applications of physics to medicine might be more appropriately presented. She knew that she was limited within her first-year course to teach basic physics, however hard she tried to add the medical context. Talking to Florence, they realised that what was needed was an advanced course in medical physics. Florence offered to donate £20 to facilitate the purchase of equipment to 'connect physics with later medical studies' [14]. This could have been an important innovation. The therapeutic applications of electricity were becoming more widespread in private practice and in hospitals. Finsen (ultraviolet) therapy and high-frequency electrotherapy were being more widely used. The diagnostic use of X-rays was by now widespread. Radiotherapy and radium treatments were being used to treat a variety of skin conditions and cancers. The optical design of endoscopes and ophthalmoscopes was worthy of exploration. Edith could have been at the forefront of modern medical technological training.

It was not to be. Increasing student numbers placed a severe limit on Edith's freedom to develop any new course, even had it been supported by her colleagues. She was frustrated that the concept of an innovative advanced course in medical physics found no support and was stillborn.

Reynolds Close

Very soon after their father's death, Edith and Florence moved into the northern suburbs. They were attracted by a new housing development north of Hampstead, the Hampstead Garden Suburb. The scheme had originated in 1906, an Act of Parliament setting the basis for the layout and planning, with Raymond Unwin as the chief planner. The intention had been that it should cater for all classes and upper income groups, including both professionals and artisans. Under the guiding hand of the architects Geoffrey Lucas and Sydney Cranfield, this high-specification development limited housing density to eight dwellings per acre. There were many trees and communal spaces, the main Hampstead Square being designed by Sir Edwin Lutyens. The house that Edith and Florence bought, 20 Reynolds Close, was on a corner plot in a quiet, tree-lined cul-de-sac on the southern side of the extension to Hampstead Heath, less than a 10-minute walk from Golders Green Station. It was an elegant three-storey brick house, facing south, with a narrowing back garden (Fig. 8.2). They sorted through the furniture that would be needed, retaining the items carrying memories of their father. The new house needed curtains and carpets. Heal and Sons in Tottenham Court Road advertised old-fashioned fabrics, glazed or unglazed chintzes, hand-printed from original peacock design woodblocks. They could get new carpets, Axminster or oriental, from Waring and Gillow in Oxford Street, who had an established reputation for supplying quality carpets and furniture to wealthy families. Modern furniture design was still influenced by several decades of the Arts and Crafts movement, which matched the Garden Suburb style, but traditional furniture designs were becoming popular again. The garden was a blank sheet, and this was where their love of gardening developed.

It was a quiet refuge from the agitation and noise of their daily lives. Cares released as they stepped into the hallway. The drawing room on the right led directly through French doors onto a veranda and the back garden. The large kitchen at the back, with its gas stove, pantry and larder, was more than sufficient for their needs. The large dining room, 16 ft by 13 ft, on the front corner, caught both the morning and the evening sun. The angled staircase led to a landing and four rooms, sufficient to have a study and a bedroom each. Open coal-fired grates heated each room, with tile surrounds of complex designs, influenced by the Arts and Crafts styling of the previous decades. The huge attic space under the roof, with its sloping ceilings and dormer windows, extended the full depth of the house, 35 feet from front to back. Here they could store their father's papers and equipment until they decided what to

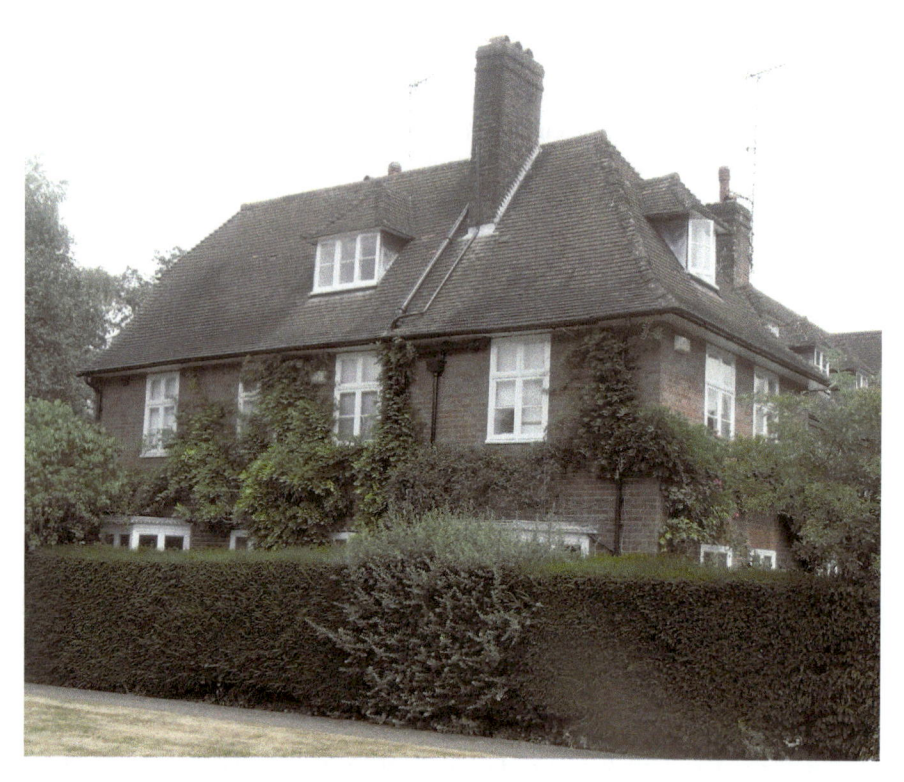

Fig. 8.2 20 Reynolds Close, Hampstead Garden Suburb

do with it all. Up here, too, was accommodation for their housekeeper Mary Kennedy. This would become their home and refuge, not only during the strikes that continued throughout the country the following spring and the increasing militancy of the suffragettes but also throughout the dark years of the war.

They bought a shiny new motorcar, parked on the road outside. Edith's enthusiasm for motoring was to last all her life, and she prided herself on not only being able to drive but also understanding car mechanics. She mastered its routine: greasing, changing the oil and adding distilled water to the battery and air to the pneumatic tyres. The acetylene lamps were similar to those on her bicycle. Edith took great pride in the vehicle, once listing her recreations as 'Driving and cleaning own motor car' together with 'gardening and reading *The Times*' [15]. 1912 had seen the launch of so-called light cars, two-seaters such as the 10 horsepower Morris Oxford and the Singer Ten, particularly popular with women motorists. In the early years of driving, the majority of drivers had been male. The main obstacle had been not driving skill, developed equally by both sexes, but the starting handle. Considerable physical strength was needed to crank the engine in order to start it, and it was only those women who were strong enough to get the car going who could be truly independent. Edith was diminutive in stature, and whilst she clearly had the determination to overcome this obstacle, obstacle it was. At last, in 1912, this final barrier was removed when Chrysler introduced the first car to include an electrical starter motor. Edith could have selected a car from a number of new models that now offered motor starting at the push of a button. Now anyone, previously dependent on a stronger person to start the car for them, could be independent and own and operate their own vehicle without assistance. For women drivers in particular, this technological advance suddenly made car ownership into a practical and liberating possibility, further emancipating women to take control of their own lives.

Florence also had her sister's enjoyment of motoring but was content to be the navigator. For a few years, the car was an exciting shared enjoyment, and the residents of the little villages in the Chiltern Hills could see the two sisters at the weekends as they explored the narrow winding lanes, sitting closely side by side in the cramped front seat of the open-topped vehicle. It was not too far to reach Amersham for afternoon tea.

A Developing Crisis

Florence's reputation and medical practice continued to grow. On the other hand, work became more difficult for Edith. In June 1912, the most recent of a succession of her part-time physics demonstrators resigned. The appointment of demonstrators was not managed with the rigour of the academic posts and was often the result of recommendation. Mary Waller, the bright young science graduate who joined Edith at the beginning of October 1912 was one such. Her mother, Mrs. Alice Waller, was one of the lay members of the School Committee, and it was undoubtedly as a result of her suggestion that Mary was appointed. Mrs. Waller (née Palmer), biscuit heiress of Huntley and Palmer, had been a student of the eminent physiologist Augustus D. Waller. They married in 1885, and Mary was their first child. His scientific standing matched that of Johnstone Stoney, though in a different field. Most famously, in 1887, he had used Lippmann's mercury capillary electrometer [16] to display, for the first time, the repeated electrical signal from the heart, detected using electrodes on the chest wall of his laboratory assistant [17], so anticipating the electrocardiogram. Their daughter Mary Waller was herself a scientist, having graduated with a B.Sc. from London University.

Funding was tight. With 22 in the incoming class, Mary was expected to work hard, but there was only enough funding for 5 hours each week at an annual salary of £30. Edith managed to increase her hours the next summer to three half-days per week. She understood that staff would not stay unless they were offered a living wage, and she made the case to Council that the rates paid were too little to make it worthwhile for a demonstrator to remain at the LSMW unless she had other means of support. Eventually four half-days a week were allowed, paying now £60 p.a. This was still not enough; Edith was not particularly surprised when Mary Waller resigned at the end of the 1913–1914 session.

The Council members did not see it quite the way Edith did, however. At the Council meeting on 24 June 1914, Mary Waller's resignation initiated a 'full discussion on the teaching and organisation of the physics department'. Whilst they were 'not satisfied with the present position, action should not be taken at the moment'. Edith did not realise it, but she was being set up to fail.

Whilst Edith had been persistent in pressing her case, she was steadily losing the confidence of those with influence, and she was on the wrong side of events and the political decision-making. Julia Cock, who had been dean for much of Edith's time at the LSMW, and so knew her well, developed breast cancer from which she died on 7 February 1914. Louisa Aldrich-Blake, who had been vice-principal under Julia Cock's leadership for a number of years, took over as dean. She and Alice Waller were both members of the University Club for Ladies, and it was most likely here that Edith's fate was sealed.

Edith had many other more important things on her mind than worrying about the internal politics of the London School of Medicine for Women. Civil war was threatening in Ireland, only prevented by the declaration of war by Britain on Germany at the beginning of August. Florence and Edith took immediate action. Edith volunteered to assist with refugees from Belgium in her spare time, while Florence started planning with the Imperial Services League to lead a front-line medical unit to Antwerp. Edith was not free to take time off from her work, as Florence did.

Returning after the summer break in 1914, it was to discover that the student numbers had almost doubled. She was faced with the need not only to replace Mary Waller but also to manage 47 students in a laboratory originally designed to hold no more than 20. She recruited a new part-time demonstrator, Marion Baxter from Cambridge, to replace Mary Waller. She secured further funding, £30 for extra apparatus for her larger class and £20 to give extra revision classes.

By January 1915, her team was nearly at breaking point. Miss Baxter said that she was overworked and asked to be relieved of some of her duties. Edith secured more funds, enough to recruit a second part-time demonstrator, May Williams. The job-share arrangement gave her almost one full-time equivalent for a total salary of £108 p.a. They just about got through to the end of term. The examination results showed the usual pattern of excellent high-flyers with a long tail of poor marks.

None of this was enough. Edith's future had already been decided behind closed doors. On 24 March 1915, the LSMW Council minutes recorded that

> the arrangements for teaching in the physics department were considered in view of the difficulties frequently before the various committees of the school in connection with the organisation of the department and the personnel of the assistant staff. It was resolved that, with deep regret and most unwillingly a change is desirable in the physics lectureship. The Dean was asked to convey to Miss Edith Stoney, M.A., lecturer in physics, the sense of the resolution previous to the meeting of the school committee to be held 5 May. The Council recorded its great appreciation of the long and loyal service rendered to the school by Miss Stoney and asked for her acceptance of the sum £300 as a token of gratitude upon her resignation of the lectureship.

So that was it, dismissed without any specific reason, except that she had continually warned the School Committee that her department could not continue to function without additional staff and funding. Such issues are not uncommon in any workplace and would not normally be seen as a reason for dismissal. Eventually the staffing need was recognised and, by 1917, long after she left, the physics establishment finally reached one lecturer and two full-time demonstrators.

The offer to pay her 2 years' salary on tendering her resignation was unprecedented. They really wanted to be rid of her. Notably, she was not removed from her post because of incompetence, nor because of poor student results. But there could have been another reason, which possibly, when Louisa Aldrich-Blake met Edith to ask for her resignation, she tried to explain.

War had changed everything. In peacetime it was possible to have some flexibility, to retain ideals and to aim for the highest performance. These had been Edith's educational watchwords during her 15 years as physics lecturer at the LSMW. She expected each new cohort of would-be doctors to have a thorough grounding in physics before allowing them to proceed to their clinical studies. Such a view had only recently been grafted on to a deep history of medical training for which the key elements were anatomy, pathology and *materia medica*. It was still required to demonstrate adequate knowledge in the basic sciences, including physics, but there was now a new emphasis, a new imperative. Male doctors were being recruited to serve in the Royal Army Medical Corps and in the growing number of civilian war hospitals that were being established throughout the land. Women doctors were going to be needed more than ever and in greater numbers to fill these gaps. The LSMW was still the only medical school in London to accept women students, remaining so until St. Mary's, Charing Cross and St. George's opened their doors in 1916. Aldrich-Blake was already making plans to further double the number of new students for the October intake in 1915. It was vital that these young women were given every chance of graduating as quickly as possible. This must include those who were weaker in physics, but would still make excellent doctors in Aldrich-Blake's view. These weaker students would risk failing, she knew, when faced with the rigorous mathematical standards that Edith set during her first-year physics examinations. That could not be allowed to happen.

It is doubtful that Edith saw her own dismissal coming, and it must have been a shock. Such an event had never happened to her before, and she had always been in control of her own affairs. The dismissal was not to take immediate effect, and Aldrich-Blake asked her to work until the end of the summer term, any replacement coming in to post for the beginning of the 1915/1916 session. The matter would be considered again at the beginning of May.

Edith did not see it that way. Within days of her interview with Aldrich-Blake, she offered her services to the Scottish Women's Hospitals, to give technical support for the all-women hospitals being established in France and Serbia. By the end of April, she had agreed to join the Girton and Newnham Unit as their radiographer, responsible for running a field X-ray department in France. Only when that was in place did she tender her resignation, giving enough notice so that it could take effect by 26 May.

The meeting of the School Committee on 5 May must have been an odd, tense affair with Dean Louisa Aldrich-Blake, Edith Stoney and Alice Waller all present. The Dean announced that she had received Edith's resignation and that she would be leaving within a month. Mrs. Waller paid a warm tribute to Edith's 15 years in the lectureship, obliquely suggesting that Edith's approach was now out of date. Then it was announced that her daughter Mary Waller, who had walked out of her demonstrator's post less than a year before, had agreed to take over as locum lecturer for the rest of the summer term.

The experience of her dismissal stayed with Edith for some while. She remained extremely sensitive to the arbitrary exercise of power. She also became very cautious about the motivations of some in the medical profession, an attitude that would sometimes sour her professional relationships over the next few years.

Mary Waller stayed and slipped in to the post of lecturer in physics the following October. She did a good job, creating her own substantial career as a medical physicist, eventually becoming reader in the University of London. She remained in charge of the Royal Free Physics Department until she retired after the Second World War [18]. She published a few papers, on skin reddening under ultraviolet and infrared radiation and on the carbon arc, and a physics textbook that was not considered to be very good. She was best known for her book of modes of vibrations of a metal plate. Of passing interest to the present story was her paper on 'The emotive response of a class of 78 students of medicine' published after she had been in post 3 years. Mary Waller tested the galvanic reflex of her physics students by measuring their skin resistance in response to a range of stimuli. She concluded that the more academically able students from her physics class exhibited a larger emotive response than did the less able, whether in response to a loud bang, bad smell or questioning [19].

No longer was the class around 20 students. A new North Wing was funded and completed by August 1917, when the incoming student group numbered 78. The enlarged 'Consuela, Duchess of Marlborough Physics Department' was in the basement with its lecture theatre, laboratories and research rooms. The Dean had certainly succeeded in expanding the intake of the School. It is difficult to imagine that Edith's style of teaching, 'mostly developing into informal talks', could never have worked with a class of this size.

References

1. Stoney EA. The terminal velocity of fall of small spheres in air. Nature. 1910;82:279.
2. Stoney EA. Approximation in method versus approximation in arithmetic. Math Gaz. 1910;86:279–80.
3. Stoney GJ. The demand for a catholic university. Nineteenth Century After Mon Rev. 1902;51 (300):263–75.
4. Stoney J. Meeting of graduates in London. Dublin University Defence. Dublin: Hodges Figgis; 1907. p. 32–8.

References

5. Stoney GJ. Preface (September 1907). In: Fournier d'Albe EE, editor. The electron theory. A popular introduction to the new theory of electricity and magnetism. 3rd ed. London: Longmans Green; 1909.
6. Turing S. Alan M. Turing. Cambridge: Heffer; 1959. p. 7.
7. Ball RS. Dr. G. Johnstone Stoney, F.R.S. The Observatory. 1911;34:287–90.
8. Trinity College Dublin archives. MS 2313/1(13). 1910 Nov 27.
9. Berry HF. A history of the royal Dublin society. London: Longmans; 1915. p. 377–8.
10. Grave site 353, St Nahi's Churchyard, Churchtown Road, Dundrum, Ireland.
11. Virgil. Georgics 2 v. 490. 29 BC.
12. Funeral of the late Mr. J. Stoney, M.A. Dublin Daily Express 1911 Jul 14.
13. Edith Stoney to Mrs Laurie. WL. TD1734/2/6/9/57.
14. London School of Medicine for Women School Committee minutes. 1912 Nov 13. LMA. H72/SM/A/04.
15. Suffrage Annual and Women's Who's Who, 1913. London. p. 366.

Chapter 9
Action and Reaction

As their father's life drew to a close, both Edith and Florence engaged more and more with national political issues, especially with developments in support of women, notably with the suffragist movement [1]. At this stage in the development of women's suffrage, women had achieved national voting rights in New Zealand (1893), Australia (1902), Finland (1907) and Norway (1908). They also had the right to vote in nine of the United States of America, starting with Wyoming in 1869. British suffragists saw themselves, therefore, at the forefront of an international fight for women's rights. Nevertheless, Edith and Florence were quite opposed to the militant methods used by Christabel Pankhurst and her suffragettes to gain publicity for the cause of women's suffrage.

They joined in the rallies and subscribed to supportive organisations. Florence was described as 'a keen constitutional suffragist' sharing in many demonstrations and processions [2]. They became members of the London Society for Women's Suffrage. Commencing with the first rally on 9 February 1907, organised by the National Union of Women's Suffrage Societies, such rallies became progressively larger and more vehement. In 1911, 40,000 demonstrators converged on Whitehall, a throng that included, according to one journalist, 'women in scarlet doctor's robes (who) sat on the steps of the deserted Government offices'. One banner celebrated Marie Curie and her discovery of radium [3]. Edith was concerned that the movement should be seen as rational and controlled. In June 1910, she wrote to Miss Pippa Strachey (then secretary of the London Society for Women's Suffrage) expressing concern about the lack of proper organisation for another proposed suffrage meeting in Trafalgar Square, fearing that it could become violent and that some accident would damage the cause [4]. In the event, the meeting went off without incident, on 11 July. Gerald also supported the movement for women's suffrage, lending his support to local suffrage meetings in Newcastle [5].

Edith joined the Conservative and Unionist Women's Franchise Association. This was a lobby group, formed within the Conservative and Unionist Party in 1908 at the suggestion of Millicent Fawcett, which attempted to return Members of Parliament who were sympathetic to women's suffrage and to oppose the rump of opposition still within the party. Many who had previously supported the Liberal Unionists had been drawn towards the Conservative party as the commitment of the Liberals to Home Rule and Asquith's personal opposition to women's franchise became increasingly clear. Florence was a member of the Women's Local Government Society, a cross-party and politically independent organisation whose aim was to expand the number of women elected as local councillors.

Edith was an avid reader of *The Times*, and, in a letter to the editor in May 1913, she signed herself as a 'non-militant suffragist' [6]. In this letter, she sets out a logical case for women's suffrage by commenting on Parliament's legislative control over the professions. Having discovered for herself how to get around the control of Cambridge University, she says that this is not an important issue: 'To many women the absence of a degree is a hindrance, but is not vital'. However, those without a medical qualification are excluded from practice by law. As she wrote, 'the fight to open the medical profession to women was arduous, painful and prolonged'. Those outside the profession, even those like herself with highest honours from Oxford or Cambridge, are prevented from using 'our knowledge for anything of such practical help to others, and especially to poor women, as medicine'. She continues 'If, however, the medical profession is now open by some roads to women, this is not true of either of the great legal professions' (that is, barristers and solicitors). As she points out, 'Women have taken high honours in the law schools of the Universities and can then proceed no further'. Women were able to consult a member of their own sex in medical matters, but 'The huge blessing, ... of being able to obtain legal advice from one of their own sex is denied them'. Her case for women's emancipation was to prevent men, who had the vote, from maintaining 'the excluding protection of an Act of Parliament which is supposed to be impartial in its care of those with votes and those without'.

The British Federation for University Women

Edith played a central role in the British Federation for University Women (BFUW) from its early days. As early as 1901, the Irish Association of Women Graduates had been formed in Dublin although, in spite of Edith's Irish heritage, there is no evidence that she was involved with this organisation. A British group was first convened in Manchester in 1907, and this became the foundation of the British Federation. It had the following aims:

1. To act as an organisation which shall afford opportunity for the expression of united opinion and for concerted action by University Women on matters especially concerning them
2. To encourage independent research work by women
3. To facilitate intercommunication and cooperation between women of different universities
4. To stimulate the interest of women in municipal and public life

Eleanor Sidgwick, who was still Principal of Newnham College, agreed to be the first president. The first Executive Committee meeting took place on 9 October 1909 at 36 Russell Square in London. There were only three women present, and it was managed by two scientists who had both been students at Newnham, the chemist Dr. Ida Smedley, who was then working at the Lister Institute and was the honorary secretary, and the physiologist Dr. Winifred Cullis who took the chair at the first meeting. Like Edith, Winifred Cullis had considered medicine but instead had joined the staff of the LSMW where she eventually became Professor of Physiology.

Edith was clearly known and well respected through her professional and Newnham connections by three of the key women who set up the British Federation. She was invited to take charge of the finances and was appointed as honorary treasurer, in her absence, at this first executive meeting [7]. She held this position for 6 years, only stepping down in 1915 when she left for Europe during the war. By this time, the membership was approaching 1000, predominantly from the 3 main centres in the north, Leeds, Manchester and Liverpool.

Florence became a member of the London Branch, though she was never on the Executive Committee. Nevertheless, her involvement with her sister's activities was close. It was Florence, and not Edith, who, on 7 July 1911, signed the cash account in preparation for the executive meeting the following day. This was because their father had died only 2 days before, and Edith was focussed on the arrangements for his cremation and the funeral in Dublin the following week. Once more the supportive bond between Florence and Edith is apparent.

Edith's involvement with the BFUW extended her range of contacts. She met the engineer Hertha Ayrton, one of the first vice presidents of the Federation. Significantly, she overlapped briefly with Frances Ivens, an early executive committee member. Miss Ivens had been one of the star students at the London School of Medicine for Women, graduating M.B.B.S. in 1902 during Edith's early years there as a lecturer. Following her move to Liverpool, Frances Ivens became 'a protagonist in all our feminist struggles. She was the leader of our younger medical women whom she never ceased to spur on to further achievements. Much fighting for hospital posts was necessary then, and Miss Ivens proved a magnificent leader' [8]. A lengthy report on the difficulties in securing hospital posts by women doctors was prepared for the Federation in 1914 by Dr. Mildred Powell. She reported that with good progress being made in London, 'any agitation should at present be confined to the north of England'. As will be told, the war would bring Edith and Frances Ivens into very close contact.

Smedley and Cullis, together with Phoebe Sheavyn from Somerville, have been seen as the main driving forces in the formative years, with Eleanor Sidgwick being primarily an important but passive figurehead. Edith's actions have gained less prominence. Nevertheless, after her father died, Edith became increasingly engaged with the political lobbying of the Federation. Indeed, it can be claimed that Edith was responsible for more serious initiatives during the years 1912–1915 than the other executive members put together. At the executive meeting on 19 October 1912, she proposed the names of two members for a subcommittee to secure the passing into law of a bill to enable women to become barristers, solicitors or parliamentary agents. The arguments against women barristers were well rehearsed and were even published by the National Union of Women's Suffrage Societies so that they could be refuted. These included that 'a woman advocate would be irresistible to a male jury', 'the male advocate would be prejudiced in his work by a chivalrous feeling not to press the woman opponent' and 'judges would insensibly incline more favourably to a woman lawyer' [9]. The war got in the way of this legislation, which eventually was enacted within the Sex Disqualification (Removal) Act of 1919. Edith was also aware of at least two occasions when the opinion of male legal council had blocked female advancement. The first was when she was little, and her father had received legal instructions to decline Edith Pechey's application to enter Queen's University. More recently, the all-male Council of the Royal Society had chosen to interpret its statutes in such a way as to deny both Marian Farquharson and Hertha Ayrton the award of fellowship.

At the same time, Edith chaired another subcommittee to press that women should be enabled to become higher officials in prisons. The meetings of this subcommittee were held, not at the offices of the BFUW at 36 Russell Square, but at her sister's consulting rooms at 4 Nottingham Place. In this, she had more immediate success. Edith was charged with task of approaching Adeline Russell Dowager Duchess of Bedford, a lifelong campaigner for prison reform, for support. The request was taken seriously by the Home Secretary, and, in 1914, Dr. Selina Fox was appointed to the prison service as Lady Superintendent and Deputy Medical Officer at the detention centre in Aylesbury. She became governor in 1916 [10].

Edith was also concerned about challenges to the established position of women in academic positions at this time. The minutes recorded that 'Miss Stoney drew attention to the fact that men had been appointed to posts at the London School of Medicine for Women and at Bedford College which had previously been held by women.' [11] Edith had in her mind her friend Miss Ellaby M.D. (Paris), whose position as lecturer in ophthalmic surgery was filled on her death in 1909 by Percy Fleming FRCS. Charlotte Ellaby had been consulting ophthalmic surgeon at the New Hospital for Women and was a respected colleague of Florence's there. Edith knew that such posts currently held by women were always vulnerable, even her own. Had she not returned to her post as physics lecturer in 1910, her male locum Mr. Brinkworth would have stepped into her shoes. At Bedford College, Alice Lee B.Sc., D.Sc., assistant lecturer in mathematics under Professor Harold Hilton, stepped aside to take up a research lectureship in 1912. The vacancy was filled by H. Bryan Heywood B.Sc., D.Sc., and it was this appointment that caused Edith's concern. The appointment was reversed, and the following year Miss M. Long, who had completed the Cambridge Maths Tripos and had, like Edith, received a BA *ad eundem* from Trinity College Dublin, took the position. A year later, in 1913, controversy flared again over the appointment of a man, George Barger, to the Chair of Chemistry at the women's Royal Holloway College, following heated discussion over the possibility of positive discrimination. Partly, as a result of Edith's initiative, a standing committee for monitoring the appointment of men to academic positions was established.

Edith's final initiative came after the war had started. She was concerned that funds should be made available to train women to take up the jobs vacated by men who entered the armed forces. At the executive meeting of the Federation of University Women on 27 March 1915, she proposed the motion 'That the FUW should collect funds to enable it to offer a few grants in aid of the higher technical training of any women who have the prospect after such training of obtaining work which before the war was done by men'. It was carried by 6 to 1. The minute continued: 'As examples, training as motor drivers or for posts in museums were instanced. The secretaries were instructed to get returns from the LAs (local associations) as to what facilities of training are being given in their districts to prepare women to take up posts held before the war by men. The secretaries were instructed also to reply to the Board of Trade mentioning that the F. (Federation) was appealing for funds for this purpose'. The changes in all their lives during the first year of the war limited the effectiveness of the Federation to take forward any political lobbying, and this sensible initiative was never pursued.

Militant Suffragettes

Both Florence and Edith became increasingly concerned as the level of suffragette militant action escalated. They were appalled when they heard that the suffragette Mary Richardson had entered the National Gallery, stood in front Valázquez's *Toilet of Venus* and then hacked at the canvas using a small axe that she had secreted under the left sleeve of her jacket. This attack, in the morning of Tuesday 10 March 1914, was followed by a number of copycat attacks on other paintings in other galleries. The official backlash was inevitable. The National Gallery closed its doors. Elsewhere, whenever the sisters wanted to enter a museum or gallery, they were met with a rule that prohibited muffs, wrist-bags or sticks. The British Museum established a rule that women could only enter if accompanied by a man or could show a letter of recommendation. Always opposed to militancy, they knew that such attacks had become counterproductive, hardening the public opinion against the suffrage cause. A spokeswoman for the NUWSS deplored 'the spirit of revenge which has so poisoned the minds of a few of the supporters of the noblest and purest of all causes' [12].

Edith was sensitive to the causes of tragedy in some women's lives. In April 1914 she wrote a brief letter, full of irony, to the Editor of *The Times* that was published under the headline 'Women and the "fascinating brute"' [13].

> Sir,—In your witty article on Petruchio up-to-date you refer to the "proved popularity with women of the hero whom the men take to be an unutterable bounder and brute".
>
> It is quaint to turn from the mirror on the stage to the real life shown on another page of the same issue of your great journal—where we read of a woman of 34 who took her own life and that of her baby rather than face for herself or her child the constantly recurring drunkenness of her husband.

> The jury of men at the inquest apparently agreed with the humour of the writer of your article as to the type of man a women ought to admire, for they brought this woman in "as of unsound mind".

The militancy of the suffragettes grew to a crescendo during the pre-war years, polarising opinion. Imprisonment led to hunger strikes and forced feeding. Members of the medical profession, especially women doctors, were drawn in, including Florence's friend Agnes Savill (1875–1964). Dr. Savill was one of the handful of women doctors who, like Florence, were practicing radiology at the time. She had completed medical training in Glasgow in 1898, and was awarded her M.D. in 1901, when she married Dr. Thomas Savill. Having moved to London, she gained an appointment at the 35-bed St John's Hospital for Skin Diseases in 1904. She became an honorary physician there, very unusual for a woman at that time, and developed an interest in electrotherapeutics, provided by the Electrical, Light and X-ray Department [14]. X-ray equipment was installed in 1906, 'although somewhat costly', when it was being used for the treatment of ringworm, rodent ulcers and lupus. Many other skin complaints were being treated, including acne, warts, eczema, psoriasis and superfluous hair, and by 1908, they had added ultraviolet light and high-frequency therapy. She subsequently became honorary physician in the skin department of the South London Hospital for Women.

Agnes Savill's main use of X-rays before the war was as a dermatologist. As Robert Knox stated 'No greater testimony to the value of X-rays in the treatment of diseases of the skin could be given than the fact that all skin hospitals have an X-ray department, and that nearly every specialist includes a more or less perfect installation in his armamentarium' [15].

Savill was a well-respected member of the medical community. In 1912, she took the lead in organising a petition against the forcible feeding of suffrage prisoners, signed by 117 medical practitioners [16, 17]. Force-feeding had been first used for a suffragette in September 1909 and by this time was a widely used procedure. Her reports provide a vivid insight into the traumatic experiences endured by imprisoned suffragists on hunger strike.

> During the struggle before the feeding, prisoners were held down by force, flung on the floor, tied to chairs and iron bedsteads. As might be expected, severe bruises were thus inflicted ... forcible feeding by the oesophageal or nasal tube cannot be performed without risk of mechanical injury to the nose and throat. Injuries to the nose were particularly common... The prisoners were usually flung down or tied and held while the tube was pushed up the nostrils .... In most cases local frontal headache, earache and trigeminal neuralgia supervened, besides severe gastric pain, which lasted throughout the forcible feeding, preventing sleep. ... After each feeding it (the nasal pain) gets worse, so that it becomes a refinement of torture to have the tube force through.

It is quite possible that her political trigger was an extraordinary misogynist outburst in a letter to *The Times* by the eminent physician Sir Almoth Wright on 6 April during the discussion in the Commons of yet another unsuccessful Conciliation Bill concerning women's suffrage. Even for its time, the language was inflammatory from beginning to end, starting by stating that man 'is not a little mystified when he encounters in (a woman) periodically recurring phases of hypersensitiveness, unreasonableness, and loss of sense of proportion'. He blamed this on not enough sexual intercourse. 'The recruiting field for the militant suffragists as the half-million of our excess female population—that half-million which had better long ago have gone out to mate with its complement of men beyond the sea' and so on. He could barely be taken seriously, and Agnes Savill dismissed him as a man who 'always affords amusement to the average public'.

Irish Home Rule

Edith and Florence worried deeply about another political development during these years, the unresolved question about Home Rule for Ireland, and its possible effect on their relatives still living in Ireland. Their aunt Frances was still in Dublin with her children, as was George Fitzgerald's widow Harriett. Their cousin Maurice was in Belfast, having retired as Professor of Engineering at Queen's University in 1910, although he was on the point of moving back to Dublin. To the sisters' heightened concern, predictions for civil war in Ireland were steadily moving towards reality.

Political opposition to Asquith's Home Rule legislation had been steadily eroding, and, by Whitsun 1914, in spite of stalwart opposition in the House of Lords, the Home Rule Bill passed the Commons for the third time, pending the passage of an Amending Bill to resolve the question of the northern, largely Protestant, counties of Ulster. The key stumbling block to progress was Carson's insistence that the Ulster counties in the north must be excluded from the provisions of the Home Rule Bill, with no time limit. On 23 June, the House of Lord's ensured that all nine counties of Ulster, including those with Catholic majorities, were to be excluded.

Edward Carson's Ulster Volunteers were now outnumbered by the Irish National Volunteers, and there was open gun running to build caches of arms on both sides. The first blood was spilled in mid-July, when a group of National Volunteers attempted to organise a gun-running exercise near Dublin that ended with the army killing 3 nationalists and injuring 38 others. Outright conflict was only prevented by the postponement of the Amending Bill, as Asquith's government faced a far greater challenge, war in Europe.

During these tense weeks, Florence and Edith had discussed with one another how they might be able to help if war broke out in Ireland. The particular skill they had, they recognised, was expertise in medical radiology. They started to make plans how they might transport some of Florence's X-ray equipment over to Ireland to operate a radiology service to help the surgeons operate on any military or civilian casualties of the conflict. Edith could set up and maintain the X-ray equipment and operate the dark room. Together they could carry out radiographic procedures. Florence could report, interpret and guide the surgeons. They knew it was possible and waited for the expected conflict to start.

References

1. The Suffrage Annual and Women's Who's Who. London; 1913. p. 366.
2. Florence Stoney OBE, M.D. The Vote. 1932 Oct 28:345–246.
3. Fara P. A lab of one's own. Oxford: Oxford University Press; 2018. p. 66.
4. Letter from Edith Stoney to Miss Strachey. 1910 Jun 6. WL. NA488.
5. The Common Cause. 1912 Feb 29. p. 806.
6. Stoney EA. The value of work: women and the professions. The Times. 1913 May 16.
7. British Federation of University Women Executive Committee minutes book. WL. 5BFW/02/01.
8. Chisholm C. J Med Women's Federation 1945 p41. Quoted in Crofton. p. 239.
9. NUWSS. WL. 2NWS/C4/2/30.
10. History of the British Federation of University Women 1907–1957. p. 18.
11. British Federation for University Women Executive Minute book. 1912 Oct 19. WL. 5BFW/02/01.
12. Bostridge M. The fateful year. England 1914. London: Penguin; 2014. p. 53.
13. Stoney EA. Women and the "fascinating brute". The Times. 1914 Apr 9.
14. Russell BF, editor. St John's hospital for diseases of the skin, 1863–1963. Edinburgh: Livingstone; 1963.
15. Knox R. Radiography and radio-therapeutics part II. London: Black; 1918. p. 444.
16. Savill A, Moullin C, Horsley V. Forcible feeding. Br Med J. 1912 Jul 13:100–1.
17. Savill A, Moullin CM, Horsley V. Preliminary report on the forcible feeding of suffrage prisoners. Br Med J. 1912 Aug 31:505–508.

Chapter 10
Florence's War

The Great War

The First World War with all its grim tragedy and large number of casualties put a considerable stress upon medical services in general, and on radiology in particular, with the necessity for quick and accurate diagnosis and for the localisation of foreign material such a bullets and shrapnel [1, 2]. There was an urgent need for doctors and radiologists, and Florence rose to the challenge. The use of radiology in war surgery was well established, and military surgeons were fully aware of its value [3]. Dr. Mabel Ramsay (1878–1954) as president of the MWF wrote of Florence, 'her practice was given up without regret, because she believed she could help England in her need'. Florence was committed to the British cause, and Ramsay continued, saying, 'When work was slack she always impressed on us that England must win the War, because the world needed the British guidance'. There was a healthy interaction between Florence's Britishness and her Irish identity, and she was described as 'British to the core, yet she will always remain in my memory as a very courteous and kindly Irish lady' [4]. There were voices that spoke against the folly of war, and Mabel St Clair Stobart (1862–1954) (Fig. 10.1) spoke at a meeting on 4 August 1914 at which many women contributed. In an article 'Women's protest against War. Great Peace Rally in London. Representative Voice of Europe', Stobart said 'Many distinguished women, each representing one or other of the largest women's organizations in this country and in Europe, spoke last night at the great meeting in the Kingsway Hall, which had been called four days before, as a peace demonstration, but was in tone (so quickly have events moved) almost a last rally of peace forces and common sense' [5]. There were many well-known speakers, and it was resolved, 'Whatever its results the conflict will leave mankind the poorer, will set back civilisation, and will be a powerful check to the amelioration of the condition of the masses of the people on which the real welfare of nations depends'. The women's demonstration against war failed, as did the entreaties of Pope Pius X. The nations wanted war, and nothing would now stop them.

Fig. 10.1 Mabel St Clair Stobart (1862–1954) (from McLaren B. (1917) Women of the War. London: Hodder and Stoughton)

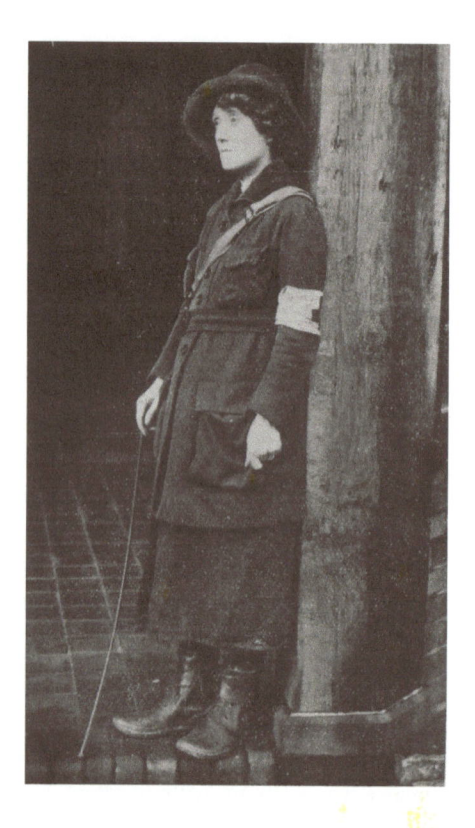

The War Office and Sir Frederick Treves

In the spring of 1914, Florence and her sister Edith had a complete portable X-ray installation prepared and ready, including the new Coolidge tube that Florence had acquired in the United States. So on 4 August 1914, which was the day that Great Britain entered the First World War, Florence and Edith Stoney were able to offer both their services and that of their portable radiology apparatus to the British Red Cross at the War Office in London (Fig. 10.2). At that time, having such apparatus was not common, and the sisters had acquired it following the suggestion of Field Marshal Lord Frederick Roberts (1832–1914) that 'medical women might be of especial use in the event of an outbreak in Ireland' since many were anticipating a civil war in Ireland [6].

On 5 August, a group of women met in St James's Street in London and set up the Women's National Service League (WNSL), with Mabel Stobart as director and Lady Muir McKenzie (Kate Brenda Blodwen Jones) as subdirector. The aim of the WNSL was to offer service both at home and abroad, and Foreign Service and Home Service Divisions were formed. The Foreign Service Division included women doctors, trained nurses, cooks, interpreters and all the personnel that would be needed for a wartime hospital. The executive committee comprised of Mabel St

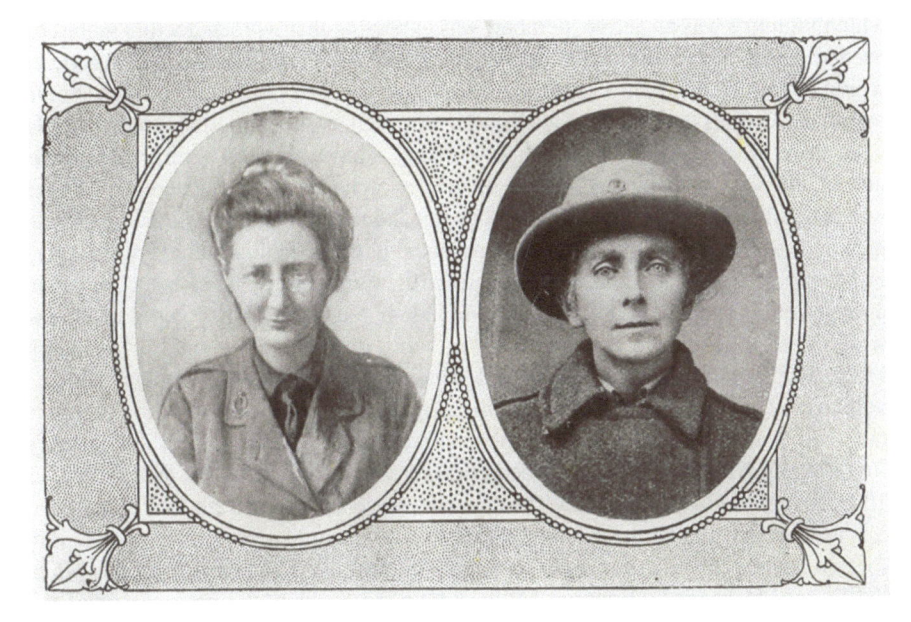

Fig. 10.2 Dr. Florence Stoney and Miss Edith Stoney (from McLaren B. (1917) Women of the War. London: Hodder and Stoughton)

Clair Stobart, Lady Muir Mackenzie, Dr. Florence Stoney, Miss Louis Fagan, Miss E M Stead (Hon. Secretary) and Mrs. Gilbert Samuel (Hon. Treasurer). The group immediately began fundraising and recruiting and within a fortnight had raised £1200 for equipment. Annie Pearson, Viscountess Cowdray (1860–1932), supported the WNSL and generously contributed an X-ray apparatus. Lady Cowdray was an ardent suffragist and philanthropist and is most remembered for her financial patronage of the Royal College of Nursing and her promotion of district nursing. She was President of the Women's Liberal Federation and the Honorary Treasurer of the Liberal Women's Suffrage Union.

Mabel Stobart on behalf of the WNSL approached Sir Frederick Treves (1853–1923) who was Chairman of the British Red Cross Society. In spite of being reminded of the Woman's Convoy Corps in Bulgaria, Treves rejected the offer saying that there was no work that was fitted for women in the sphere of war.

As far as Florence was concerned, she had 13 years of experience in radiology and was very experienced. Her offer of service was declined by Sir Frederick Treves 'because she was a woman' [7]; however, it is worth considering his reasons. Certainly, Treves was well aware of the value of radiography in military surgery, and he had seen its practical applications at first hand during the Boer War. Treves was also aware from his clinical experience of the bravery that women showed and said 'a woman is, in my experience, as courageous as a man, although she may show less resolve in concealing her emotions' [8]. Women were also accepted in medical practice by that time. The Association of Registered Medical Women (ARMW), of which Florence was an active member, was expecting that women doctors would be needed on the home front since many men would be serving abroad and vacancies would be created. Certainly, there was a feeling in the War Office that women should be protected from the horror of war, and it was seen as shocking that women would want to be involved. However, since so many women were in foreign service as nurses and VADs, then why should medical women be treated differently? There was certainly a fear about what would happen should women be given equality with men and real responsibility, and this is reflected in the difficulty women doctors had in getting both military rank and uniforms [9]. For a professional man, a woman doctor would compete in a way that no female nurse or VAD ever could or indeed would need to. Florence was not alone in being rejected, and a similar fate befell Mary Murdoch who wrote to an old school friend on 16 November 1914 'I volunteered for the front at the beginning of the war, and then withdrew because our own War Office did not want medical women' [10]. The Queen Alexandra's Royal Army Nursing Corps expanded considerably during the Great War with over 100,000 nurses in active service. These nurses serve in all of the theatres of war, and it is noteworthy that whilst the War Office was reluctant to send female doctors into foreign service, this did not apply to female nurses. It's also noteworthy that when the Queen Alexandra's Imperial Military Nursing Service, the prececessor of the Queen Alexandra's Royal Army Nursing Corps, was formed in 1902, that Sir Frederick Treves was supportive and a member of its committee [11]. Clearly, Treves' objection to women serving overseas applied only to medical women.

Mabel St Clair Stobart and Antwerp

Florence 'wasted no time with arguments or indignation' following the rejection by Treves, and she actively cooperated with Mabel Stobart in organising a voluntary women's medical unit for foreign service with the WNSL. The Belgian Red Cross Society 'had sent out an urgent and cordial appeal for English woman doctors' [12].

Mabel St. Clair Stobart was a remarkable woman [13]. She was born Mabel Annie Boulton and married St. Clair Kelburn Stobart on 16 July 1884. Mabel noted 'The days of my girlhood ended by my entering one of the few professions that were open to women in those days—a profession that is unpaid financially, but is rich in rewards according to what you yourself put into it'. Sadly, Mabel's first husband died on 9 April 1908. Mabel became deeply interested in Spiritualism and wrote many books on the subject [14]. In South Africa, she joined the First Aid Nursing Yeomanry Corps and on returning to England in 1907 founded the Women's Sick and Wounded Convoy Corps. In the Second Balkan War, the Convoy Corps served in Bulgaria, thereby demonstrating that women could be perfectly capable of serving in a war zone. Mrs. Stobart was highly critical of the Red Cross VAD scheme believing that it 'played with women' and did not give them appropriate recognition or responsibility. Early in the war, Mabel offered the services of a women's medical unit to the Belgian Red Cross and travelled to Brussels under St John Ambulance to set up a hospital in the university buildings. However, before the hospital could be

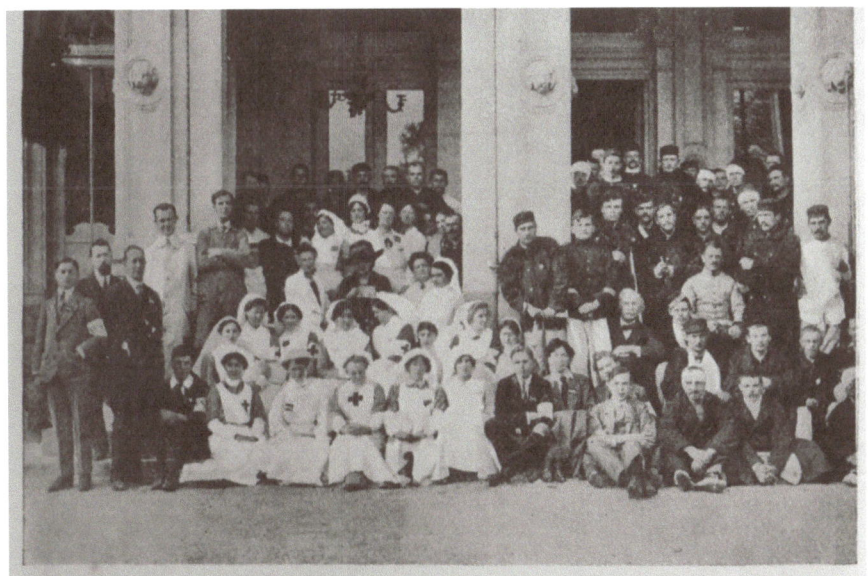

STOBART UNIT AND CONVALESCENTS OUTSIDE THEIR HOSPITAL AT ANTWERP. (Concert Hall of Société de l'Harmonie)
Mrs. Stobart showing medals presented by grateful patients. Dr. F. Stoney on her right; Dr. Ramsey left; Dr. Joan Watts, Dr. Emily Morris, Dr. Rose Turner and Dr. Helen Hanson behind. Miss S. Macnaughtan in front, centre

Fig. 10.3 Stobart Unit and their convalescents outside their hospital in Antwerp. George Mallet is seen standing with folded arms in front of the pillar on the left. (From Stobart M A St Clair (1916) The Flaming Sword in Serbia and Elsewhere. London: Hodder and Stoughton)

set up, the Germans entered the city on 20–21 August. Mabel was imprisoned by the Germans and condemned to be shot as a spy in spite of having a stamped passport; however, she managed to escape.

When she returned from Brussels, Mabel consulted with Lord and Lady Esher, and through their intervention, the Belgian Red Cross and Sir Cecil Hertslet, the British consul-general in Antwerp, invited her to take her unit to that city. This unit was established under the Belgian Red Cross and consisted of 100 (later 135) beds, 6 women doctors and surgeons, 12 trained nurses, 10 female orderlies and other staff including cooks, secretaries and interpreters. Florence organised the medical part of the surgical unit, which was predominantly staffed by women, and was the principal medical officer and radiologist, and Mabel Stobart was the administrator or directrice as she called herself. Mabel Ramsay recalled in later life meeting Florence in August 1914 and 'was easily persuaded to join a woman's hospital unit which was going to Antwerp'. The hospital orderlies included several well-known women, including the Scottish novelist Sarah Broom McNaughtan (1864–1916) [15, 16]. It was on 20 September 1914 that they went to Antwerp and set up their all woman's hospital (Fig. 10.3).

Fig. 10.4 The Zeppelin bombardment of Antwerp on 24 August 1914. Painted by R G Mathews (from "The Great War" c1914)

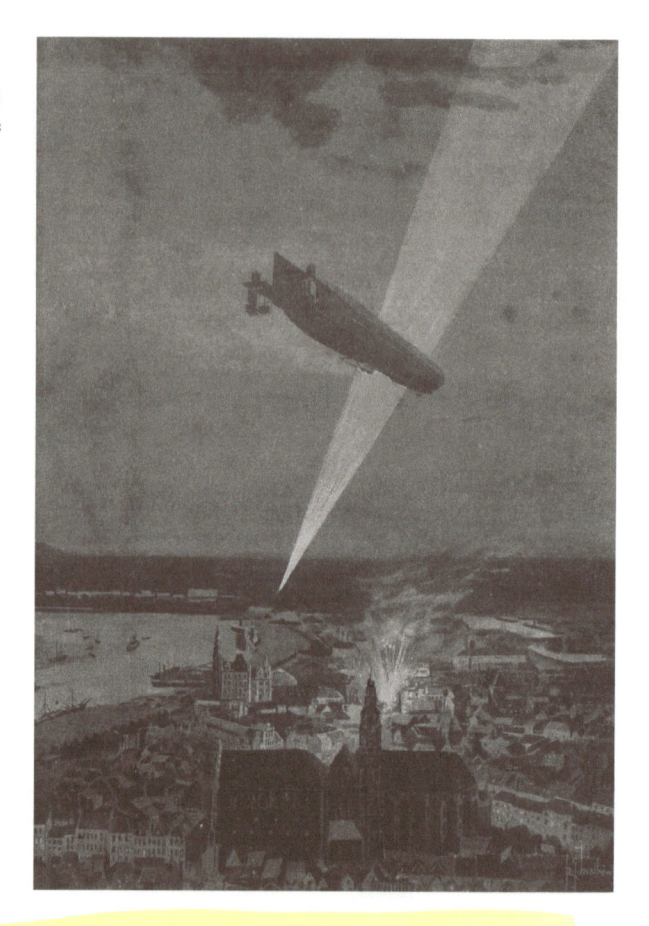

One exception to the all-woman rule was George Mallett, and Florence had included him in the group as her mechanic. He was a Londoner, born in 1891 and the son of a shipping agent. By this time, he was living with his mother and brothers in Cricklewood, not far from Florence's house in Reynolds Close. In planning the group, Florence felt that she would need the assistance of a technician, and no woman was available to accompany the group. Unfortunately, shortly after they arrived in Antwerp, George was sent back to London because 'he was of military age' [17]. As will be seen, this did not prevent him from continuing to work with Florence and then Edith, until the summer of 1917.

The situation that they found in Antwerp was never going to be an easy one. The citizens were in a state of panic, caused by the advancing German army and by aerial attacks by the Zeppelin airships. On 24 August, a Zeppelin airship sailed over Antwerp and dropped shrapnel bombs, which killed ten people including four women, and the Royal Palace was also damaged (Fig. 10.4). This attack was in direct contravention of the Fourth Hague Convention and signalled a change to the nature of war. War was now to involve the whole population with everyone at risk, not just the soldiers at the Front. The Stobart Hospital in Antwerp was located in the Summer Concert Hall in the Rue de L'Harmonie and was established before the official British Army hospitals had been set up. The Concert Hall was not entirely suitable as a hospital, and the building was flimsy and designed for summer use only. There was much to be done to convert it into a fully equipped surgical hospital with an X-ray installation. The dark room and the attendant bullet-localiser were fitted by the Belgian Croix Rouge. Within 48 h of arrival, the new hospital received 40 wounded soldiers from the trenches at Lierre, and a week later, its 135 beds were full of British and Belgian wounded. Florence wrote to Edith about the progress on 23 September and described the conditions. For a period of about 3 weeks, the unit saw many casualties arriving straight from the front, 'the maimed and shattered remnants of manhood that were hourly brought to us from the trenches' as Mabel exclaimed. Dealing with the wounded was not easy, with 50 men often arriving at one time, and usually at night. This was compounded by a blackout that was imposed after 8 pm. Although the Unit had been warned by English surgeons that the patients would object to being treated by women doctors and nurses, this proved to be mistaken, and the soldiers showed gratitude and appreciation. Indeed, no question of gender arose, and when one soldier asked where the doctors were, when he saw women in white coats, he received the reply that they were the doctors. He then exclaimed with a nod of his head, 'Ah! You are gentle; you don't hurt us like they do in other hospitals'. Sir Cecil Hertslet, the British Consul-General, wrote to his son, who was Chaplain to the Archbishop of Canterbury, shortly after the hospital opened stating 'I spent two hours at Mrs Stobart's hospital this afternoon, and had a few minutes' talk with every wounded man there. The hospital is a model of organization and, I think, the best of the hospitals in Antwerp. Everything is so quiet and well arranged. The Belgians are greatly impressed by it'.

The X-ray apparatus was the best available at the time and had been given by Lady Cowdray, and Edith had assisted Florence in choosing the equipment needed. The unit had a 12-inch coil and would work either on mains electricity or an accumulator. The electricity supply in Antwerp due to the war was insufficiently reliable for direct use and so accumulators were used. Florence had brought her Coolidge tube with her, which she had seen in America the previous spring, and she had formed a high opinion of its value. The tube had cost her £25. When she brought it over from America, there were only three others in England. Her tube was the first to be used outside of America and England, and the first to be used in wartime conditions. The doctors in Antwerp were most interested to see it in use. The tube was stable and reliable, and Florence used it for all of her work [18]. Florence saw the main value of the department in locating bullets, and she used the popular Mackenzie Davidson localiser. This allowed for the rapid localisation of the bullet, which could be extracted using a small incision. Florence freely acknowledged her debt to Sir James Mackenzie Davidson for his help and advice. Florence noted how difficult bullets were to locate without radiography. Florence was able to tell the surgeon the exact position of the bullet in relation to the anatomical structures that the surgeon could recognise. She mentioned specifically one soldier who had a piece of shrapnel lodged between the joints of the foot, and the surgeon was able to remove it in only 7 minutes. The bullets were only removed if they caused problems, either by pressing on structures such as nerve or muscle or by causing infection (blood poisoning). An infected wound would not heal if foreign material was retained. Infection was particularly a problem with retained shrapnel balls.

It had been hoped that the forts around Antwerp would hold out against the German advance and that French and British reinforcements would arrive. By 1 October, they were told by Sir Cecil Hertslet that a boat was being prepared to take to safety the British subjects. By the 3 October, the Germans were expected, and the city was in a panic with the inhabitants leaving with what they could carry. There was some hope on 4 October, since Winston Churchill as First Lord of the Admiralty visited the city; however, this was not to be the case, and by 7 October, the Germans had broken through the outer defences. On 8 October 1914, the German bombardment of the city commenced in earnest, and the hospital was under shellfire for 18 hours. The situation became desperate; however, the women 'took no notice of the shells, which whizzed over our heads, without ceasing at the rate of four a minute, and dropped with the bang of a thousand thunderclaps, burning, shattering, destroying everything around us' [19]. Unfortunately, the hospital was in the direct line of fire of the ammunition depôt, which was the German target. The American Consul-General at Antwerp wrote: 'One of the first buildings to be shelled was the hospital run with such magnificent efficiency and success by the British women doctors'. The women evacuated their patients in a calm manner 'as though they were in a Hyde Park parade', and they were either taken into the basement of a local convent or moved by lorry. The beautiful city of Antwerp was in flames, and the inhabitants now fled with whatever they could carry. The portable equipment was packed up; however, nearly all the X-ray apparatus was lost. The road out of Antwerp was described by Florence as a sad procession of fleeing peasants, troops, cattle, guns, wagons, children and carts, all moving in the same direction as rapidly as possible (Fig. 10.5).

The group started walking along the Chauséee de Malines, still under shellfire. Somewhat incongruously, they then came across three London motor-omnibuses driving at breakneck speed. They waved the buses to stop and found that they were being driven by British soldiers. The buses were carrying a load of ammunition and were rushing to cross the bridge made from boats before it was blown up (Fig. 10.6). Sixteen of them now sat in the buses on boxes of ammunition and were conveyed through the shelled and empty streets with burning houses, and they were the last to cross the bridge over the River Scheldt only 20 minutes before the Belgians blew it up.

The use of mechanical transport in warfare on a large scale for the first time enabled the rapid concentration of troops at any given point and was a major reason why there was such a large numbers of casualties. In fact as early as 1908, the War Office had hired *General* buses to experiment on their possible use for the transport of troops [20]. The buses were used to transport troops and ammunition from the railhead to the firing line and were equipped with shovels so that they could be dug out of the mud (Fig. 10.7). The glass was also taken out of the windows, which were boarded up. A large number of buses were sent to the war, such as the AEC type B

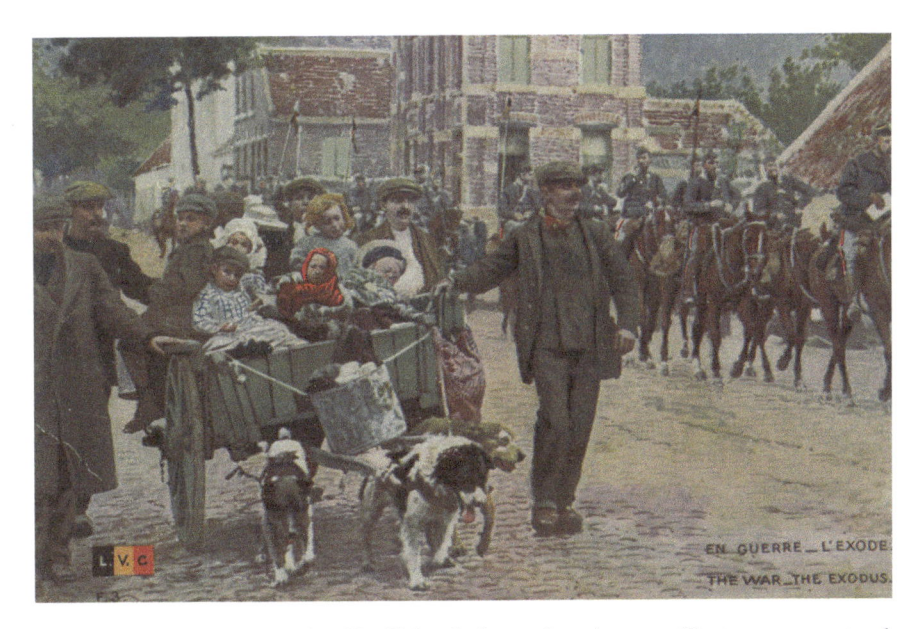

Fig. 10.5 The War—The Exodus. The flight of refugees from Antwerp. (Contemporary postcard. Unidentified publisher)

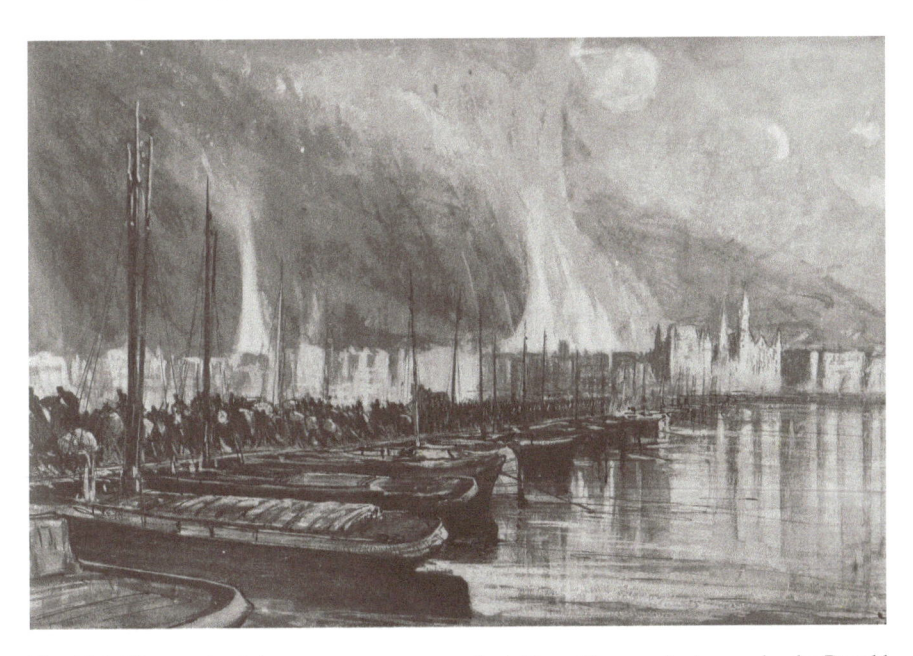

Fig. 10.6 The people of Antwerp pouring across the bridge of barges. An impression by Donald Maxwell compiled from descriptions by refugee soldiers. (from The Graphic 2 October 1914)

A LONDON 'BUS IN ACTION

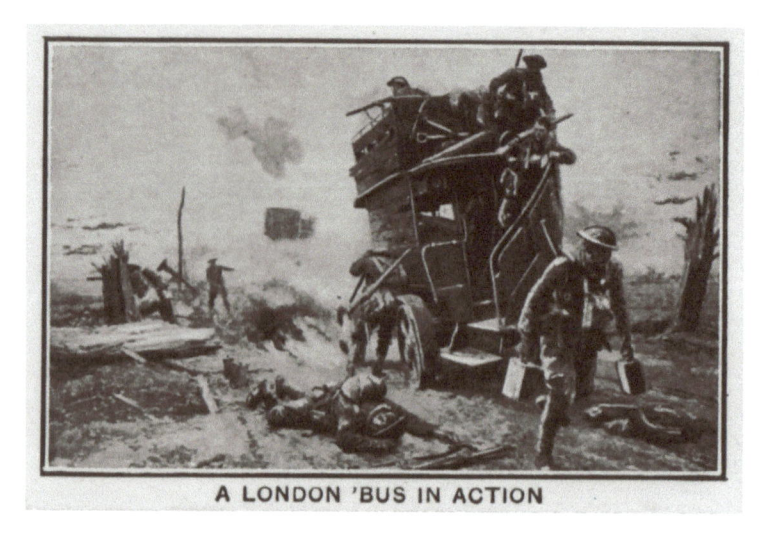

Fig. 10.7 A London bus in action, shown on contemporary cigarette card. Given with 'Triumph' (unidentified publisher)

and a similar Daimler bus, and resulted in a scarcity of buses on the streets of London.

The Anglo-French Hospital, No. 2, Le Château Tourlaville, near Cherbourg

Following the fall of Antwerp, it was not obvious what the next move would be for the unit. The WNSL again set to work collecting money for supplies and equipment. The X-ray apparatus was replaced by a generous donation from Sir Charles and Lady Parsons. Mabel Stobart accepted an invitation from the French Croix Rouge to establish a hospital in Cherbourg, and by November 1914, the corps was installed in the picturesque mediaeval Château Tourlaville, which was near Cherbourg [21]. The Château Tourlaville had been offered by Lady Guernsey as a hospital for French and Belgium wounded (Fig. 10.8). Florence's position was as 'Radiographer and Head of the Staff' at this Anglo-French Hospital, No. 2, Château Tourlaville, Cherbourg, which was under the care of the French Red Cross and the St. John Ambulance Association [22]. The unit was made up of 45 women with Florence leading a team of 6 woman doctors (including two fully qualified surgeons), 15 nurses, 10 orderlies, 3 motors and 4 motor ambulances and Mabel as the directrice. The only male element was supplied by some local French reservists who helped to draw water and to carry patients from the ambulances. The disused château was transformed into a modern hospital. The building was not well suited for a hospital, and Florence and her colleagues had to arrange for sanitation, water and

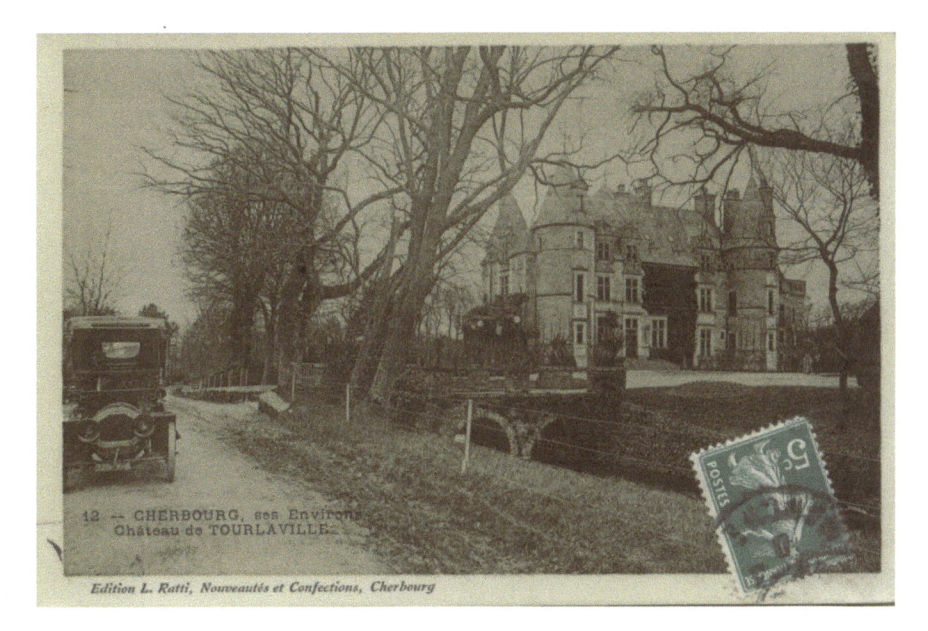

Fig. 10.8 Château de Tourlaville on a contemporary postcard (Edition L Ratti, Cherbourg)

heating, and even had to generate their own electricity, which was for lighting the hospital and for the X-ray machine. The generator was powered by a stream, which ran through the grounds. Life at the château was not easy, and whilst the doctors and nurses had more experience of human suffering and sickness, this was not the case for the orderlies who were generally from privileged backgrounds and had no experience of the terrible sights or manual work encountered in a military hospital. Stobart said that the pluck, determination and loyalty of the women could not be too highly praised. A week after reaching Cherbourg, the hospital's 72 beds were filled by the French with badly wounded casualties. At this point of the war, the French wounded were coming up by ship from Dunkirk to Cherbourg. Those with minor wounds were diverted to the south, and only the more badly wounded were retained. The casualties that they received were therefore the more serious cases, and many had septic fractures due to contamination with bacteria from the soil. Florence took radiographs to demonstrate the positions of the fractures for reduction and to locate shrapnel and bullets prior to surgical extraction (Fig. 10.9). Florence used her privately given X-ray apparatus and her Coolidge tube. Full use was made of localising devices such as the Mackenzie Davidson localising stand [23] and the Pirie stereoscope. The surgeons required as much help as possible to locate and remove small pieces of broken rifle bullets. It was whilst at Cherbourg that Florence discovered how to differentiate a sequestrum, or dead bone, from living bone by radiography.

Florence wrote "We horrified the French by insisting on fresh air, with the result that all visitors, medical as well as lay, remarked how ruddy and well our patients

Fig. 10.9 Elbow with severe injuries from shrapnel. The exact injury and foreign material are shown well and would have been difficult to assess clinically. (Stoney FA. The Women's Imperial League Hospital. Arch Roentg Ray 1915; 19:388–393. (acknowledgments to the BJR and with permission)

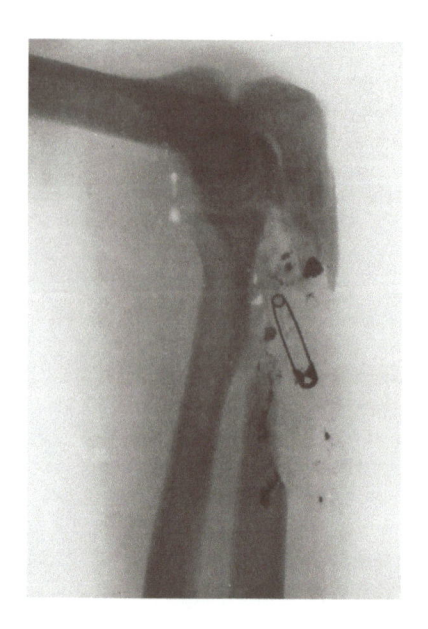

looked, unlike the white faces you see in most of the hospitals. The consulting surgeon for the whole of the Cherbourg district came to see our hospital, thinking it was a waste of time to go to a place only staffed by women doctors, but after spending a couple of hours going thoroughly round the wards he wrote 'L'hôpital de Tourlaville est très bien organisé, les malades sont très bien soignés, et les chirurgiennes sont de valeur égale aux chirurgiens les meilleurs' (The Hospital of Tourlaville is very well organized, the sick very well cared for, and the surgeons are of equal value to the best surgeons)". The patients were also appreciative and Lance-Corporal F Reynolds of the 2nd Oxford and Bucks. Light Infantry said in the Daily News of 9 January 1915 that "Lady doctors do all the work—no men at all, so you can guess I am all right. George and I were the only two spared out of six in our trench. Don't you think I had a fine birthday?'

Florence worked with one of Madame Österberg's old students at Cherbourg. This was Emma Sylvia Cowles (1881–1975), who subsequently worked in France for the American Red Cross and after the war for the Society of Friends (Quakers) Anglo-American Mission in Germany and Poland. Cowles had left the Österberg College in 1903. Cowles was a masseuse and was of the strong opinion that 'massage and medical gymnastic movements have been much used to help in the cure of soldiers wounded during this war' [24]. Cowles combined massage and electrical treatment, as did Florence. Cowles noted that 'At Le Château Tourlaville almost half the whole number of patients, all of whom came to us direct from the front, and were serious cases, had massage at one time or another, and it seems a great pity that far more massage is not being done by competent people in the military hospitals as a whole'.

In 1915, Florence visited Dr. Agnes Savill (1865–1964) at the SWH at Royaumont, which was about 25 miles from Paris. Savill had joined the staff of the Scottish Women's Hospitals, going to France in May 1915, and being placed in charge of the X-ray and electrotherapy departments, serving until the end of 1916. Savill recollected that Florence 'freely placed at my disposal all that she had learned of war radiology. Her knowledge of anatomy made her work in this department of exceptional aid to surgeons'. In her BJR, obituary of Florence, Savill said 'Always I found her the same helpful, generous colleague, reliable, thorough, persevering, accurate in all she undertook. Her charming and welcome smile, her eyes with the bright twinkle behind the glasses, her amusing and entertaining comments—at radiological gatherings we shall all miss that quiet pioneer, that little figure with a great heart'.

By the March of 1915, the steady stream of wounded going to Tourlaville had been diverted to other hospitals, and it became possible for the hospital to close and for Florence to return to England. In April 1915, Mabel Stobart led a fresh unit of volunteer doctors and nurses and travelled to Serbia where the military situation was very difficult [19]. After they arrived, a tented hospital was set up in Kragujevatz. The Stobart Unit performed magnificently, particularly during the catastrophic 'great retreat' of the Serbian Army, and the Chief Officer of the Serbian medical staff said of Mabel 'You have made everyone believe that a woman can overcome and endure all the war difficulties ... you can be sure, esteemed Madam, that you have won the sympathies of the whole of Serbia' [21]. Serbian affection for the British nurses remains fresh to this day.

Fulham Military Hospital, Hammersmith

In March 1915, Florence was one of five women doctors who were accepted for full-time work under the War Office by Sir Alfred Keogh. She was appointed as Head of the X-ray and Electrical Department of the Fulham Military Hospital (FMH) and when she took up her post was the first woman doctor to work under the War Office in England, taking up her post about a fortnight before Louisa Garrett Anderson opened the Endell Street Hospital in London. For a long time, Florence was the only female member of the medical staff at FMH. During the war, 265 women doctors served the War Office under a definite contract, and of these, the majority served in home hospitals [25]. The Scottish Women's Hospital units and the Stobart Unit were never attached to the British RAMC.

The mood of the nation had changed by 1915 from the enthusiasm of August 1914. It had initially been believed that the war would be short, and therefore there was no real preparation for either a prolonged conflict or for coping with the large numbers of casualties. The voluntary hospitals responded to the need; however, more facilities would be needed. Whilst the voluntary hospitals could look after both civilians and soldiers as patients, this would not be possible for the Poor Law workhouses, even though the workhouses had a medical role their communities.

The workhouses engendered a feeling of dislike and fear as a place of last resort for the very poor, and if they were to be used for war work, then the workhouse infirmaries had to be taken over completely. This proved to be the case in Fulham, and on 15 March 1915, the Fulham board of Poor Law Guardians were told by the Local Government Board that the War Office wanted to requisition the workhouse and infirmary.

In 1884, the Fulham Union Infirmary had been opened in Dunstan Road and was situated north of the workhouse. The infirmary was large, catering for 486 chronically sick workhouse inmates and had a staff of 2 doctors and 31 nurses. Initially, the patients were medical in nature; however, as time passed, the proportion of surgical cases increased. An operating room was installed in 1905, and a nurses' home was opened. There had been an X-ray department at the workhouse infirmary, and in 1914, before the war, it was stated that with improved apparatus 50 skiagrams (radiographs) were made, as well as a large number of fluoroscopic examinations.

The workhouse inmates were transferred in 1915 for the changed role of the site, and the new hospital was named the Fulham Military Hospital, although still remaining under the control of the Board of Guardians. The buildings were capacious and accommodated 1130 beds, but all beds were for other ranks and none for officers, and this is presumably why Florence had been appointed. It could be questioned if Florence would have been appointed to an officer's hospital, and one would suspect that the answer would be an emphatic negative. In November 1915, Syon House in Brentford, which was the home of the Duke of Northumberland, was attached to the FMH as an auxiliary hospital for officers. King George V and Queen Mary visited many war hospitals, and in December 1915, FMH was visited by Queen Mary. The medical staff of the infirmary was supplemented by staff from the RAMC. There were visiting consultants, and some were distinguished, such as Samuel A Kinnier Wilson (1878–1937) who provided neurological consultations.

The department was busy, and in the 6 months leading up to January 1916, 5530 radiographs were taken. Florence both took the radiographs and reported the results to the referring clinicians and also set up a small treatment department where she treated both 'nerve' and goitre cases. Florence was using nerve stimulation to assess the degree of trauma to nerves and to exclude functional paralysis. Florence had a staff of VAD assistants and trained two of them to take over some of the radiographic work. The X-ray facilities needed to be expanded in 1917. Florence personally examined over 15,000 cases, and the use of the fluoroscope added considerably to her radiation exposure. This was also the case for Marie Curie whose radiation injuries are partly attributable to her war work.

Foreign bodies could be located either using a purely radiographic technique or else be located fluoroscopically. In the fluoroscopic technique, the patient is placed on a stretcher, and an under-couch tube is used. By moving the fluorescent screen and using a simple parallax technique, the depth of the foreign body may be determined. The fluoroscopic technique had the advantage of speed and the avoidance of processing of X-ray plates; however, there was a higher radiation dose to the operator. The apparatus of the period was now powerful enough to diagnose chest injuries [26, 27], and the use of stereoscopy was commonplace as recommended by

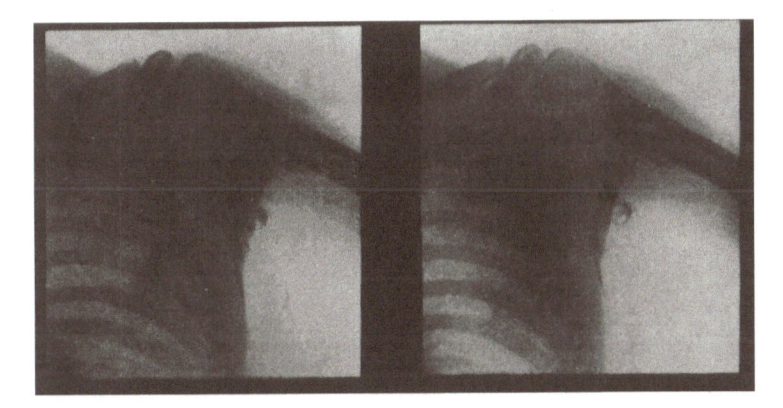

Fig. 10.10 A stereographic X-ray examination of a soldiers injury in 1915. (from The Graphic 18 December 1915)

Sir James Mackenzie Davidson (Fig. 10.10). Florence also emphasised the need of looking at fractures in two projections and the inadequacy of assessing a fracture on a single radiographic plate [28].

Florence's work was particularly concerned with localization of bullets, and her knowledge of anatomy greatly helped the surgeons. This was particularly illustrated in a case described by John Lee who was an Australian RAMC surgical colleague at FMH. Lee describes a soldier who had developed an intracranial abscess with retained shrapnel [29]. Lee had tried unsuccessfully to extract the shrapnel with an electromagnet, and then it occurred to him that it might be possible to see and remove it under X-ray fluoroscopic guidance. Lee discussed the patient with Florence, and on 9 November 1915, a surgical operation was performed. With Florence's assistance, it was possible to see both the probe and the fragment and their relation to each other. The fragment had been pulled by the magnet and was lodged in the cerebral substance. Forceps were then passed to a depth of 4 in and the shrapnel was removed. This is an early example of radiologically assisted intervention, and Lee recorded his indebtedness to Florence.

A somewhat more curious case at FMH involved a 42-year-old patient with asthma [30] (Fig. 10.11). He was admitted in December 1917 with a neck wound and chronic asthma. He had previously had a neck injury but now presented with rheumatism, asthma and a swelling in the neck. On radiography, Florence was surprised to see a paediatric tracheostomy tube, which was shown by stereoscopy to be in the trachea. His mother recounted that he had suffered from 'bronchitic croup' in 1877. The surgeon John Lee was again involved, and apart from the superficial abscess, a child's tracheostomy tube was removed. There was rapid healing, and the asthma and hoarseness disappeared.

The FMH held regular fortnightly clinical meetings when interesting or difficult cases were presented, and Florence actively contributed. There were discussions about the management of complicated fractures, and in one case, Florence suggested that chronic pulmonary changes in a patient with syphilitic laryngitis were more

Fig. 10.11 Paediatric tracheostomy tube revealed in the radiograph. (from Stoney F. Two Skiagrams. Arch Rad Elect. Ther. 1920 24:352–354 (with permission BJR))

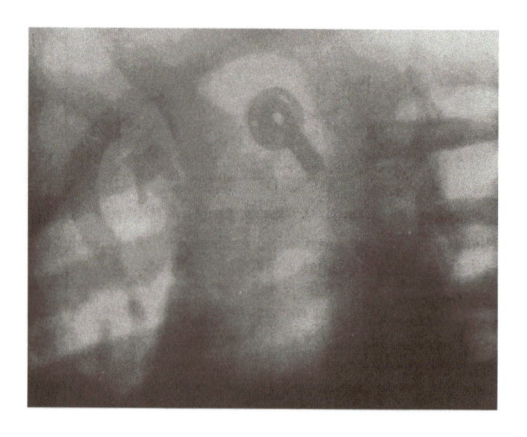

likely to be related to syphilis than to tuberculosis. Syphilis was a significant problem with British soldiers in France, and pulmonary tuberculosis was also common. Daniells and Dachtler writing in 1911 [31] described a series of patients and gave the radiographic and clinical features. That Florence suggested this diagnosis is evidence of her wide knowledge and general reading and a time long before radiologists specialised in defined clinical areas.

She also was able to identify the presence of sequestra (dead bone), and the removal of this greatly aided the healing of these injuries. A total of 18 other hospitals and camps sent her cases for skilled X-ray localisation of bullets and for treatments using both X-rays and electrotherapy. Florence describes six cases that she had seen at Cherbourg and Fulham at a meeting of the electrotherapeutic section of the RSM on 18 February 1916 [32]. Two of the cases were of sequestra following fractures, and Florence wrote that 'there are two fragments: one throws a normal shadow and is living bone, and the other throws a denser shadow, and was diagnosed as a sequestrum (confirmed at operation)'. Major Maurice G Parsons, the officer in charge at FMH and previously of the South African Medical Corps, fully recognised the debt that the surgeon owed to the X-rays and to the work of Florence, as did Major John R Lee the Officer in Charge of the Surgical Division.

Elizabeth Garrett Anderson died on 17 December 1917 at the grand age of 81, having contributed so much durting her long life to the women's movement in medicine. A memorial service was held at the church of the Military Hospital in Endell Street on 22 December 1917. In his address, the Bishop of Stepney spoke of 'the great work of medical women, and their swift triumph over the forces of reaction'. Elizabeth Garrett Anderson 'whose energy and fortitude had done so much to break down barriers and increase the opportunities of service for women'. The service was well attended with representatives from many organisations to which she had contributed, and many individuals were present including Louisa Martindale and Florence Stoney [33].

Florence's contributions and those of Fulham Military Hospital were considered of national significance since, with additional work by Capt. H E Gamlen, a collection of radiographs, called 'skiagrams, many of them of great merit', were included in the Army Medical Collection of War Specimens held at the Royal College of Surgeons of England [34]. Harold Gamlen (d1943) was a radiologist from the Royal Victoria Infirmary in Newcastle and was major in the RAMC at No. 11 General Hospital BEF and consulting radiologist to the Indian Expeditionary Force. The collection was started in November 1914 by Lieutenant General Sir Alfred Keogh (1857–1936) who was Director General of the Army Medical Services. The aim was to provide a collection of war specimens that would be useful to the RAMC. The collection went on display on 11 October 1917 being opened by Keogh in three rooms of the then vacated Hunterian Museum of the Royal College of Surgeons of England, and the radiographs were displayed in room 3. The display of specimens of recently deceased soldiers whilst the war is still in progress may seem to us as rather inappropriate or macabre. Certainly, there has been a discussion of the ethics of collecting and displaying such material, and Alberti has stated 'The work that went into the collection and the post-war debates about the ownership of these specimens demonstrate the value of human remains in medical museums in the early twentieth century' [35]. The ethical issues of displaying radiographs will obviously be different from those of displaying bodily parts. The contributions that Florence made to the War Office collection was of use to the great anatomist Sir Arthur Keith (1866–1955) who was writing describing a familial bony condition that became known as diaphyseal aclasis [36]. Keith described several patients and said, 'For a third case, also added to the War Office Collection, I am indebted to Dr Florence Stoney. In this case the man was aged 29 and the modelling process had been much less retarded than in the two younger men. In Dr Stoney's case a brother and four maternal uncles were affected with the same disorder. A survey of recorded cases shows that about half the subjects have one or more relatives similarly affected, and that the disorder is Mendelian in its incidence' (Fig. 10.12).

At the end of the war, there was a world pandemic of Spanish flu, and FMH was affected like so many other institutions with many staff and patients becoming ill and dying in November 1918. It is poignant to reflect on the position of those who had survived hostilities only to succumb to illness. The military use of FMH came to an end in 1919, and it was renamed Fulham Hospital. Ultimately, the hospital was incorporated into the Charing Cross Hospital group.

Soldier's Heart or DAH

Florence was interested in Soldier's Heart or Disordered Action of the Heart (DAH) and believed that some cases were related to hyperthyroidism. DAH was discussed at the regular clinical meetings at FMH, and there were many examples in the hospital. The topic of heart disease in soldiers was an important one, and there was a large contemporary literature. There was an interesting paper by Carey Coombs (1879–1932) in December 1915 when Coombs was a captain in the RAMC (Territorial Force) [37]. Coombs was a distinguished cardiologist and described the characteristic heart sound that is heard when the heart is affected by acute rheumatic fever. Men were needed in the army, and determining the exact nature of any cardiac

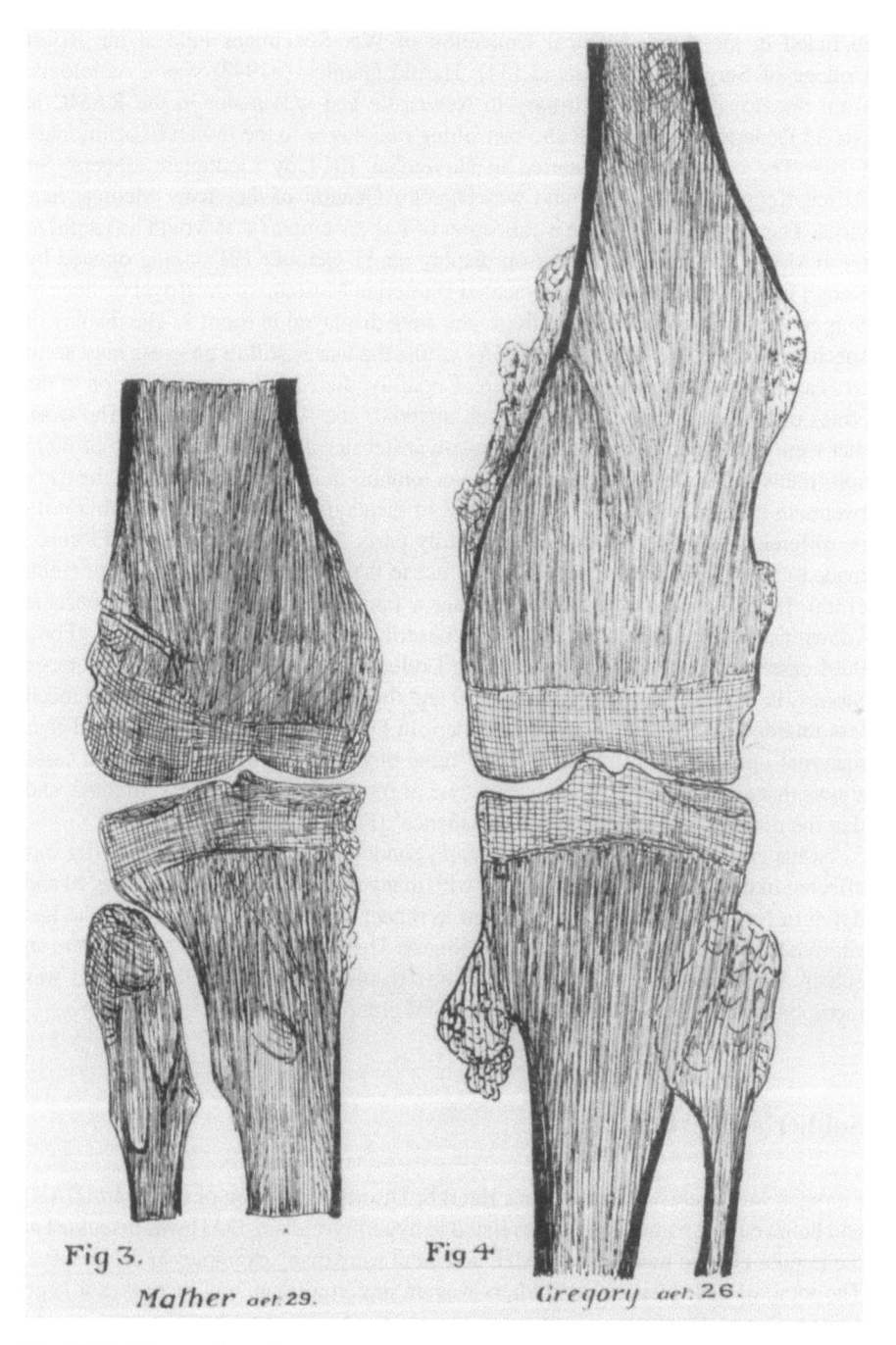

Fig. 10.12 Florence Stoney's case used by Sir Arthur Keith. (from Keith A. Studies of the anatomical changes which accompany certain growth-disorders of the human body. J Anatomy, 1920; 54 (P2–3): 101–115)

abnormality that was found on medical assessment was important. Men with significant heart disease would be discharged from the army; however, they might be fit for work on the home front. Men with milder disease such as aortic regurgitation or mitral stenosis may still be useful in service in England or in the training of recruits. Coombs thought that the symptoms experienced were more important than any signs elicited by the doctor and that every soldier should be judged individually. There was a large group of soldiers with DAH, and many more were seen than were commonly encountered in civilian practice. The average age of patients suffering from DAH was 24, and they were usually slender in build. For some reason, DAH was commoner in those who had served in Gallipoli than in Flanders. Coombs thought that nervous stress could release a toxin and that 'the nervous factor is by far the most important'.

Florence wrote in the *British Medical Journal* of 13 May 1916 [38] that Sir James Barr had proposed the hormonal cause for soldier's heart, and Francis Hernaman-Johnson and Percival White had thought that the cause might be Graves' disease and that therefore X-ray treatment may be helpful. Florence presented her results for the X-ray treatment of DAH, and since she had cured a number of cases, she felt that the association was proven. There was a well-known relation between hyperthyroidism and heart disease, and at least superficially, the symptoms of thyrotoxicosis may resemble the agitation and nervousness seen in shell shock or NYDN (Not Yet Diagnosed [Nervous]) as the army doctors were then instructed to call these suspected mental disorders. Sir Arthur Hurst had considerable experience of the medical diseases of war and had worked in Salonica in the Great War [39]. Hurst believed that soldiers should not have attention drawn to the heart, and so the term effort syndrome was introduced by Sir Thomas Lewis in 1917. Hurst agreed with Florence and stated that in a small proportion of cases of DAH, there was overactivity of the thyroid and also the adrenal glands due to prolonged nervous strain. He believed that thyroid hyperplasia was rare in soldiers and also noted that occasionally men took thyroid tablets to avoid enlistment.

However, in addition to her war work, Florence was able to continue with some aspects of her civilian work. In December of 1917, Florence published a paper showing the good results that she had achieved in the treatment of uterine fibroids with X-ray therapy [40]. Florence had seen the patient in the February of 1917. The patient was a married 42-year-old woman who had significant symptoms from her fibroids. The patient received eight X-ray treatments over a 3-month period, and following treatment, the patient's menstrual periods ceased, and the uterus significantly decreased in size. The patient's symptoms were relieved, and Florence said that the patient was well and strong and was very pleased with the final result. This patient was the fourth patient with fibroids that she had treated. Currently, we do not commonly treat benign disease with radiotherapy; however, at that time, knowledge of radiobiology and the long-term consequences of such radiation treatment was only poorly understood. However, Florence's work prefigures contemporary nonsurgical treatments for uterine fibroids such as noninvasive MR-guided focussed ultrasound ablation and angiographically guided therapeutic embolization.

Florence was generous of both her time and money where there was a need, and a record is made of her contribution of one guinea to a fund for the reimbursement of a Dr. J H Bell for his legal expenses, two guineas to the Belgian Doctors' and Pharmacists' Relief Fund and one guinea to help support two scholarships for women in commercial chemistry.

The First World War changed many things, both in social attitudes, and also in medical practice. Vincent Cirillo has demonstrated the importance of the war for the development of the medical speciality of radiology [41]. The army surgeons had become accustomed to working as part of a team in cooperation with radiologists, and this continued after the war. After the war, the number of radiologists steadily increased, and with the introduction of the Coolidge tube, the X-ray equipment became easier to use. Radiography was also developed, and the Society of Radiographers was founded in 1920. The First World War legitimised the discipline of military radiology if indeed there had been any lingering doubts.

References

1. Anon. Wizardry of the X-ray, how the radiograph tracks down bits of frightfulness. The War Budget. 1916;7:15.
2. Hampson W. Localising simply and immediately. Arch Roentg Ray. 1914;14:200–3.
3. Thomas AMK. The first 50 years of military radiology 1895–1945. Eur J Radiol. 2007;63:214–9.
4. Ramsay M. The Times. 12 October 1932.
5. Daily News and Leader 4 August 1914.
6. Obituary. Florence Stoney. Lancet. October 1932;15:871.
7. Leneman L. Medical women at war, 1914–1918. Med Hist. 1994;38:160–77.
8. Treves F. The elephant man and other reminiscences. London: Cassell; 1923.
9. Leneman L. Medical women in the first world war, ranking nowhere. Br Med J. 1993;307:1592.
10. Malleson HA. Woman doctor. Mary Murdoch of Hull. London: Sidgwick & Hackson; 1919.
11. QARANC History. https://qaranc.co.uk/history.php. Accessed 25 Jan 2019.
12. Votes for Women - Friday 21 August 1914.
13. Stobart MA St Clair. Miracles and adventures, an autobiography. London: Rider; 1936.
14. Stobart MA St Clair. The open secret. London: The Psychic Press; 1947.
15. McNaughtan SB. A woman's diary of the war. London: Thomas Nelson and Son; 1915.
16. McNaughtan SB. My war experiences on two continents. London: John Murray; 1919.
17. Mabel L Ramsay. Notes and diary from 16 September to 14 October 1914.
18. Florence A Stoney. The Stobart hospital in Antwerp. Votes for Women - Friday 06 November 1914.
19. Stobart MA St Clair. The flaming sword in Serbia and elsewhere. London: Hodder and Stoughton; 1916.
20. Kidner RW. The London motor-bus 1896–1975. 5th revised ed. Dorset: The Oakwood Press; 1975.
21. McLaren B. Women of the war. London: Hodder and Stoughton; 1917.
22. Stoney FA. The women's imperial league hospital. Arch Roentg Ray. 1915;19:388–93.
23. Davidson JM. A method of localization by means of Roentgen rays. Arch Roentg Ray. 1897;2:64–8.
24. Cowles S. Massage in a French war hospital. J Sci Phys Train. 1916;23(8)
25. Medical Women of the War. Globe. 12 November 1919.

References

26. Rea RL. Chest radiography at a casualty clearing station. London: HK Lewis; 1919.
27. Borzell FF. Some observations on the radiographic findings in a series of 333 chests examined at a base hospital in France. Amer Jn Radiol. 1919;6:573–4.
28. Metcalfe J. J Roy Soc Med (Elect Ther). 1919;12:72–5.
29. Lee JR. Removal of intracranial foreign body under X rays. Br Med J. 1916;1:447.
30. Stoney F. Two Skiagrams. Arch Rad Elect Ther. 1920;24:352–4.
31. Daniells RP, Dachter, HW. Syphilitic manifestations in the lungs resembling pulmonary tuberculosis with report of cases. In: Proceedings of the 12th annual meeting, American Society of Roentgenology 1911:97–106.
32. Stoney F. J Roy Soc Med (Elect Ther). 1916;9:93–4.
33. Memorial Service for Mrs. Garrett Anderson. Common Cause - Friday 28 December 1917.
34. The Army Medical Collection of War Specimens held at the Royal College of Surgeons of England. Br Med J 1917;ii:531–34.
35. Alberti SJMM. The 'regiment of skeletons': a first world war medical collection. Soc Hist Med. 2015;28:108–33.
36. Keith A. Studies of the anatomical changes which accompany certain growth-disorders of the human body. J Anat. 1920;54(P2–3):101–15.
37. Coombs C. Cardiac disease and disorders in warfare. Bristol Med Chir J. 1915;33:149–56.
38. Stoney FA. The "soldier's heart" and its relation to thyroidism. Br Med J. 1916;1:706.
39. Hurst AH. Medical diseases of war. 2nd ed. London: Edward Arnold; 1941.
40. Stoney, FA. Fibroid uterus treated by X-rays. Br Med J, 1917;ii:723. (Br Med J 1917;2:723).
41. Cirillo VJ. The Spanish–American war and military radiology. Am J Radiol. 2000:1233–9.

Chapter 11
Chateau de Chanteloup

During the months of Florence's absence, first in Belgium and then in France, Edith had much time on her own to consider how she might best support her country, now at war. The newspapers were filled with dire warnings about future Zeppelin raids, following the bombardment of Scarborough by three German battleships on 16 December, and the first enemy bomb dropped from an aircraft on Dover a few days later. As might be expected, Edith did what she could to support her sister. She assisted in the organisation of supplies through the London office of the WISL and helped Florence with the X-ray equipment in Cherbourg. But she was frustrated that she was unable to play anything other than a supporting role, watching as the men she knew volunteered to join the armed forces, and admiring her professionally qualified younger sister for her ability to make a contribution as a radiologist. And the war, which was imagined to be over by Christmas, was clearly going to last very much longer.

Not long after Florence escaped from Antwerp, they heard from Australia that their brother Robert had died at the age of 48 on 9 November. He had suffered from tuberculosis for many years, and his death had been long anticipated. The three sisters shared their memories of their brother, wondering how his children, their nieces and nephews, would manage. It was typical of Florence that she immediately wrote suggesting that the four children should be sent to London to complete their education. It was an emotional and unrealistic offer. Gertrude remembered them as the little ones she last saw 5 years earlier. In reality, Archie was now 20 and had a scholarship to take him through his university engineering degree in Australia, whilst the youngest, William, was by now 15 and would soon be finished at school. Their Australian grandmother and uncles would take care of them. Once the war was over, they thought, they should keep in touch by writing regularly and perhaps even by making a visit.

As Belgian refugees flooded into Britain as a result of the German advances, Edith joined the Hampstead Garden City Belgian Relief Committee. This organisation converted a local club into a home for 40 Belgian refugees, where they stayed whilst the committee members found work and permanent accommodation for

---

The original version of this chapter was revised. A correction to this chapter is available at https://doi.org/10.1007/978-3-030-16561-1_19

© Springer Nature Switzerland AG 2019
A. Thomas, F. Duck, *Edith and Florence Stoney, Sisters in Radiology*, Springer Biographies, https://doi.org/10.1007/978-3-030-16561-1_11

them in the area. She helped to set up a VAD Hospital at 4 Lyndhurst Gardens, Hampstead, not far from where she now lived. Searching for a particular way to help, she volunteered to drive her car for the Medical Commandant [1].

When the sisters had volunteered their support the previous August, no one had any idea what a horrific and lengthy conflict the war would become, and they surely believed that their assistance would be required for a few weeks or months at most. Florence only arranged a 6-month leave of absence from her post at the New Hospital for Women to work in Antwerp. Now, after over 6 months of war with the forces already bogged down in the trenches of Northern Europe, there could have been no illusions in Edith's mind when she committed herself to following in her sister's footsteps. Edith appears to have made a decision to engage more fully with radiology at the end of 1914, when she became a member of the Rontgen Society, a large multidisciplinary organisation devoted to medical radiology. Florence had joined in 1903 when she had become the Medical Electrician at the Royal Free Hospital. Now Edith decided to become a member also, implying that she intended to become much more involved with the practice of radiology, stimulated by her sister's war efforts.

The Scottish Women's Hospital for Foreign Service

Very shortly after Edith was asked to resign from the LSMW in March 1915, she contacted the Scottish Women's Hospitals for Foreign Service (SWH) to offer her skills to this organisation. The SWH was arguably the most successful all-women hospital service to operate during WWI. This organisation had been formed at the outbreak of war by the Edinburgh graduate Dr. Elsie Inglis to give medical support in the field of battle. Their first military hospital had already been set up under the French *Croix Rouge* in the *Abbaye de Royaumont*, about 35 miles north of Paris, and it had opened as *Hôpital Auxiliaire* 301 on 13 January 1915 [2]. It became the longest-standing hospital under women's leadership to operate in France during the war. Eventually the SWH established other hospitals in France, Serbia, Corsica, Russia, Salonika, and elsewhere, in which all the medical, nursing, and administrative staff were women. Vigorous and successful fundraising, raising in total over £500,000, supported the operation. The funds for Royaumont were raised by the London Branch of the National Union of Women's Suffrage Societies, so the resulting hospital unit was often referred to as the London Unit.

Edith knew of this fundraising on behalf of the SWH by the NUWSS, so it would not have been a surprise to hear that her old Cambridge College had launched a similar fundraising initiative. Towards the end of 1914, a joint Committee of Girton and Newnham Colleges had been formed, following a suggestion from a Mrs. Jacob, a past Newnham student, to raise funds to equip a hospital unit for service in Western Europe [3]. By then the SWH had already raised funds not only for the Royaumont Unit but also for a second one bound for Serbia. It was initially agreed to set a target of £1000, split between appeals through each of the two Cambridge colleges, which would have been sufficient to equip a new SWH hospital of 100 beds. It would be given the name 'The Girton and Newnham Unit'. It turned out that the SWH Committee in Edinburgh was already planning a third hospital, and the Scottish organisation made an urgent request that the colleges gave a guarantee of the funds with as little delay as possible. The appeal exceeded expectations, and by the beginning of 1915, £1809 12s 5d was handed over to the SWH, raised from present and former students of Girton and Newnham Colleges. (Approximately £4160 was raised by the end of the war. This would be worth about £300,000 today but would have purchased considerably more than that in terms of labour and materials at today's prices.)

Initially there had been discussions that the Unit would be assigned to a hospital at Creil, at an important railway hub not far from Royaumont, which was being prepared to treat an outbreak of cases of typhoid, or enteric, fever. Such a unit would have had no particular need for a specialist X-ray department. However, such was the dynamic nature of wartime medical care that, by the time the wards had been prepared, the epidemic had subsided, so an expansion of 100 beds at Royaumont was considered. Nevertheless, the funds raised had far outrun the original target, making a larger and more ambitious project possible. By the end of April, the French War Office indicated to the SWH Committee that it would be willing to accept a field unit under canvas close to the front line, a decision that had General Joseph Joffre's personal approval. This was when Edith had been recruited, and the task was given to the Girton and Newnham Unit [4]. Unlike Royaumont, which operated under the direction of the French *Croix Rouge*, this closer association with the military was a new venture for the SWH and much depended on its success. As the French Army authorities under General Joffre knew, but was surely hidden from the SWH, a major summer offensive was being planned in Champagne Region in an attempt to break the trench-bound stalemate that had already become established across Eastern France. French casualties were already high from several battles in this area, and any hospital support would have been welcomed.

Within a month of being asked to leave the LSMW, Edith was recruited to run the X-ray department at this new SWH unit in France [5]. At the end of May, Edith attended her last executive meeting of the British Federation for University Women and told them she would shortly be off to France. Whilst her initial contract was for 6 months, in common with all other SWH staff, she would not permanently return to England until 1919.

Edith brought an unusual set of skills to the SWH, and her new colleagues took a long time to understand, and use effectively, what she could offer to the organisation. For the immediate future, they really wanted a doctor who could do radiography. In reality, there were very few women who had any radiological experience at this time, and even fewer who would be willing to leave their medical practice and go to France. On the other hand, Edith had more than a decade of practical experience with X-ray equipment, starting in 1902 when she was tasked with the care of Florence's 'Rontgen Ray apparatus' at the Royal Free. She now saw herself as a technical consultant in radiography and medical electricity, with sufficient awareness of the clinical applications, learned from her sister, to enable her to work in a hospital as a radiographer. As the war progressed, Edith and her senior colleagues worked out her role as they went along, but the clash of expectations would result in a great deal of irritation to both Edith and some of her SWH colleagues. Nevertheless, Edith looked like a good bet at the time, and they took her on.

The role that Edith eventually created for herself was quite new and would later be known as a medical physicist. But no such function had yet been named, let alone created, and the formation of the Hospital Physicists' Association was still nearly 30 years in the future. The role included the specification, procurement and maintenance of equipment, its clinical use when needed to support surgeons and physicians and the training of others in new and advanced techniques. In the absence of a suitable job title, the Newnham College record of war service gives Edith's role as 'Head Radiologist and Engineer with rank as Specialist Doctor', a pragmatic description that recognised her lack of formal medical qualification, whilst emphasising the importance of her technical and scientific ability. Sometimes she was referred to as an electrician or as a radiographer, a term widely used to refer to anyone who took X-ray pictures, whether they had medical training or not. The distinction between radiologist and radiographer was yet to crystallise and was only fully defined in Britain with the formation of the Society of Radiographers after the war.

Florence discussed with Edith the importance of having a technical assistant for the X-ray service, and Edith gained the agreement of the Committee to this appointment during a visit she made to Scotland in mid-May. In principle, Edith would have preferred to have recruited a woman to be her technician. Not only would that have been in line with her own view, that women were capable of filling any role filled by men in peace-time, it also was completely aligned with the central tenet of the Scottish Women's Hospitals as an all-women outfit. Florence had not been so principled when she recruited George Mallett as her mechanic in Antwerp and Cherbourg. Florence pointed out that she had trained Mallett in X-ray technology that he was reliable and competent, and, moreover, he was available and keen to find another post that would postpone his recruitment into the army. Edith appreciated that her alternative, to accept an untrained orderly once she arrived in France, would be considerably less satisfactory, took a pragmatic decision and proposed Mallett's appointment to the Scottish Committee. He was recruited, and Edith found him to be a 'clever, delicate, artizan lad' [6] (Fig. 11.1). By accompanying Edith to Troyes it was tacitly understood that George could avoid call-up by associating himself in another way with the war effort. He stayed with Edith until June 1917, and his later SWH war record identifies him as a radiographer. Otherwise, apart from a couple of male drivers, the staff in the Girton and Newnham Unit was entirely female.

Edith was not the only woman physicist to offer her services to radiography at this time. In France, Marie Curie was raising funds for more X-ray ambulances (see Chap. 14) and was also planning to set up her school of radiography in Paris to provide the skills required to operate X-ray equipment. In July 1915, just as Edith was setting up her own X-ray equipment in France, and on the other side of the battle lines, the outstanding Austrian nuclear physicist Lise Meitner had also volunteered as an X-ray nurse-technician in the Austrian army [7]. She left Vienna on 4 August,

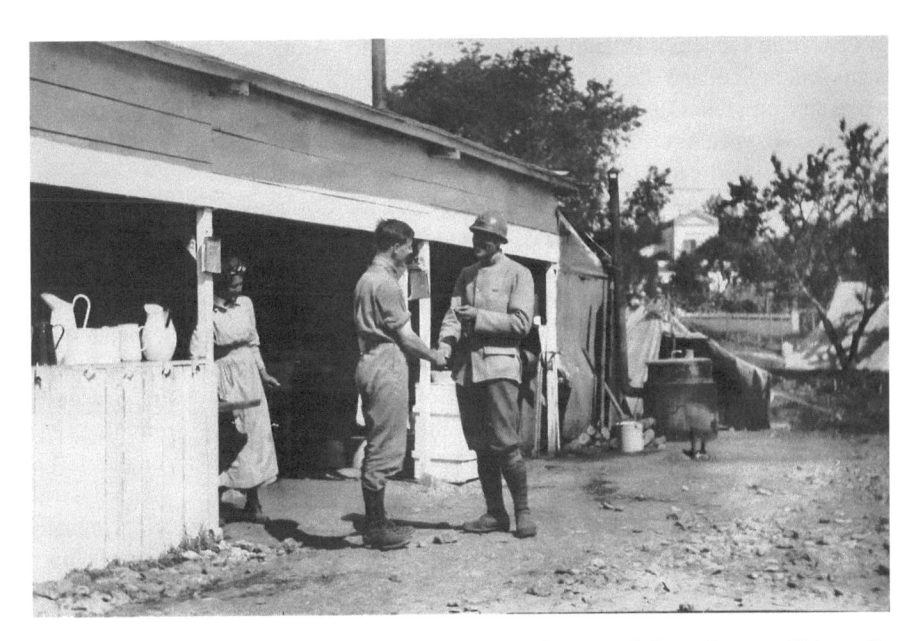

Fig. 11.1 Edith Stoney's assistant George Mallett greeting one of the patients at *Château De Chanteloup*. (University of Glasgow)

assigned to a military hospital in Lemberg on the Russian front (now Lviv in Ukraine), where she remained until early in 1916. Meitner worked in military hospitals for a year but then returned to Berlin to continue the experimental studies on beta decay of radium series for which she became internationally renowned. Each woman had become swept up within her own country's efforts to support the wounded, wherever they were.

Edith 'was probably the most brilliant of those who joined and certainly one of the most outstandingly useful' of those who offered their services to work for the SWH [8]. This statement from a senior medical colleague must be remembered, to be set against the personal criticisms of Edith from some of those who managed the SWH during the next few years. She made plans for her own X-ray department based on the experience that Florence had gained in Antwerp and in Cherbourg. She soon discovered that her own clear ideas were at odds with those of the organisation she was joining. Edith considered that she was bringing unique knowledge about modern X-ray equipment and techniques. She and Florence had detailed knowledge of the newest developments in X-ray technology and knew from experience that there was no fundamental reason why these could be put into operation even in a tented field hospital. Indeed, Edith looked forward to the unique challenge that was being presented to her. The officials in Edinburgh did not see it that way. For them, X-ray equipment was only one item to be purchased in the logistical challenge of implementing a new hospital overseas. They had a simple precedent. When setting up their first two hospitals, 6 months before, one at the Abbey of Royaumont north of Paris and a second, ill-fated, hospital in Serbia, they selected the standard pre-packed system from Frederick R. Butt and Co, designed for Army field operation. For the managers in Scotland, this was a very convenient, low-cost way of dealing with the necessary provision of X-rays, which required a minimal level of technical understanding. It was, for them, no different from buying an operating table or an ambulance, good value for money and was designed for the job.

This was not how Edith saw it, and she told the Committee so in no uncertain terms. Her position was completely misunderstood in Edinburgh, partly because of Edith's tendency to be rather abrupt in placing her case. Mrs. Jessie Laurie,[1] the Honorary Treasurer, who later became Edith's greatest confidant and supporter, was completely confused, thinking that Edith was arguing that she did not want an X-ray system at all. On 12 May she wrote 'I have all along understood that all the hospitals were more than anxious to get the benefit of our X-ray apparatus' but went on to observe that 'if this is the attitude Miss Stoney goes out in—of grumbling, and nothing being good enough—I think it is a pity that she has been taken on the staff at all'.

Edith wanted high-quality equipment and viewed the Committee as technically unsophisticated. She was able to draw on Florence's experience in setting up a radiological service under conditions of war. She wanted better tubes, concerned that the low tube ratings would result in long exposure times. The sisters may also have been concerned, even then, about the lack of provision to protect the operator from being harmed from exposure to radiation, a matter that would become of considerable significance by the end of the war.

There was also a question of cost. The set-up cost of several hundred pounds that was needed for a complete X-ray system, even a modest one, constituted a relatively large capital outlay for an organisation that fully depended on charitable donations. Whilst the committee fully accepted that a modern military hospital could not operate without an X-ray department, they were not prepared to consider the limitations that a low-cost system would impose.

Finally it was probably a matter of familiarity and confidence. The equipment that Edith took with her at this stage was not so different from that which the SWH was offering. The coils were both 12-inch, the interrupters were similar. However, by taking her own equipment, Edith was both following Florence's lead and making her own statement. She was independent of any constraints that might be imposed from Scotland. Instead of accepting the standard X-ray system that the SWH Council was prepared to authorise, she set about getting together her own system, as Florence had done the previous year. This was possible partly because Florence had been able to bring her equipment back from Cherbourg when she returned in March, and it was not needed in London. Any gaps were filled with new items that she bought herself. Her decision to invest a large amount of her own funds independently from the purchasing and management structures of the Scottish Women's Hospitals was to cause considerable conflict as time went by.

---

[1]Jessie Laurie was a non-militant suffragist, and a member of the Executive Committee of the Scottish Federation of Women's Suffrage Societies.

Amongst Florence's equipment was a 12-inch spark induction coil with condenser, a gift from their family friend Lady Margaret Parsons. They had a MacKenzie-Davidson mercury interrupter and a control board with ammeter. These precious and essential items were packed into specially designed boxes for transport. Other items were placed during June ready for dispatch to France [9]. Edith used three London suppliers. Most of the X-ray apparatus came from Schall & Sons, Electromedical Instrument Makers at 71 & 75 New Cavendish St., with the remainder from Newton & Wright, 72 Wigmore St. Over £170 worth of equipment was delivered to their home in Hampstead, to be dispatched onto France once Edith had satisfied herself that the hospital was ready to receive it. It comprised X-ray tubes, a fluorescent screen, a tube stand, a stereoscopic viewer, accumulator cells, intensifying screens, viewing boxes and a variety of meters and control boards. Aware of the need to protect herself from radiation, protection, she ordered diaphragms to limit the size of the beam and a lead protection box to cover the X-ray tube. Edith also included an oscilloscope tube, an addition that allowed her to display the electrical pulse across the X-ray tube and so to troubleshoot any malfunctioning of the total X-ray circuit, including the interrupter and diode valves. The Wehnelt radiometer, with its flat silver strip alongside a wedge of aluminium, mounted in front of a fluorescent screen, would allow Edith to judge the hardness of the X-ray beam. In addition, X-ray plates, chemicals and darkroom equipment for film processing were ordered from Jonathan Fallowfield, Central Photographic Stores, 146 Charing Cross Road. Edith later estimated that the total value of the equipment she had provided was £231:17:0, somewhere between £15,000 and £20,000 at today's prices.

Chateau de Chanteloup, Troyes

The 200-bed tented hospital where Edith was headed was in Troyes, the ancient capital of the Champagne district, surrounded by vineyards, about 100 miles southeast of Paris, and a similar distance south of the front line. From the beginning of the war, Troyes had become a true *Ville-hôpital* (hospital city). The French army health service had set up some 20 temporary hospitals there, mostly in schools in the city. In total, these military hospitals housed about 4000 beds [10]. The SWH hospital was the first tented hospital to be established in Europe during the war and as such caused considerable interest both from the soldiers and the authorities. The hospital rapidly gained a reputation for its high standard of nursing and medical care, giving confidence to those planning similar tented hospitals elsewhere.

Edith arrived towards the end of June, her departure from London slightly delayed, owning to residual commitments at the LSMW [11], and attendance at her last executive meeting of the British Federation for University Women on 19 June. Her first view of her new home was quite favourable. She was met at the station by the administrator, Mrs. Katherine Harley (1855–1917), who had transferred in the latter part of May from the SWH unit at Royaumont as part of the advance guard. They were picked up by the Australian *chauffeuse*, Olive Kelso King, who had accompanied Mrs.

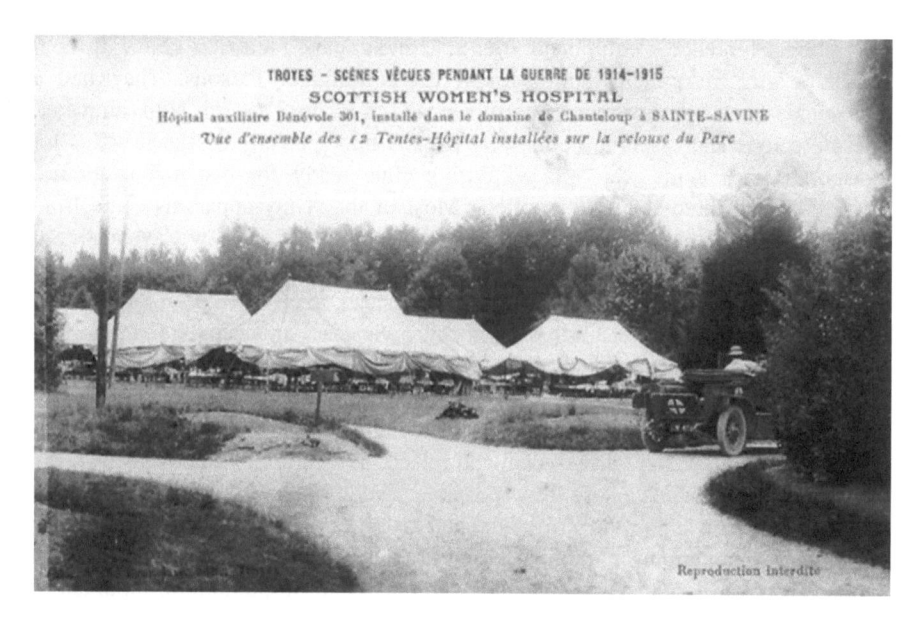

Fig. 11.2 The medical and surgical tents in the Girton and Newnham Unit Hospital in the grounds of *Château De Chanteloup*, Troyes. (Francis Tailleur)

Harley from Royaumont in her own 3-litre Alda. In just over a mile, they reached the *Château de Chanteloup* in Sainte-Savine, now an Eastern suburb of Troyes. The two large iron gates were open, flanked by the French *Tricolore* and the Union Jack. Above, in bold letters, were the words 'Scottish Women's Hospitals—L'Hôpital auxiliaire bénévole 301'. To the right, Edith could see the long main building, with its large windows, a chateau in name only, bright and airy and with enough accommodation for all the administrators and some of the medical and nursing staff. A line of large palms in tubs gave it a semi-tropical feel. In the middle of the park, about a hundred yards from the house, a double row of 12 marquee tents, 16 beds in each, had been erected to accommodate the patients (Fig. 11.2). Each bed was covered with a pink counterpane, and each had its own bedside table. She could see wooded walks through large trees, reminding her of the woods back home in Hampstead. In the meadow beyond, there were a few more tents for the night nurses and some of the doctors. Some new buildings had been recently added, a field kitchen in wood and red brick, a wooden bathroom block and a separate shed for dressing septic wounds. The operating theatre had been set up in the orangery [12].

Edith took stock of the women who would be her intimate colleagues, with whom she would face the unknown challenges in the months and years ahead. Several had arrived with the first contingent of medical and nursing staff that had set off from London on 2 June [13] (Fig. 11.3).

First and foremost, Edith was pleased to find a common heritage on meeting the surgical head of the unit, the Irishwoman Dr. Anne Louise McIlroy (1874–1968) (Fig. 11.4). Initially she felt confident with her 'ready wit and great natural charm', attracted by her 'charming low voice with a touch of a soft brogue'. Beyond their

Chateau de Chanteloup, Troyes

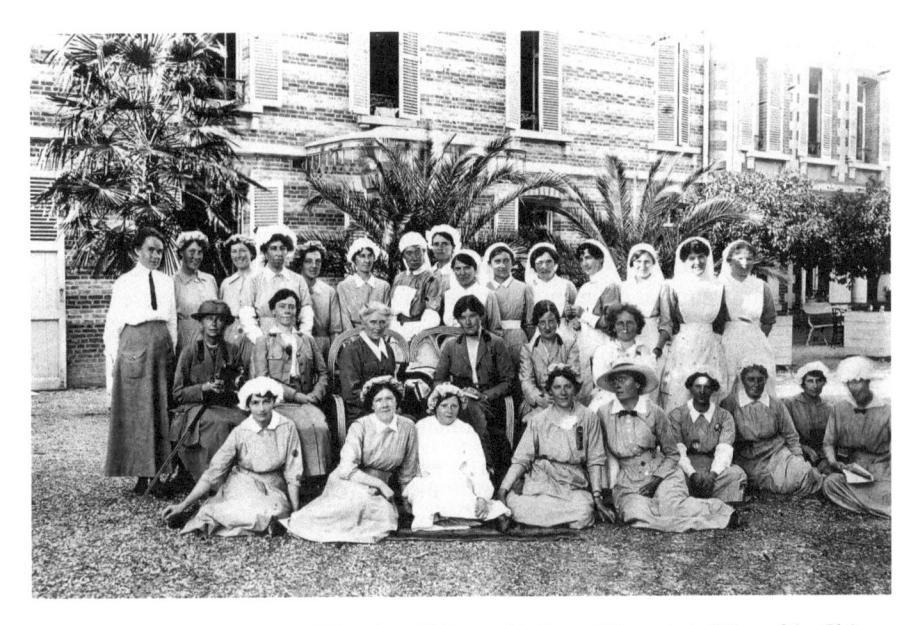

Fig. 11.3 Staff of the Girton and Newnham Unit posed in front of the main building of the *Château De Chanteloup*. Top row left Honoria Keer, second row from left Edith Stoney, Jean Gordon, Katherine Harley, Louise McIlroy and Isobel Emslie. Edith holds her camera, preparing to take her own group photograph. The unit was entirely female, except for two part-time male drivers, and Edith Stoney's technical assistant George Mallett. (Dany Peuchot)

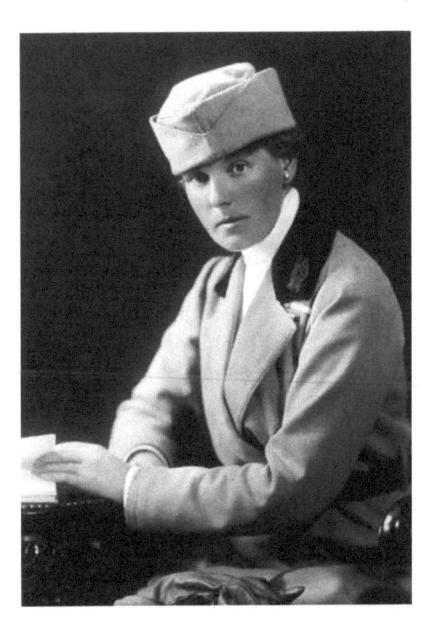

Fig. 11.4 Louise McIlroy, Chief Medical Officer of the Girton and Newnham Unit

background in Ireland, however, there had little in common. Five years younger than Edith, Louise McIlroy had been born in the north, in County Antrim, eldest daughter of a medical practitioner. She had studied medicine at Glasgow University, obtaining her MB ChB in 1898 and MD in 1900. Following experience in several European medical centres, she had returned to Glasgow to become gynaecological surgeon at the Victoria Infirmary and then senior assistant to the Muirhead Professor, Munro Kerr. From the outset, McIlroy relied strongly on Edith's advice as her technical expert. As early as June she had asked Edith to select and order a cystoscope with electrocautery for her.

Edith's other surgical colleague was the younger Canadian-born doctor Honoria Keer (1883–1969). Commonly attired in masculine clothes, her steady skill as a surgeon was more important than her appearance. As Edith was not one for idle chat she found Keer's serious, reserved character and her old-world manners quite easy to deal with. It was a joy when Keer occasionally came out of her shell, showing a sly wit that they all enjoyed.

Edith soon realised that the woman who met her at the station, Katherine Harley, carried a sense of seniority that challenged Louise McIlroy's authority. Mrs. Harley, the Unit Administrator, was known by all the French as *Madame la Directrice*. Edith was immediately struck by the beauty of this slight, graceful, older woman, with her 'well-chiselled nose, pale-blue piercing eyes, and hair that looked neither grey nor fair'. Born into an aristocratic, wealthy and well-connected family, she had been widowed when her husband George was killed in the Boer War. Her value to the unit was considerably enhanced by being the sister of Field Marshall John French, who was at that time the commander of the British Forces in France. She always wore full uniform and 'wore an ancient hat with a tattered red veil wrapped round it'. Her previous appointment as the administrator at Royaumont had ended over major disagreements with both Miss Isobel Tod, the ageing matron, and with Frances Ivens, the Chief Medical Officer, over who was in charge. She brought strong suffragist credentials: her sister, Mrs. Charlotte Despard, had been arrested several times and ended up in Holloway prison for taking part in a pitched battle with police following a suffragette demonstration.

A new member of the medical staff arrived in August. Edith understood, but did not share, this younger woman's support for the militant suffragettes in pressing the cause. She also found it difficult to believe that Isobel Emslie (1887–1960) (later Isobel Hutton) was old enough to be a fully qualified doctor let alone one with experience as a children's and mental health physician. Edith soon learned to respect her scientific ability. Being the most recently trained of the doctors, she had the most up-to-date knowledge of recent developments in bacteriology and medical laboratory science. She was able to take over the well-equipped bacteriological laboratory, which had been set up by Dr. Ellen Porter, who had left to join the Serbian unit. Unlike the other three physicians, Isobel Emslie remained with the Girton and Newnham Unit as physician and bacteriologist when the unit moved on from Troyes.

Edith rarely made comments on her colleagues in her letters and reports, but Isobel Emslie did. She penned some delightful little character sketches, extending from a few lines to over a page in length, from which the following quotations have been drawn [14]. Perhaps surprisingly, the longest was of Edith, and it is worth quoting this extensively, as it gives a one of best descriptions of her from this time.

Miss Edith Stoney was our scientist, and had charge of the radiography department, a most important factor in war surgery. She also arranged the electric lighting plant, and presided over her installation in the stables of the Château. She was one of those who added greatly to the efficiency of the unit, and was probably its most brilliant member. A mere wisp of a woman, she gave the impression of a reed that might snap in two when the wind blew; her ankles were the slimmest I have ever seen. With rubber overall, thick rubber gauntlet gloves, spectacles at the end of her nose, her fair hair streaked with grey gathered tightly into a top-knot on the summit of her head, her whole mind centred on her work and serious as a judge, she certainly looked a venerable scientist. Then she would speak in a clear young voice with perfect enunciation and the purest English, and look up with periwinkle-blue childlike eyes, and you would wonder if you were talking to a vivacious girl of seventeen. Her physical endurance was marvellous, for she was really rather fragile; yet I have seen her carry huge loads, scramble up tent-ropes, and sit astride the ridge of tents in the biting wind repairing electric lighting wires. I have seen her swim powerfully in a heavy sea, and work almost day and night and be none the worse.

The question remained: how effective could they be as a team? And certainly there were many who doubted that any hospital staffed entirely by women could ever operate satisfactorily, let alone one in a war zone under canvas in a foreign land. Isobel Emslie remarked how her friends had said 'Oh, you'll all be quarrelling with each other the whole time, and the show won't last very long; these shows run by women never do'. To be fair, to use a modern idiom, they were largely women 'with attitude', and the potential for flash points between such intelligent, single-minded and strong-willed women was considerable. Before what they referred to as 'the show' was over, Louise McIlroy would need all her leadership skills to build and maintain the respected field hospital that the Girton and Newnham Unit of the SWH would become.

Casualties soon arrived, and by 20 June, Mrs. Harley reported that they had already accepted about 60 patients. But, in truth, the next couple of months were a bit of a honeymoon, without the surge of dreadfully damaged casualties they would later experience. The unit was getting used to operating as a team, and most surely the French Military authorities were keeping a close eye on these British women to ensure that they would be able to cope effectively under more arduous conditions. There was some coming-and-going of staff, but, on average, there were approaching 60 members of the unit at any one time, of which about 40 were nurses and orderlies. The remaining staff included four physicians, two surgeons, a pharmacist and two cooks. The absence of a named anaesthetist is notable. Only simple anaesthetic techniques, either using oxygen and nitrous oxide or ether, were used, often administered by one of the nurses.

In these quiet formative months, Edith was able to join the others as they explored the war-torn countryside around them, to observe first-hand the devastation that had already resulted from a year's warfare in Eastern France. Isobel Emslie reported how they saw 'whole villages razed to the ground and the countryside absolutely barren of vegetation'. They had travelled towards the front line near Verdun, passing through the hamlet of Sermaize-les-Bains where they found the greater part of the population living in cellars or little shanties set up by the Society of Friends. It would

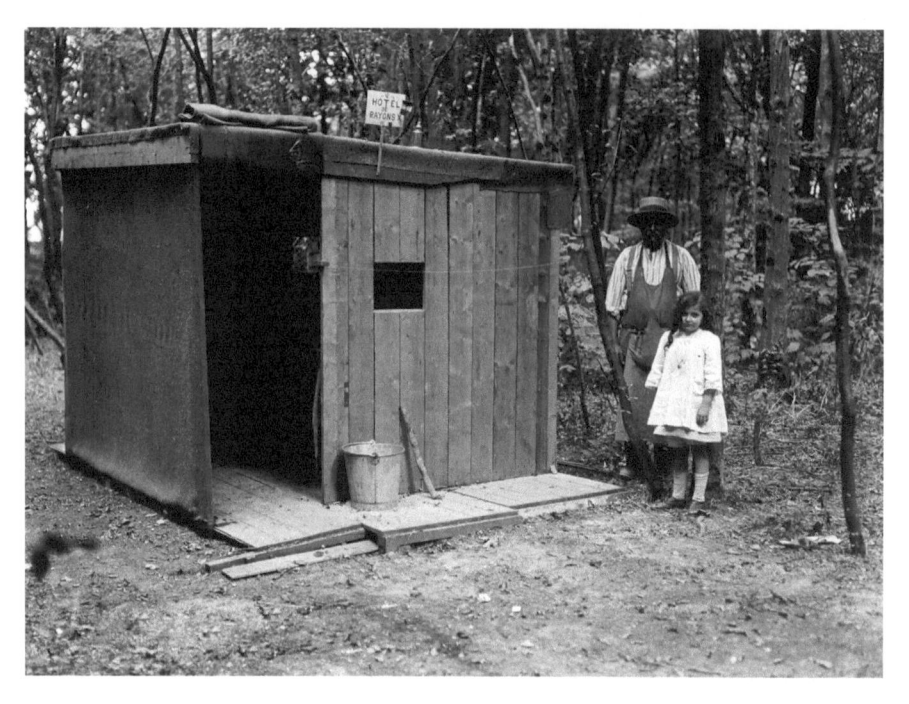

Fig. 11.5 'Hôtel de Rayons X', Château de Chanteloup, Troyes. (Francis Tailleur; Roger-Violet)

have been comforting when Edith returned to *Château de Chanteloup*, with its civilised meals, modern sanitation and electric light.

Shortly after she arrived, Edith connected the 110 V electric supply from the Chateau to provide lighting for the tented wards, obviating the need to use smoky, hazardous oil lamps. She brought another cable into the saddlery where she set up the X-ray equipment. With the help of George Mallett, she improvised and constructed a small, windowless wooden hut, which they labelled *Hôtel de Rayons X*, to be their darkroom to develop the X-ray plates (Fig. 11.5).

A straightforward X-ray image was of considerable importance to the surgeons to learn about the presence and general position of any bullets or shrapnel embedded in a wounded soldier's limbs, body or head. The severity of fractured bones and the positions of bone fragments could also be ascertained. Only then could a suitable operation plan be agreed. At that stage, what the surgeon wanted to know was where to cut, how deeply and in which direction. This could not be achieved from a single-plane X-ray image, and a more precise means of localisation was needed. Details of the various techniques that Edith would have used are set out in the Appendix at the end of this book. Louise McIlroy later remarked that she 'never failed to find pieces of projectiles in wounds which have been photographed by Miss Stoney's stereographic process' [15]. Continually inventive, Edith also worked with Honoria Keer to develop a microphonic method for locating foreign bodies, using a telephone earpiece whilst probing for the bullet with a fine needle [12]. A similar approach became popular with French surgeons during the war. The commercial version used a small coil in a fingerstall to act as the detector [16].

Edith was keen, perhaps assertive, in demonstrating that she was able to interpret the radiographs with as much understanding as her medically trained colleagues. Much can be read into a newspaper article by Louise McIlroy in which she described the operation of the X-ray department. 'The "saddlery" makes an excellent X-ray department, and it is here that some of the most animated discussions among the staff take place. It is generally ceded, however, that the opinion of the radiologist—who is also a physicist—is infallible in the interpretation of the photographs under discussion' [17].

Some of the wounded soldiers who arrived at Troyes during these first formative months were already infected with gas gangrene. During the early part of the war, 70% of those who became infected with gas gangrene died. Edith realised that X-rays had the potential to give an rapid diagnosis, leading to earlier treatment or surgery. She observed that interstitial gas created a natural radiological contrast with the surrounding tissues, in a similar manner to that provided by gas in the lungs. More details of the use of radiography in the diagnosis of gas gangrene are given in Appendix.

Sunlight was considered to have important healing and therapeutic value. The practice of heliotherapy had been given considerable publicity 10 years earlier by Auguste Rollier, who had established his 'Sun Clinic' at Leysin, high in the Swiss Alps, in 1903. This sanatorium was largely intended for the treatment of tuberculosis but, once war broke out, Rollier promoted the further value of sunlight in the treatment of wounds [18]. Whilst the therapeutic action of sunlight was yet to be fully understood, there was by this time an appreciation of the combined bactericidal and heating effects of sunlight, and a belief in its analgesic effect [19]. At Troyes, 'sun baths' were given in the morning and followed specific dosimetry prescriptions as advised by Rollier, under which the wounds were exposed to sunlight for a definite period of time, before being redressed. Damp gauze was laid over the open would to keep it protected and hydrated. Florence had taken an interest in heliotherapy in her medical practice even though the climate had undoubtedly inhibited its use in Britain. Sun treatment was supplemented, especially in northern latitudes, with electric lamps, and in due course Edith added electric lights to her own range of electrotherapeutic equipment.

The hospital prepared for a further influx of casualties. The allies had initially planned to launch an offensive in Champagne in August, but it took longer than anticipated to build the supply lines. The planned attack was delayed until 8 September and then delayed again. Whilst Edith waited, during the night of 8–9 September, bombs dropped on Golders Green, not far from her home, at the start of the first Zeppelin raid on central London. When the airships returned to Germany they left behind 22 civilian dead and 87 wounded.

In France, rumours started to circulate that the French Military authorities had other plans for the Girton and Newnham Unit of the SWH. Orders to move were first received on 13 September and the tents dismantled ready to go. During the previous 3 months, they had treated over 1000 patients. Three of the four physicians left, and about one-third of the nurses and orderlies were leaving, some simply because they were reaching the end of their first 6-month contract and did not wish to travel further than France, and others because they were too young or not strong enough for the challenge of working in these conditions. Louise McIlroy and Honoria Kerr returned to Britain to recruit replacements. Those left behind heard plans for the forthcoming winter. There was some talk that they would be temporarily relocated to Bizerte, near Tunis, to help to care for French casualties from the Dardanelles, returning to Troyes the following spring when the tented hospital could be re-erected. Other rumours swirled—that they were going to Rhodes, or to Alexandretta (now Iskenderun in Turkey).

Orders to Move

Then, without warning on 23 September, the orders to close were reversed. They were instructed to re-erect the tents in preparation to accept up to 200 casualties from the Second Battle of Champagne, directly from the front line. The battle started 2 days later. 'The station had been mined, and we heard the heavy guns ever going at night time' [6]. On one occasion they were faced with the arrival of 174 soldiers at once, making irrelevant the neat division into surgical and medical beds [20]. For 12 days the unit worked under intense pressure, made worse by the absence of the two senior surgeons, recruiting back home. They had become a small but important cog in one wheel of a much larger war. To place these efforts in context, the recorded French casualties between 25 September and 7 October totalled 143,567 men. At the end of the battle, the greatest advance achieved by the French army was 2.5 miles.

Edith Stoney was by now middle-aged and had spent her whole life until then as an academic teacher of mathematics and physics. The summer months with its steady flow of wounded and sick soldiers acclimatised her to the challenge of military radiography. During these intense days in September, the need to deal rapidly with traumatically injured soldiers under extremely pressured working conditions was acute. It could have crushed a weaker character, but there is no sense of weakness either in her own or in others' reports.

Finally, on 4 October, when they were still full of wounded from the front, they received instructions that they were to join the 'Armée d'Orient'. Their all-women's hospital was to be assigned to the French Expeditionary Force in Serbia, in support of a 1000-bed French military hospital in Salonika (Thessaloniki).

This conflict has not been called a World War without good reason. Bigger intersecting wheels of war were turning. Fighting was breaking out on many fronts simultaneously, as each country and alliance attempted to force its own gains as far as it could. Germany and Austria had been planning an attack on a weakened Serbian army throughout 1915 and, on 7 October, commenced their advance across the Drina and Sava rivers, crossing the Danube and securing Belgrade 2 days later. On 14 October the Bulgarian army attacked Serbia from the East. The allies had vacillated in their support of Serbia but now were forced into action, to try to prevent the German-led forces gaining access to the Mediterranean. The Girton and Newnham Unit was being gathered up into these rapidly unfolding events.

Very speedy planning would be needed to prepare for the move. Within 2 days the remaining patients had all been moved on from *Château de Chanteloup*. This left only 4 or 5 days to dismantle the hospital and complete the planning and packing. It was anticipated that an even larger capacity would be needed, and 50 extra beds were ordered. Apart from the need for last-minute organisation, it was hard physical work for the women to pack up the whole tented hospital, weighing a total of 300 or 400 tons. Recruitment had been successful and 23 new staff sailed from Liverpool under the care of 26-year-old Dr. Barbara MacGregor, recently graduated from Glasgow together with the nurses Miss Culbard and Miss Toache.

Edith launched herself with dedication into the next phase. By now it had been made clear to her that any major new equipment to be bought by the SWH would have to be approved first. She wished to deal with two issues, and time was not on her side. In a series of letters to Edinburgh, she requested that the induction coil donated to Florence by Lady Parsons, and her sister's circuit interrupter, should be replaced, so that they could be returned to England. This was approved [21].

More contentious were her requests for two new items. She had managed to set up a temporary lighttight shed as a darkroom in Troyes but had no confidence that this would be possible at their destination. Borrowing one of the standard hospital tents was not an option, because the thin canvas was insufficient to create the complete darkness needed for film processing. She raised this problem and requested a tent with sufficiently thick canvas to keep out all the light—quite a tall order. In the event, this request was not followed up, and Edith had to improvise once the unit had arrived, first in Serbia and finally in Salonika.

One item was essential, however, and that was a secure source of electricity. An engine and dynamo were absolutely necessary, and HQ in Edinburgh was well aware of this. Indeed the Equipment Committee instructed that a telegram should be sent, authorising the purchase of an engine if the unit was moved to Bizerte (31 August), and 2 weeks later, it was again minuted that Edith should be authorised to get an engine. In Edith's own words,

> I feared (and it proved to be true) that the Serbia we were probably going into was by now a war-swept country, and that, in any case, the hospital would fail as a surgical hospital, *bien installé*, if we were located where the X-rays could not be worked.

However, by this stage, Edith's challenging and independent attitude had upset Dr. Marian Erskine, the newly appointed chair of the SWH Equipment Committee. Marian Erskine (1870–1942) was just 6 months younger than Florence and traced her medical lineage to the pioneer of women's entry to medicine, Dr. Sophia Jex-Blake. Erskine was one of 33 women who had completed medical training in the Edinburgh School of Medicine for Women, which had been run by Jex-Blake from 1886 to 1898. This achievement allowed her to gain a Licentiate of the Royal Colleges of Physicians and of Surgeons of Edinburgh in 1894 and so to practise medicine. She worked for many years as a physician at the Edinburgh Hospital for

Women and Children, where she became head of the X-ray and electrical departments [22].

Erskine vetoed the funding for the purchase of the generator. The reason why she changed her mind on such a fundamental piece of equipment tells us more about the sources of Edith's irritation in dealing with her colleagues. In a revealing letter to the Honorary Treasurer, Mrs. Laurie, Erskine gave no logical reason for her veto and the tone of the letter makes clear that it was caused by a personal antipathy towards Edith [23]. Edith had no negotiating skills, and if she disagreed with someone, she said so. Erskine had been offended by Edith's tone: 'I've had lots to put up with in her letters to me'. She was also of the view that Edith had already set her sights too high and needed to be controlled. She wrote that if she (Erskine) had been on the committee she 'would have protested against spending so large a sum in one department of a small temporary hospital'. She seems unaware that the 'large sum' came from Edith's own pocket. Erskine added that 'Stoney is always comparing us to our detriment with the War Office Hospitals' presumably a reference to the Fulham War Hospital where Florence was able to specify equipment at the top of the range.

A final comment is perhaps the most revealing in Erskine's plan to establish her authority. Erskine pulled rank. 'Of course I think it was a mistake to appoint anyone as radiographer without any anatomical or medical knowledge'. Erskine clearly had no sense of irony, seemingly confident that her medical degree assured a deep competence in modern X-ray physics. The clash between these two women epitomised the potential for conflict that Edith experienced in her interaction with her colleagues. As opportunities for higher education for women had opened up in the latter decades of the nineteenth century, Edith had taken an academic route, whist Marian Erskine and Florence had gained a vocational training in medicine (Erskine never obtained an MD). Radiography drew on both disciplines. Edith may well have reminded Erskine that, as a Cambridge-educated physicist, she had a deeper and more technical understanding of the equipment than did Erskine, who was only a radiologist. Such professional tit-for-tat underpinned the difficult and competitive relationship between these two women throughout their contacts during the war.

The abrupt about-face could have had another explanation, however, which Erskine would have kept hidden behind her objections to Edith's position. By the summer of 1915, three further SWH units were in preparation for Serbia, to add support the one at Kragujevac that had been set up at the end of 1914 with Elsie Inglis as the CMO. Dr. Erskine had taken responsibility for the new X-ray equipment. In July, only a month after Edith was ordering most of her own radiological equipment, Dr. Erskine had travelled from Edinburgh to London to sort out similar equipment for Serbia. This was shipped in September. Serbia was now the priority, led by Elsie Inglis, and what happened to the Girton and Newnham Unit was a side issue, considered to have no further need of large purchases. If there were limited funds to go round, it is fairly clear which way Erskine's decision would go, whatever reason she chose to give. The SWH added three hospitals in Serbia in 1915, at Valjevo and at Mladanovac in May and at Lazarevac in August. By November, all

Orders to Move

four Serbian hospitals had been overrun by the Austrian advance, all staff taken as prisoners-of-war and all the equipment had been lost.

As far as Edith was concerned, events were already taking over. It really did not matter now whether she had confirmation from Edinburgh for the engine or not, because there would still have been a delay in delivery of 3–5 months, such was the wartime demand for portable power for wireless communication and lighting. So she simply ignored any instructions to the contrary and proceeded to find one to buy, using her own money.

Edith accompanied Mrs. Harley on the overnight train to Paris, where her colleague had to make the final transport and administrative arrangements for the move. Meanwhile, for Edith,

> luck brought me across a beautiful little portable engine-dynamo (one and a quarter horsepower [1 kW]) weighing some two hundred pounds, already half-packed for someone else. I sat on the engine for a couple of hours till I could shew the sceptical French manager that I could take it to pieces and work it. I speak villainous French, alas! but I have a generous drop of disreputable Irish blood in me, and that engine was mine! War does not make for honesty! To my sober Scotch uniform I owe it that the bank manager cashed at sight my cheque for £150.

The Lister petrol engine and dynamo that she had bought, although the smallest in their range, would be one of the unit's heaviest items of equipment. But, as she pointed out to her more sceptical colleagues, 300 or 400 pounds (weight) added to 300 or 400 tons is of no importance. The contemporary Lister design used a single cylinder engine with a flywheel. The gravity-fed fuel would have been held in an associated tank, with a belt-driven dynamo mounted alongside. Edith would need to become quite an expert in engine design during the years of the war.

Back in Troyes, Edith was irritated to find that George Mallett (who she refers to here as *my* orderly) had been commandeered by others to help with their packing. She quickly redirected him to the careful packing of her more delicate instruments, leaving him to accompany the unit when it set off southwards. She herself returned to Paris to collect the engine, gain permits to travel, and to take it to meet the others in the port of Marseille. She also needed chemicals and other smaller items. In her claim letter to the SWH treasurer, Mrs. Laurie, she was pleased to point out that she was able to get 25% off by paying cash because she was working for a hospital directly under the French War Office [24]. Edith planned to take enough consumables to last 3 months, especially photographic plates and chemicals. Some items were in very short supply: her preferred developer, metaquinone, could only be found in small expensive bottles. Sulphuric acid was needed so that she could transport the accumulator batteries dry, to be refilled on arrival. The consignment from London had been filled before dispatch, and this suggests that there had been some previous spillage in transit. Edith was very conscious of the need for protection from the deleterious effects of exposure to X-radiation. She explained in her claim that a protective lead glass plate, used during fluoroscopy, had been broken and needed to be replaced. In justifying this expense, she says 'I am sure that the committee would not wish me or my assistants—and much less the doctors—to work without this ordinary protection', nicely implying that the use of lead glass protection was widespread and common practice.

Florence, at home in Reynolds Close, passed on her claim and acknowledged payment of £3.8s.6d at an exchange rate of 27 francs to the pound. Nevertheless, the greatest out-of-pocket expense was for the engine/dynamo. Negotiations over the recovery of this expense were protracted and became acrimonious, particularly because Dr. Erskine's biased opposition was shown by Edith's action to have been a misjudgement. Florence also wrote to Edinburgh at the end of October on Edith's behalf, making the case for the purchase of the engine, reinforcing the importance of X-rays in hospitals for the military wounded [25].

During her brief shopping trip to Paris, chatting to equipment suppliers, Edith became more aware of how her own role fitted into the broader perspective under which French military hospitals operated at that time. This reinforced her understanding of the central role that technology and physics were playing in the management of military casualties as the war progressed. Notably, each of the main French military hospitals had set up combined departments of radiology and electrotherapy. Furthermore, her knowledge of developments in these areas made Edith realise that those appointed to be heads of these departments were the same men (and they were of course all male) who had already made serious contributions to the use of electricity and X-rays in French medicine. Indeed (and the terminology would have caused the physicist in Edith some excitement) three of them were also professors of *Physique médicale*.

Medical physics had a very much longer history in France than in Britain. The first professor of medical physics and hygiene, Jean Hallé, had been appointed at the *École de santé* in Paris well over a century before [26]. Protected by national statute, the position of Professor of Medical Physics had been retained in the Faculty of Medicine in Paris throughout the nineteenth century, and, as new medical schools were established, each appointed its own professor. Armand Imbert had been appointed as medical physics professor in Montpellier in 1889 and, after contributing to the use of X-rays in their very early days, had devoted his attention to occupational medicine and safety in the work place. Joseph Cluzet was professor in Lyon, and his recent textbook on medical physics was widely used [27]. Most prolific for his scientific and technological contributions was Jean Borgonié in Bordeaux. When Paris was in great danger of being overrun by the German advance in the early stages of the war, it was Borgonié who Marie Curie approached to take custody of her radium, for fear that it might fall into enemy hands. Amongst the other heads of radiology, Edith and Florence would have known also of Antoine Béclère, the dominant force in Parisian radiology, at the Val de Grâce, the military hospital in Paris, and of the published contributions of Hyacinthe Guilleminot in Bourges and Stéphane Leduc in Nantes. There was nothing in Britain to compare with this breadth of committed knowledge and competence throughout France, so clearly linking academic excellence with clinical need. The formal integration of radiology and medical electricity was a model that entirely fitted with the way in which Florence's career had developed, and with Edith's view of how she could best contribute to the function of the Girton and Newham Unit. She now found that it was also entirely

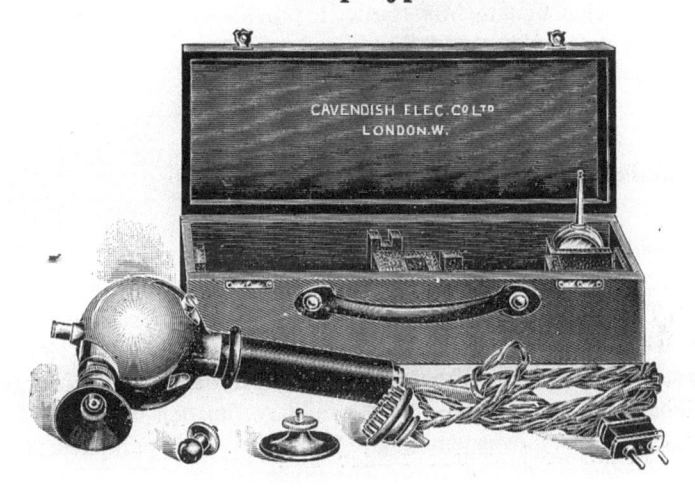

Fig. 11.6 Electro-massage unit

congruent with the structure that had been established within French military hospitals.

On her sister's advice, she had brought electrical massage equipment with her from London. On this second visit to Paris, she arranged to have the equipment converted from the alternating 110 V supply that she had specified for use at Troyes, so that it could be operated using her new dynamo and batteries. Electrical vibrators were quite commonly used for massage at this time. These would typically consist of a small motor, connected through a flexible drive shaft to the massage head, which contained an eccentrically mounted revolving weight (Fig. 11.6). A rheostat controlled the voltage and hence the force of the vibration.

Having dealt with this detail, she had a day or so before she had to leave to join the main unit again, and she had some more shopping to do. Her next purchase demonstrated an astonishingly imaginative confidence in her new role in the Newnham and Girton Unit. Edith was aware that a fully equipped department of electrotherapy offered much more than electro-massage and was thinking ahead to how she could make herself more useful in whatever conditions lay ahead. She had already suggested to Louise McIlroy that she should make a request for some high-frequency therapy equipment, the latest development in medical electrotherapy, a request that had, not surprisingly, been rejected by the equipment committee. So, encouraged by what she was learning of the French way of doing things, she headed off to the sixth Arrondissement to visit the premises of the large French manufacturer of electromedical equipment, Gaiffe, at 40, *Rue Sainte-André-des-Arts*. Here she selected and bought her own high-frequency unit, typically picking the larger and more expensive of two alternative models. The manufacturers' catalogue gives its surgical uses, electrocoagulation and fulguration, and its therapeutic uses including spark treatment, deep heating and auto-condensation. She arranged for the equipment to be shipped on to Salonika, together with the other stores including some stoves that had been bought by Mrs. Hartley to provide welcome warmth in the tents against the anticipated winter cold.

Off Towards Serbia

The main band left *Château de Chanteloup* in the afternoon of 13 October, with mixed feelings, walking into the centre of the deserted town to join the train for Marseille at Troyes station: sorry to be leaving their French friends but excited at the prospect at what lay ahead. Edith met up with them in Marseille at the Hotel Regina, having travelled independently from Paris. Looking through Sunday's *Le Temps* on the train, she could read a review of the military situation in the Balkans. This reported that the allies, now assembling in Salonika, would not hesitate to march to the defence of *fidèle et héroique Serbie*. The article was accompanied by a little map showing the Austro-German forces north of the Danube at Belgrade and also, more ominously, the potential threat from the Bulgarian army to the East.

During the next few days, the equipment and cars were taken on board the Messageries Maritimes steamer *Mossoul* (Fig. 11.7). They left Marseilles on

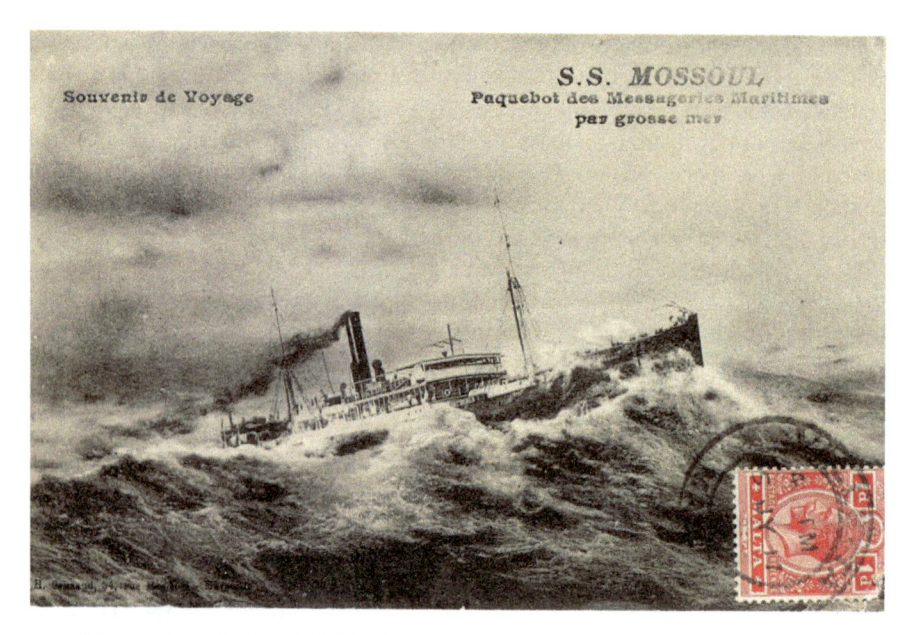

Fig. 11.7 SS Mossoul. (Francis Tailleur)

20 October at 6.00 a.m. on a grey misty morning, singing *'La Marseillaise'* in response to the French solders' *'God Save the King'*. The *Mossoul* was slow and very heavily loaded, carrying eighty French infantrymen, whom Edith referred to by the French nickname *poilu*, with their ammunition stacked alongside the hospital's supplies. It was so crowded that many decided to sleep on the deck. They also had some advance notice of the deteriorating situation in Serbia, meeting some English nurses returning to the Paget and Wimborne Hospitals there. Operating under the Serbian Relief fund, the first of these hospitals had been set up by Lady Leila Paget, a diplomat's wife, in Skopje late in 1914, a 330 bed hospital staffed by 4 doctors and 16 nurses. The closer they got, the worse became the news from the war zone ahead.

It took them nearly 3 weeks, sometimes escorted by destroyers, on a circuitous route through the Mediterranean to avoid the threat of submarine attack, via Malta (Oct 25), Athens (Oct 30) and Mudros Harbour on the Island of Lemnos (Nov 1). The weather had been initially very calm but after leaving Malta the *Sirocco* wind from North Africa had raised a storm that left most of the unit very uninterested in food. On reaching Mudros Harbour, Edith visited the Australian Hospital on Lemnos, where the island's one X-ray facility was able to continue work because they were not dependent on the intermittent local electricity supply, having installed their own generator. Edith would have been reassured and pleased and with her own similar purchase in Paris.

The situation in the harbour was chaotic. The French and British had secured the "loan" of Mudros Harbour from Greece, still neutral, so they shared the harbour with large numbers of dreadnoughts, super-dreadnoughts, battle cruisers, destroyers, torpedo boats and submarines of the combined allied fleet, the Eastern Mediterranean Squadron. Here was a different sort of war from that in France. The port was entirely dependent on imported water, extremely hot with flies everywhere. It was full of wounded and seriously ill men from the fighting in the Dardanelles, waiting for care, whilst the troop carrier Mauretania, with 20 doctors and 80 nurses aboard, lay idle in the bay because of red tape.

Edith first saw Salonika appearing out of a misty morning on 3 November. Initial impressions were vivid, with its long rambling fort and minarets known previously only from the pages of *Arabian Nights*. Salonika had been a Turkish town within the Ottoman Empire until 3 years before, when Greece had invaded during the First Balkan War. At the end of the Second Balkan war in 1913 Macedonia was divided, when the southern part including Salonika was ceded to Greece. The town was now crammed with soldiers, mostly from the Greek army that was in the process of mobilisation. Donkeys and bullock carts added to the chaos: the only motor vehicles were those that had arrived with the French Expeditionary Force earlier that year.

In preparation for the departure towards Serbia, all the women cut their hair, much to the distress of many; though not Honoria Keer, whose cropped hair had always set her appearance apart from her colleagues. They stayed for 5 days, looking for the lost stores that had been dispatched separately. They never did find the stolen tent poles.

References

1. Sharply EM, Archer-Hind L. War work 1914–18. Cambridge: Newnham College.
2. Ivens F. The part played by British medical women in the war. British Medicine in the War, 1914–17. London: British Medical Association; 1917. p. 117–20.
3. Newnham and Girton Colleges Hospital Unit. Newnham College Letter. 1915 Nov 6.
4. The Girton and Newnham Unit, Ch 1 Troyes and Salonika. McLaren ES, editor. A History of the Scottish Women's Hospitals. London: Hodder & Stoughton; 1919.
5. The Common Cause. 1915 Apr 30.
6. Stoney EA. The Girton and Newnham Unit of the Scottish Women's Hospitals for Foreign Service, National Union of Women Suffrage Societies. 1916 Dec 12. Newnham Letter Jan 1917.
7. Sime RL. Lise Meitner. A life in physics. Berkeley: University of California Press; 1996. p. 59.
8. Lawrence M. Shadow of swords. A biography of Elsie Inglis. London: Michael Joseph; 1971. p. 103.
9. Troyes X-Ray. ML. TD1734/6/2/3/8.
10. Francis Tailleur, private communication.
11. London School of Medicine for Women Council minutes. 1915 May 14. LMA H72/SM/A/02/03/01.
12. Tailleur F. 1915 Chanteloup L'hôpital des Dames écossaises. Sainte-Savine: Coopérative scolaire de l'Institut Chanteloup; 2015.
13. The Common Cause. 1915 Jun 4.
14. Troyes. In Hutton IE. With a Women's Unit in Serbia, Salonika and Sebastopol. Chapter 2. London: Williams and Norgate; 1928.
15. Testimonial from Louise McIlroy. 1916 Aug 8. ML. TD1734/2/6/9/69.
16. Van Tiggelen R. Radiology in a trench coat. Brussels: Academia; 2013. p. 71.
17. Claire Keohane. Private Stoney family Cuttings album, undated, with an added handwritten note 'written by the head surgeon'.
18. Rollier A. Le pansement solaire: héliothérapie de certaines affections chirgicales et des blessures de guerre. Paris: Payot; 1916.
19. Rollier A. Heliotherapy. London: Frowde; 1923.
20. Report by the Newnham Committee. Newnham and Girton Colleges Hospital Unit. 1915 Nov 6. Newnham College Letter. 1915.
21. These letters have been lost, but reference is made to them in the Equipment Committee minutes, and in Dr Erskine's later correspondence.
22. Obituary of Marian Erskine. Edinburgh Evening News: 1942 Jun 1.
23. Mrs Erskine to Mrs Laurie. 1915 Sept 23. ML. TD1734/2/4/1/19.
24. Edith Stoney to Mrs Laurie. 1915 Oct 23. ML. TD1734/2/6/9/5.
25. Florence Stoney to Mrs Laurie. 1915 Oct 24. ML. TD1734/2/6/9/7.
26. Duck FA. Physicists and physicians: a history of medical physics from the Renaissance to Röntgen. Ch 6. Jean Hallé and the definition of medical physics. York: IPEM; 2013. p. 70–86.
27. Cluzet J. Précis de Physique Médicale. Paris: Octave Doin et fils; 1913.

Chapter 12
Serbia and Salonika

On the evening of 7 November 1915, the Girton and Newnham Unit of the Scottish Women's Hospitals boarded the night train from Salonika towards Serbia and the advancing Austrian and Bulgarian forces. They now knew that their destination was to be Gevgheli, about fifty miles north, just over the Serbian border, where the French were planning their main army hospital in Serbia. Edith's anticipation of what lay ahead made the uncomfortable ride tolerable, and the women reached their destination in the early hours. Their destination was a small village housing a chaotic mix of local peasants and large numbers of Greek and Serbian soldiers. The existing medical facilities consisted of a mere 100 beds in the local military barracks, where the conditions were appalling, in utter contrast to the conditions they had left behind in France. There was no attempt to separate soldiers with dysentery from others, no disinfection, no instruments, no anaesthetics, and no electricity. The following day Edith started to help to set up their hospital, which was to be part of the larger French military hospital complex. Their accommodation was to be an unused, unheated, draughty silk factory. Edith was assigned a small windowless room on the ground floor as her X-ray room, alongside the operating theatre and Isobel Emslie's laboratory. At night she had to climb to the dormitory in the loft, with some 60 ill-fitting shutters over glassless windows: others had to make do with the balcony. The stalwart dispenser Minnie Baughan (1868–1950), previously a lady of leisure from Aberdeen, who remained with the unit until the end of the war, arranged her pills and potions on the landings. There was a frustrating delay of about 10 days in setting up the ward tents on the adjoining piece of flat land, whilst French engineers obtained tall trees to replace the stolen tent poles. Still positive, Edith added that 'the views of the hills around, and over the Vardar… were very lovely and the air was keen and bracing'. But the contrast with the relative comfort of *Château de Chanteloup* could not have been more extreme.

Edith concentrated on setting up the electric supply with her assistant George Mallett, whilst the others watched her agility on the rafters in some amazement. By the very first evening, she had the dynamo going, and several 50-candlepower lamps were illuminating all floors and the open-air kitchen. She was delighted to demonstrate how right she had been in the purchase of the engine. Even before the tents were up, they were taking radiographs. It turned out that three X-ray sets had been provided for the French hospital complex, but only one of them was operating, powered by a dynamo similar to Edith's. It was run by Charles Géneau, a characterful professor of physics from Paris with a high-pitched voice who 'bulged in all the wrong places and had spectacles on the tip of his nose'. He had been teaching in the Faculty of Sciences in Paris, where he was *préparateur de physique PCN (physique, chemie et science naturelles)*. His course was preliminary for those wishing to enter medical school with otherwise insufficient formal science qualification. It thus had a very similar purpose to Edith's course in London, so the two would have had much in common in their backgrounds, and these two medical physicists formed a mutually supportive bond which continued until Edith left in the summer of 1917. Edith compared favourably what her colleagues could accomplish with the guidance of her X-ray equipment with the surgery in other hospitals she visited in the area without it, where she saw the 'unavoidable horrid search for bullets which X-rays should have localised at once'. Her workload was about ten patients each day, an example of 2 days' workload being four chest cases, two wounds in the head and two in the abdomen, eleven leg cases and three arm cases [1].

The weather steadily deteriorated, but the stoves that Edith had obtained in Paris were sufficient to give some warmth in the tents. The operating theatre was lit with only two lamps, 'a tiny room into which all of us who were needed could hardly fit'. The patients, about 100 at any one time, filling the tents that had finally arrived, were mostly French and Senegalese soldiers, some with frostbite and others with severe blast and shrapnel wounds to their lungs or head. Edith thrived on the challenge, when even George Mallett succumbed to illness for a couple of weeks. In her report home, Edith said:

> The electric light was needed in the Pharmacy until they had finished, and it was often late before I could stop the little engine and pack it up warm for the night. The 'dark room' could not be used while the engine worked, so that my photography came later. The dark room was partly in the flue of the tall factory chimney, and the blizzard streamed through the outhouse, where I was, and up the chimney. My solutions had to be warmed, then froze, and were warmed again. When I creaked up the ladders in stockinged feet to the loft where 54 of us now slept, there could be no thought of washing with ice already in the jug. Instead of undressing one piled on every scrap of extra clothes one had, and put one's waterproof under the mattress to stop the draught up through it.

Less than 200 miles to the east, the British and French forces were bogged down on the Gallipoli peninsula following the disastrous failed attempt to enter the Dardanelles, capture Istanbul and remove the Ottoman Empire from the war. The bitter weather that Edith was experiencing in Serbia had also blanketed the Gallipoli trenches with snow, with many soldiers suffering from frostbite. On 7 December the British cabinet made the decision to evacuate the Gallipoli bridgeheads, and the final troops left Turkey on 9 January 1916.

The Girton and Newnham Unit was on the southern flank of a losing battle for Serbia against the Austrian and Bulgarian forces. As the battle turned, Gevgheli became progressively more crowded and more disorganised. Edith reported that 'The civil population poured in their hundreds past our camp towards Greece all day long; women, children, old men, donkeys laden with queer goods.... The tots of four or five were left behind in those mountain villages, too heavy to carry, too wee to walk'. Packs of stray dogs raided by night, stripping dead animals to the bone. Special care was needed to protect the mortuary. The main street collapsed under the strain, the sewer becoming an open drain. For 3 days they were assailed by the icy wind known as the Vardaris, straining and tearing at the tents and howling through the accommodation. Many of the women had brought insufficiently warm clothing, not expecting such dreadful conditions. Edith felt that she was herself well equipped but even so her feet ached till midday, recalling an old Macedonian saying that the Vardar wind can blow though nine thicknesses of flannel.

Evacuation from Gevgheli

Finally, on 4 December, they received the order that Gevgheli was to be evacuated, leaving Serbia to her fate as an occupied country. So, less than a month after their arrival, George Mallett was again helping Edith to carefully pack all the X-ray and electrical equipment. Everything was completed within 2 days, evacuation of the remaining patients, dismantling the tents, clearing personal possessions and burning anything that could not be removed. They left Gevgheli at 2.00 a.m. on 6 December and were in Salonika by 9.00 a.m., evacuated down the single-track railway, leaving the silk factory burnt and blown up as they left. The Allied Armies under General Sarrail were not far behind, setting fire to Gevgheli and destroying the railway as they went, reaching the Greek border on 11 December.

On arrival back in Salonika, Edith found the situation chaotic; all available accommodation was already overfilled, swamped with French, British and Serbian troops and with civilian refugees. Greece was still neutral at this stage in the war, remaining so throughout Edith's stay, and so there were also numerous German and Austrian observers noting all the military activity. After one night in a filthy casualty evacuation tent, Mrs. Hartley arranged for some of the women to move in to some empty barracks on the outskirts of town on low swampy land by the sea, undrained and uninhabited except for a pig farm. The region had already been earmarked for the French temporary hospital No 4. A few lucky ones were housed temporarily on board the *Manquo*, lying in the harbour. By 11 December, Edith moved with the others into their new little green ridge tents, which felt luxurious in comparison with the conditions they had experienced during the past week. Fresh water supply was installed, and ditches dug to help with drainage, although that did not prevent Edith's tent being flooded on at least one occasion. For the first time, the Unit had to accommodate all the staff under canvas.

The first casualties straggled in to the hospital on the 18 December, before it was really ready for use, 55 emaciated Serbian soldiers too weak to walk unaided, a small remnant of the part of the army that had not retreated westwards across the mountains into Albania. The first German air raids occurred before the end of the year, shrapnel from the defending guns proving to be much more dangerous than the attacking aircraft.

The retreat from Gevgheli and the following few weeks in Salonika nearly destroyed the Girton and Newnham Unit. The Committee in Edinburgh had already learned that all their Serbian units had been overrun and that the CMOs including Elsie Inglis and Alice Hutchison and their staffs were now in captivity. They could obtain no clear overview of the situation in Salonika. Irrespective of the view from Scotland, local negotiations with the French authorities were taking precedence over any instructions from Edinburgh, filtered through inadequate communications from 2000 miles away.

As the Chief Medical Officer, it was up to Louise McIlroy to make judgements about the best course of action for her unit. Whilst Mrs. Harley negotiated with the French medical authorities to set up the new site for their hospital, McIlroy had to work out what new medical service they could best deliver in these highly fluid circumstances. What kind of casualties might they expect now that the major attack from the north had stalled and once the Dardanelles had been evacuated? Was there going to be a role for their small unit in the planned multinational medical complex in Salonika? Indeed, once Greece joined the war, would Salonika itself be overrun? She was also aware that her staff were mostly on 6-month renewable contracts and that there was a need to deploy them correctly and to clarify each person's future intentions.

It was in these conditions of extreme uncertainty that an event occurred that caused Edith considerable distress and coloured her future relationship with the Scottish Women's Hospitals. Shortly after they had arrived in Salonika from Gevgheli, Louise McIlroy had an interview with Edith, in which she explored her future role in the unit. When they had left Troyes, several of the physicians had returned to England because the expected future need was for surgeons near the front line. Now, McIlroy told Edith, the medical needs were changing again. The patients they would be treating in Salonika would be very different from the front line casualties they had dealt with in France and Serbia. These new patients would be mostly admitted suffering from dysentery, typhus, malaria and malnutrition, for which X-ray diagnosis would not be required. Mallett could look after the electrical supply and the few radiographs that would be needed. Louise McIlroy had a high respect for Edith's practical contributions to the unit both in Troyes and in Serbia, writing later 'her work is a long way ahead of any of the men I have seen out here with their very expensive outfits' [2]. But now, Edith could leave. The only opening that she offered was to help to set up new X-ray units in more remote hospitals. Edith later referred to this suggestion as being 'sent up country'.

Edith, tense and uncertain, reacted very badly to the interview. In a less stressful environment, these matters could have been resolved without conflict. But these were not normal times, and both women were exhausted and emotionally drained by their experiences in Gevgheli and very worried about their uncertain future.

Louise McIlroy had not yet had to face the full depth of Edith's steely determination when faced by a challenge, whether this was academic, practical or personal.

Edith had not expected to be asked to leave and felt that she was being abandoned [3]. Not only that, she believed that she would have to leave all her own X-ray and electrical equipment behind, letting George Mallett take her place, and that she would be left to make her own way back to Britain at her own cost. This made her very annoyed and very frightened. Her reaction was also coloured by the recollection of her recent dismissal by Louise Aldrich-Blake from her lectureship at the London School of Medicine for Women. Whilst much had happened since, the memory of a doctor forcing her resignation without apparent good cause was still fresh and raw. And there is no doubt that Edith considered herself the professional equal of all her medical colleagues and reacted very badly to any implication of seniority that was based only on the possession of a medical qualification.

The immediate outcome was that the storm cleared as quickly as it had arisen, and for the moment the matter seemed to have been resolved. Having clarified Edith's wish to stay, Dr. McIlroy immediately assigned a senior member of the nursing staff to help with the X-ray work and encouraged her introduction of electrical therapy enhanced by the high-frequency surgical diathermy equipment that Edith had bought in Paris. No further action was taken, and Edith set about the task of setting up her department. Unfortunately, from then on Edith became highly defensive about her role and position in the unit, adopting a much more aggressive negotiating stance when challenged, leading to a widely held view that, however brilliant Edith was at her job, she could at times be very stubborn and difficult to work with.

Electrotherapy in Salonika

Edith's first task in Salonika, as in Gevgheli, was to set up the engine/dynamo and to install electric light throughout the accommodation tents, both for staff and patients. Next she needed to set up her X-ray room. Everything was up and running by 1 January, even procuring a replacement for a broken Schall X-ray tube and some other equipment that had been damaged by water. Edith had hoped to be able to use the local mains electricity supply, but it was not possible to make arrangements for this to be connected, so the hospital continued to rely on Edith's little engine for a considerable time. A leaking wooden hut acted as the operating theatre, and Edith set up in an adjacent hut, whilst waiting for a new tent for the X-ray processing. In this way she was able to carry out the accurate localisation of embedded bullets with the patient lying on a mobile canvas-topped operating table, which was immediately moved next door into the operating theatre, where the surgeons carried out a guided and therefore quick removal. It is remarkable that, in spite of the chaos surrounding them, these women had the foresight to plan an integrated X-ray imaging and operating facility. Elsewhere in this apparently primitive hospital, there were other examples of up-to-date medicine. The tented laboratory, for which Isobel Emslie was now the bacteriologist, housed modern incubators and instruments for cutting sections, and autogenous vaccines, blood cultures and typhoid agglutinations were all carried out. No matter how dire the situation appeared to be, Edith's intentions to create a well-equipped X-ray and electrical department sat well with the aspirations of the unit.

Edith was settled again, with a secure focus for her work. For the first few months, the hospital in Salonika remained only about half full, with about 120 casualties at any one time. As Louise McIlroy had anticipated, relatively few of the new patients needed X-ray investigations, and Edith found her radiological workload reduced to only about ten investigations each week. In the general uncertainty that prevailed for the first couple of months of 1917, other hospitals in the vicinity initially delayed installing X-ray equipment, relying on Edith to deal with their more urgent cases. These included, during the first 6 weeks, four British soldiers, three naval officers and eight French soldiers. At times Edith's workload may have reduced to the 'mule-kicks, football injuries and slips in the dark' reported by one RAMC officer working in a mobile X-ray unit in Salonika [4]. They were in the vanguard of a development that would see Salonika becoming host to a vast network of Allied hospitals, as those at Alexandria, Mudros and Malta became swamped with casualties.

Both Edith and the French Professor Géneau rapidly gained their own reputations amongst the local military and medical networks. For Géneau it was his attempts to make equipment to improve sanitation that gained most prominence, though not necessarily for the right reasons. As Isobel Emslie remembered 'he had very enlightened views on sanitation, and he had all sorts of original schemes which theoretically were wonderful, but which did not seem to work out as well in practice' using as one example how he demonstrated his patent self-emptying latrine, with graphs to illustrate how it worked.

Edith's reputation was much more firmly based on her outstanding skill in practical radiology, not only now an expert in the wartime medical applications of X-rays but also deeply knowledgeable on the practical aspects of the equipment. She was pleased with her own set-up, which was capable of giving a tube current of 12 mA from a new 16-inch coil, allowing exposure times to be relatively short. With no local engineers to install and service the equipment, her knowledge and skill were essential if the radiology service was to be maintained. On two occasions she was called on to visit British hospital ships in order to get their X-ray equipment back in to working order after it had been dismantled or damaged, on one occasion having to request technical information from Britain to effect the repair. The naval men had heard of this brilliant woman who might be able to help and were delighted to find that that the fact lived up to the reputation.

With time on her hands, a supply of electricity, and with Louise McIlroy's support, Edith set about establishing her own electrotherapy department, including electrotherapy, mechanotherapy and heat therapy. She was very confident that she could develop this new field, recalling that she 'had fortunately been in close contact with massage and electric treatment for several years from home circumstances'. This refers to Florence's clinical training in and knowledge of electrotherapy, commencing when she was appointed as the medical electrician at the Royal Free Hospital in 1901. Edith learned from her sister how she was using electrotherapy in her private medical practice, so knew in general terms how to expand her activities in line with those found in the other French military hospitals. This included

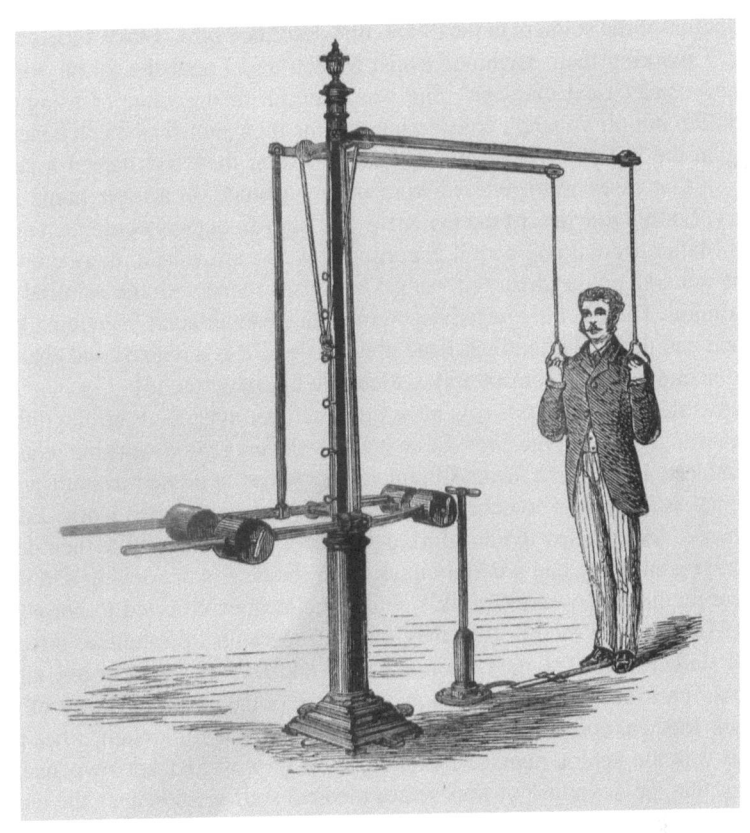

Fig. 12.1 An example of Zander apparatus which could have been easily improvised by George Mallett for use in Salonika [29]

widespread use of hot air and radiant heat therapies. Here Edith had to improvise. She reported that 'our ingenious X-ray lad (Mallett) made us up hot-air baths we could work from the engine out of old petrol tins', and on another occasion a hot lamp was constructed with a shade made out of an old cocoa tin.

Edith also used her high-frequency apparatus at the highest powers for surgery, for which the high current could be safely used for cutting and cauterisation. This replaced the older hazardous method in which a direct current was conducted through a fine wire, usually made of platinum, causing it to become white-hot. It could be used, for example, to remove and cauterise small growths or cysts, typically for ear, nose and throat surgery. Such was her local reputation that both British and French doctors used both her high-frequency cautery and hot lamps in their work.

Neither did she restrict herself to electrical equipment when she saw a need that challenged her innovative skills. She had knowledge of the system for controlled muscular exercise, working over pulleys against weights, known as the Zander apparatus (Fig. 12.1). Very early in their stay in Salonika, and with the help of George Mallett, she improvised a similar system and used it for the muscular rehabilitation of the soldiers in their care. She described how 'I take 4 men at a time and put 3 working their machines whilst Mallett and I treat the fourth with high-frequency or electrical massage'. She was doubtful of the value of using another method, the 'hot-air douche', considering that the men gained as much benefit from basking in the hot sun. Word got around, and soon they had gained a sufficient reputation that cases were referred from other hospitals. In a letter home in early February, Edith wrote describing her X-ray and high-frequency equipment and what she and Mallett were doing with it, reporting how 'we are quite a merry crew over it all'. She remarks on the stream of visitors and visits to tea with the Admiral and the Rear Admiral. There is little negative comment in the letter apart from remarks about poor food and that she often feels dead tired at night. It is a relaxed and chatty letter from someone who has comfortably settled into her new role [5].

Meanwhile, another major row blew up which demonstrated the fragility of the staffing arrangements in the Unit. Edith had developed a good working relationship with Kathleen Harley, the Unit Administrator, whose approach to hard work and operational organisation matched Edith's own approach to her work. Edith had accompanied Mrs. Harley to Paris during the frantic few days prior to their departure from Troyes, and they had worked out together the details of packing and shipping that were required. However, Edith's clinical colleagues objected to her autocratic manner. Less than a month after they had set up camp in Salonika, three senior medical staff, Mary Alexander, Honoria Keer and Barbara MacGregor, all threatened to resign over who was, ultimately, in charge of the unit. They, naturally, sided with their medical colleague Louise McIlroy. Mrs. Harley maintained her position that she was the senior manager. Louise McIlroy proffered her own resignation knowing that the departure of four senior medical staff would cause the closure of the unit. The compromise agreed with Edinburgh was that Kathleen Harley would not be forced out but that her contract would not be renewed when it expired in May. She left for England on 21 May 1916.[1]

Conflict with Edinburgh

Edith's observation of the way that her medical colleagues had dealt with Mrs. Harley reinforced her own feelings of insecurity. If her colleague could be removed, simply because she had upset the doctors, how should Edith feel about her own future? The spark that ignited her offensive to protect herself arose from negotiations about the purchase of the engine from her. Louise McIlroy approached Florence without letting Edith know. By this stage McIlroy recognised the necessity of the engine to provide lighting and power for the X-ray and electrotherapy equipment and wished to place its purchase on a correct footing. Having experienced Edith's

---

[1]Mrs. Harley was tragically killed a year later in Serbia, dying instantly when a shard of metal from a bomb penetrated her skull on 7 March 1917.

emotional reaction to her earlier approach, she decided to negotiate with her sister Florence in London, who she considered could approach the matter in a calmer and more reasonable manner. Florence knew that Edith had already written to Edinburgh, informing them of her purchase and asking whether the SWH would now buy the engine, so she had no reason to block the arrangements. When the news reached Edith, she was even more annoyed, seeing evidence that her position was being further undermined.

On 10 March, Edith composed a long letter to the head of personnel, Mrs. Russell. She goes on the offensive, demonstrating she was capable of determined and self-righteous aggression if she thought that she was in the right. It is an emotional outburst, written by someone who feels angry, threatened and aggrieved, written when her heart rather than her head was in charge. She lets rip, flooding the pages with her frustration and irritation.

First she deals with the purchase of the engine, a matter that was not strictly anything to do with the head of personnel. Having got that off her chest, the rest of the letter is a long diatribe about the argument with Louise McIlroy the previous December. She made clear her wish to stay attached to the Girton and Newnham Unit but that, if she were to leave, either of her own volition or because her contract was not renewed that she would take all her equipment with her. This was a logical and clear position to take and one that Edinburgh needed to be aware of in order to plan for the future of the unit and of Edith's place within it.

She reveals her sensitivity over her lack of medical qualification, asserting, quite unreasonably, that Dr. McIlroy thought that she could bully her as a result, claiming that her long university training gave her 'far higher degrees than a doctor'. She also complains that she has never received acknowledgement or appreciation for the fact that she 'saved this corps from *utter* inefficiency as a surgical corps in Serbia'. This was as much a comment on poor management style than on her own feelings, suggesting that McIlroy's reputation for being tough but fair did not extend to positive reinforcement of contributions and achievement.

Edith was beginning to realise that bonds between women were overridden by professional allegiances and status. She had inherited a view from her father that achievement in the academic world was a sufficient goal. In reality, she had been unable to capitalise on her initial success in Cambridge, and 15 years teaching first-year medical students would have felt a poor reward for all that effort.

It is worth exploring further the comparison between her situation and the employment conditions of her medical colleagues. Like all her medical colleagues, Florence knew that, as a qualified and respected doctor, she would have no problem re-establishing her practice on her return from war service. On the other hand, in common with many science graduates, men or women, Edith was in no such position, and there was no independent professional career for her to re-enter if she were to return to Britain. There were others, albeit in more junior positions, who were in the same boat, especially the orderlies. Although she never mentioned them, there is good evidence from her past that she was well aware of the importance of the conditions of service in providing secure employment for women. Edith had spoken up for her assistants at the LSMW and would do so for the orderlies in the SWH. Her letter to the head of personnel in Edinburgh, a qualified doctor herself, was in part a statement that conditions of service that might be appropriate for doctors and nurses could not be assumed to be so for other staff.

Edith also raised the question of George Mallett. It would have been in her nature to be concerned for his future security as much as for her own. She makes much of the fact that he had been initially recruited and trained by Florence, and she certainly felt responsible for looking after him on her behalf. They had formed an effective working partnership, and she was already developing a strategy for moving on in which he could have formed a part, especially if it had been in a military post. Feeling under threat of losing her job, Edith claims that she had already received an offer from the South of France. Using an academic model, she pointed out that specialists often took their assistants when they moved. She seemed unconcerned that her insistence that he should leave the unit with her would probably result in military conscription, an outcome that eventually proved to be true.

By suggesting that Louise McIlroy was a bully because she was a doctor, she had set herself on a collision course with Beatrice Russell, who was bound to react by closing ranks with her medical colleagues. Whilst working relationships in Salonika were seemingly resolved, the damage that Edith had done to herself with the Edinburgh committee cannot be overstated and was never mended. Memories are long, and from then on she had an established reputation in Scotland as being a difficult woman, and subsequent events did nothing to alter this view.

Does the letter give greater insight into Edith's character and ideas? An interesting theme starts to emerge, one that is easily hidden in the emotion of the moment. Edith presents herself as disenfranchised, powerless and under-appreciated. She interprets her experience as the arbitrary exercise of power by a self-appointed autocracy: they happened to be doctors, but she would have opposed them in whatever guise they appeared. She marshals her own weapons to defend herself, her academic standing, her ownership of essential equipment and her rescue of the surgical services of the unit. She also identifies with others who she sees as vulnerable, specifically George Mallett, speaking on his behalf as his self-appointed protector. She was an independent spirit and expected the organisation she worked for to give her the freedom to act on her own initiative, a right she saw exercised by many of her medical colleagues. She also expected them to value and recognise as equals the contributions of all those who were part of the enterprise.

These private battles did not detract from the positive reports in public about Edith's work. A brief article in *The Common Cause*, 'The Organ of the Women's Movement for Reform', noted the importance of Edith's work. 'We have had several letters lately, all of which speak of the excellency of the X-ray department (in Salonika) and the capital way in which Miss Edith Stoney came to the Rescue of the Unit while at Gevgheli.' A letter from Florence was published in full and gave a detailed report on the events in Gevgheli that she had gleaned from Edith's own letters home [6].

Summer by the Mediterranean

We now return to the conditions in the Salonika hospital in 1916 as spring turned in to summer. The winter had been relatively quiet, but summer brought new problems. It was said to be the hottest summer for 20 years, and they were plagued with ants, flies and mosquitoes. Professor Géneau demonstrated his inventive powers once more. He filled boxes with a mixture of earth and beer, with the intention of attracting the flies to lay their eggs there. Once the eggs hatched, the boxes were burnt: 'La voilà, chéres collègues, vous n'aurez pas une mouche'. Unfortunately the technique did not appear to have lessened the actual numbers of flying insects.

However hard they tried to maintain cleanliness, most of the staff suffered from illness of one sort or another. Several of the medical staff, including Louise McIlroy, needed sick leave. Even Edith, who largely avoided eating with the others in local restaurants, had to take some time off with a bout of diarrhoea. She felt very tired but recognised that was true for them all. The hospitals were swamped by a huge increase in patients, suffering from dysentery, sunstroke, malaria, sand-fly fever and infective jaundice. Their hospital expanded once more, this time to 340 beds. The throughput of patients was about 1000 each month, the beds being emptied and refilled as each batch arrived at the hospital. Edith's nurse assistant was needed elsewhere, and Mallett was unable to work for 4 months with an infected foot, leaving Edith to look after everything herself. She was self-contained, focussed on her work, and this kept her going. It was tragic when first one and then a second nurse died. But Edith, perhaps deliberately, kept herself emotionally detached, moving on to the next practical challenge, not dwelling on local events over which she had no control. The one emotional tether that kept her sane was the regular correspondence from Florence, sane, sensible Florence, giving regular advice and news. Florence, at least, understood the importance of what she was trying to do.

They received a steady flow of visitors, many of whom were very complimentary of the work of the unit and of Edith's X-ray and electrotherapy department. The letters of one particular visitor have left a clear record of how enigmatic and unusual a figure she appeared at this time. On Monday 17 April 1916, the hospital was visited by an eminent Canadian, John Mackenzie, Professor of Pathology and Bacteriology at the University of Toronto [7]. Mackenzie was slightly older than Edith and was spending some time serving at the thousand-bed No. 4 Canadian Hospital, one of several Allied hospitals that had been set up in Salonika by this time. He was interested to find out how this unusual all-woman hospital functioned. In a letter to his wife, he expressed his approval: 'I was very much taken with them' he wrote, 'They seem earnest, capable women'. And that was all he said about the hospital itself. He did not mention Louise McIlroy or even the bacteriologist Isobel Emslie and her well-equipped laboratory. Edith was the only person he mentioned, and she seems to have really attracted his attention. He recognised the name Stoney and wondered if she was a relative of Johnstone Stoney, although he did not ask her directly. His wife Margaret confirmed that she had a family connection: her godmother was Edith's aunt. He was interested that she had degrees from Trinity

College Dublin, his own father being Irish and that she had lectured in physics at the LSMW. He described her to his wife as a 'funny-looking frowsy old maid with untidy grey hair and large blue eyes'.

A week or so after John Mackenzie's visit, Edith received a letter from her Dublin cousins. Several of her family still lived there, including their ageing aunt Frances, Bindon's widow, their cousin, the engineer Maurice FitzGerald and his sister-in-law Harriett. They had been following Edith's progress with considerable interest, and Harriett had even collected a small amount of money to help her buy more equipment [8]. Now they had alarming news of their own to tell her. Spectacles on her nose, she opened the letter, read and reread their news. There had been a revolution in Ireland: rebels had taken over the General Post Office on O'Connell Street—the army were on the streets. A very large number of civilians had been killed, not the small number that Edith may have read in the press. Furthermore, the rebels had hundreds of machine guns. She was reading first-hand accounts of the events of what has become known as the Easter Rising, which started on Easter Monday 24 April, a week after Mackenzie's first visit. Edith's life had been embedded in Irish politics, being effectively a refugee from her native Ireland, and she knew to expect this as the inevitable next stage in the ongoing battle for Irish Independence. If civil war was to break out, as they had expected to happen before the war, should she return to take an X-ray service there with Florence, as they had planned 2 years before?

Edith could think of nothing else, and so she was very pleased to pour out her concerns when John Mackenzie returned a couple of weeks later. His second visit was ostensibly to find out more about the typhus cases that they had treated at Gevgheli. His letter home makes no mention of this, though, and again he writes of no one else in the hospital apart from Edith, with whom 'he had a long talk about Ireland'. Edith explained to John Mackenzie that she was a Unionist and that she was very agitated about the Sinn Fein rebellion. She was very pleased to express her worries to someone who she felt might have some sympathy, although he might have wondered if her estimates of machine guns and civilian casualties were a bit exaggerated. Her Dublin relatives had certainly over-egged the rumours about the machine guns. Whilst the British Army were equipped in this way, the Irish rebel forces had only a few Mauser semi-automatic pistols and no machine guns. On the other hand, the reports of civilian casualties were broadly correct. The Easter Rising was over in 5 days, by which time there had been 485 deaths, of which 260 were civilians.

Mackenzie finished his letter to his wife with a phrase that encapsulates the effect Edith had on some who met her for the first time: 'She is a most weird old person'. How unlike is this description of Edith to that of Isobel Emslie! Her words of description included 'Serious as a judge', '(like) a vivacious girl of seventeen', 'fair hair streaked with grey' and 'periwinkle-blue childlike eyes'. Similar but so different, the same woman seen through different eyes, both noting the grey hair and blue eyes, but one seeing an old maid and the other a girl of seventeen, one seeing her as weird and the other as serious. The difference is so marked that it demands comment. Both descriptions say as much about the writer as they do about Edith. The woman's view is highly complementary about her looks, character and intelligence. The man's view is coloured by his expectations of a woman's place in society. Mackenzie seems to have been simultaneously attracted to and unnerved by her. He found her intellect attractive, but intelligent women were also supposed to be feminine, and he had rarely met a woman with such strongly voiced opinions. Professor Mackenzie fell back on the only opinion that fitted with his world view. She was not like other women he knew, and so was weird, and he did not find her easy company, so he labelled her as old. The fact that she was 5 years his junior seems to have passed his notice. Still, the apparently derogatory description was not intended for public view, so was perhaps lightly meant.

By August, Edith was quite exhausted from her efforts during the previous year. With little need for radiography, she planned to leave Salonika and return home at the end of September. All seems to have been forgiven between her and Louise McIlroy, who composed a glowing testimonial for her in response to her resignation. In it, she noted that she had 'never failed to find pieces of projectiles in wounds which have been photographed by Miss Stoney's photographic process'. In a closing remark she regretted that 'she (Edith) has seen her way to sever her connection with this hospital owing to the cessation of active warfare and therefore the lack of surgical work' [9].

Such are the unanticipated fluctuations during wartime however that, shortly after deciding to leave, further wounded arrived from the battle for Ostrovo and Monastir (now Bitola) in Serbia. There was now more work to do, and Edith temporarily withdrew her resignation. In early September she had time to set up a generator for the electrical supply at the newly formed SWH America Unit at Ostrovo in Serbia, established under the leadership of the New Zealand doctor Agnes Bennett and named from its source of funds. By this time she was able to obtain a more suitable French generator, the Ballot Groupe électrogêne, a single cylinder petrol engine directly connected to a dynamo giving 9 A at 110 V.

Home and Rest

Nevertheless, the delay in departure was short-lived. By the end of September, she was home to take a long and well-deserved holiday that extended into sick leave, to make a full recovery from her 16 months away. As she explained to Mrs. Laurie, 'It is my nerves which want rest—Don't think me hysterical or anything of that sort—but my pulse runs up and I get breathless and cough when tired in the silliest way' [15]. Mallet's salary was raised by £2, in recognition of his added responsibility whilst Edith was away.

As she left, Edith would have been aware that the unit was still not secure. Marion Erskine, still chair of the Equipment Committee in Edinburgh, visited with another committee member Agneta Beauchamp, arriving in Salonika on 27 October. They were primarily there to carry out an inspection of the Salonika hospital, but there were also concerns about the new America Unit in Ostrovo and about Mrs. Harley's semi-independent 'flying column' of vehicles. The visit did not get off to a good start when they were not met off the boat when they arrived. The unit was not receiving many patients and was relaxing. Edith described this time in Salonika in retrospect as 'easy and luxurious' after the difficulties in the heat of the summer. She was a strong swimmer, and the Mediterranean beach close by offered warmer water than that of the Irish Sea at Bray or Hampstead Ponds. Erskine noted that all the staff were healthy and well fed. But this did not prevent her from being very critical about a unit for which she felt no sympathy. What she saw was not a unit taking a well-earned rest but one in which there was 'an atmosphere of frivolity'. She was unhappy about Louise McIlroy's management ability, appointing Mathilde Laloe, who had arrived in January as a cook, as administrator. She compared unfavourably the unsanitary site in Salonika with that at Ostrovo 'an almost ideal site amid surroundings of the greatest natural beauty' and recommended that the Edinburgh committee should consider withdrawing the unit. Salonika was beginning to look like a dead end [10].

Nevertheless, Edith remained highly committed to Salonika and very supportive of Louise McIlroy. The clash between her own devotion to the Girton and Newnham Unit and the central plans emerging from Edinburgh as the war developed would be the cause of further arguments and distress during the next few months. During her autumn break in London, there was continued correspondence about the future of both Salonika and Ostrovo, including the suggestion that Edith could supervise both X-ray units. Edinburgh knew that the main front line need was at Ostrovo and wanted Edith's skills and knowledge to be exercised there. Once more, Edith refused to be forced out of her comfort zone. At last, on 20 February 1917, in a frosty interview with Mrs. Russell, Edith absolutely refused to be posted to Ostrovo, and it was agreed that she would return to Salonika to complete her current 6-month contract [11].

Edith's antipathy to the Scottish organising committee was not unique, though perhaps she felt more confident than others in being open about her criticisms. In a private letter written from the Serbian Unit at the time they were in Gevgheli, one of the doctors complained 'I would like to send out here some of the good ladies who sit smugly by their fires and forbade us to take fur coats etc. etc., and gave us great coats that are almost useless and blankets made of paper and tents that let in the rain' [12]. Edith was not prepared to keep quiet about those aspects of her responsibility that she felt could be improved.

Edith's immediate concern during her time in London had to do with a new X-ray ambulance that was being planned for Salonika or Serbia, the fruition, as Edith saw it, of her own argument in favour of a mobile X-ray van, raised as soon as she had become involved with the SWH back in April 1915. The sorry story of this ambulance is told in the next chapter and will not be repeated here. Edith expressed her concerns and could then only leave it with the Committee to address at least some of these before they shipped the van. She had other things to do. As soon as she returned to London after inspecting the van in Glasgow in mid-October, she gave a fundraising talk to the Girton and Newnham subscribers and a second whilst having a well-earned rest in Bournemouth 'illustrated by the lecturer's own excellent lantern slides ... of the Hospitals at Troyes, Gevgheli and Salonika ... also X-ray photos taken of fractures, a bullet in the heart, and pieces of shrapnel embedded in wounds' [13]. Fresh from an active war zone, one can imagine the impact she would have had on her audience, not least that she would have been introduced as a past graduate of Newnham, so 'one of ours'. Not surprisingly the organisers of the London lecture asked her to write up her talk for the *Newnham Letter*, an account from which much of the background to this and the previous chapter has been drawn [14].

Edith needed a thorough rest, and this, together with the unresolved decision about her posting, delayed her departure until February. This period of recuperation allowed her to recover her enthusiasm and clarity of thought on how she could best contribute to the work back in Salonika and perhaps also in Ostrovo [15]. She wanted to find out how much longer the Girton and Newnham Unit would be staying in Salonika under Louise McIlroy (in the event they stayed until after the end of the war) and whether Agnes Bennett was staying in Ostrovo (she stayed for a year, to be replaced by Isobel Enslie). It is doubtful that she would have learned any more, not least because the Salonika Unit was now under the direct control of the French military. It was Edith's personal view that one reason for their local popularity, and why they would probably not move, was that they 'have many visitors and there are few Englishwomen and many Englishmen!'. She also hoped to meet Marian Erskine in London, presumably to discuss the problems with the X-ray van and some new electrical equipment that she wanted [16]. In between times, since Florence was having a fairly slack time during the winter lull in the conflict in France, they would have been able to spend some pleasant relaxing times together at home in Hampstead.

Edith was still at home in February 1917, waiting for papers and clearance to travel [17]. Unknown to her, the debate about her future continued behind her back. One suggestion was that both she and Mallett might be posted to Ostrovo. As part of this rearrangement, and to prevent the debacle over ownership of equipment that arose previously, she reluctantly agreed to sell her high-frequency diathermy unit so that it could stay in Salonika, at a price of £33-13-9. There was no depreciation included in the calculation—quite the opposite. Edith added a 15% 'war increase' to the list price of 800 francs!

Still, she had caused considerable irritation to those in the head office in Edinburgh, and voices were being raised against her reappointment. Back in May, Mrs. Russell, still smarting from the rather extreme letter that she had received from Edith, advised against lending her to the Serbia forces, writing, 'if you want to be kind to the Serbian army in Salonika, please do not propose this, she is an extremely difficult women to work with' [18]. Even those who had benefitted from her expertise in the past expressed concern about her sometimes erratic behaviour. McIlroy referred to her 'habit of writing numerous contradictory letters without much expenditure of brain power'. In fact, if there was any general fault in her letters it was that they were repetitive rather than contradictory. Louise McIlroy also thought that it would be a pity 'if she was allowed to come out at all, as she is so complicated, and will only cause trouble in the unit if she elects to stay in' [19].

At the same time, Louise McIlroy was still looking for guidance from Edinburgh about the future of her unit. It turned out that she was asking the wrong people, and, however the Edinburgh committee wanted to manage things, there was a higher authority that took precedence. The future of the Girton and Newnham Unit was being negotiated between the French and British armies. For 2 brief weeks in February, control of the unit was taken over by the British War Office, only to be firmly returned to the French in March. So McIlroy's unit was in yet another state of flux, and she would have been concerned that she would not be able to manage Edith's undoubted talents in a unit undergoing yet more change. Edith had demonstrated stubborn stamina each time she had been required to establish an X-ray department in a newly challenging environment, tented Troyes, freezing Gevgheli and then swampy Salonika. But McIlroy had seen a deeper side to Edith's nature and realised that Edith might be better employed in a less uncertain environment.

Return to Salonika

Edith finally left London with seven others on the 24 February 1917, travelling *via* Paris, to leave Toulon on the Sunday night boat. Before she left England, however, she received some very good news. The Serbian authorities had been so appreciative of the work of the SWH Unit that they had honoured several of the staff, including Edith, with the award of the Order of St Sava (Fig. 12.2). The Serbian authorities thought highly of Edith, even if Mrs. Russell did not. In addition, the French authorities had awarded her the Medaille des Epidemies.

She found strange comfort in returning to her own tent in Salonika. This had been her home and refuge ever since they set up the hospital in January 1916. In this small space, her own space, she set out her possessions again, organised her clothes and placed her belongings where she knew she could find them. This was where she had lived, slept, dressed and undressed and where she had read letters from Florence, written reports and her own letters home. Power for the electric lamp came from her own little engine. She ordered several electric fans to offset the stifling summer heat that would come. She rarely looked back on her life, but in the quiet late evenings, the stars in the Mediterranean sky recalled the times when she viewed the rings of Saturn with the Newnham students and showed Miss Beale the craters on the moon in the night sky of Cheltenham. Memories of her father inevitably followed, and she realised that in the summer it would be 5 years since he had died.

Edith may have been stubborn, but she was no fool, and she understood that she was becoming *persona non grata* in some quarters of the SWH. Before leaving England she approached the War Office to determine whether there might be openings for her in electrotherapy or radiology departments in either France or Malta [20]. This approach was well accepted in London, and Edith was interviewed by the radiologist Major (later Sir) Archibald Reid and the physicist Captain (later Major) Charles E. S. Phillips before she left. Reid was at that time still working as the radiologist at the second London General Hospital in Chelsea, close to the Fulham Military Hospital where Florence was working. He had instituted a course of lectures for RAMC orderlies working in military X-ray departments around the country in

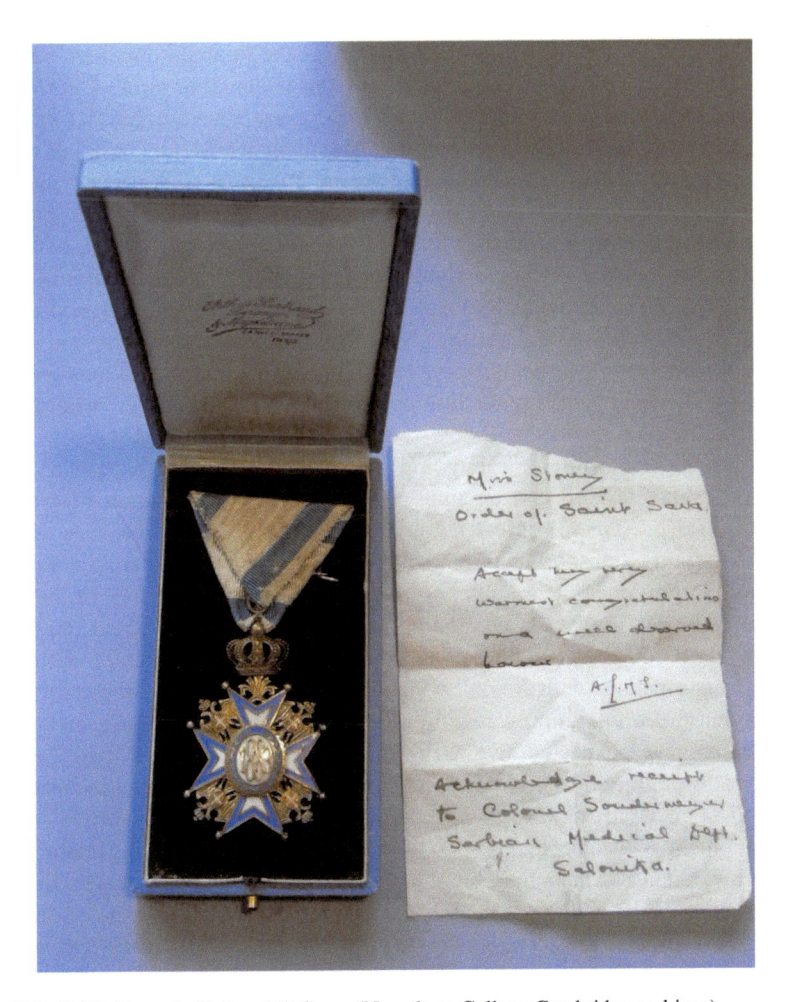

Fig. 12.2 Edith Stoney's Order of St Sava. (Newnham College Cambridge archives)

which Charles Philips gave the physics lectures with Dr. Russell J. Reynolds giving the clinical instruction. The inclusion of the physicist Charles Phillips is significant, emphasising the integration of physicists with the development of military radiology. Phillips was a man of private means with a driving interest in science, who had made pioneering contributions to radiology in its early years, compiling the first bibliography of X-rays, which he published in 1897 [21]. He had been President of the Röntgen Society from 1909 to 1910. Later, Phillips was to become one of the very first hospital physicists when he was appointed as honorary physicist at the Cancer Hospital in London. These two men, Reid and Philips, would have taken great interest in Edith's views on such matters as the optimum methods for X-ray localisation and the practical design of X-ray vans suitable for military use.[2]

When she arrived back in Salonika, Edith received several pieces of news that were relevant to her future. She was told that they would not be transferred to Ostrovo after all, simply required to oversee the operation of the X-ray unit there. She was told that the practice of physiotherapy and electrical massage had been transferred to the care of a nursing sister Elizabeth Ogilvy and her assistant, Hilda Gray [22]. And, of greatest importance, a letter was waiting for her from the War Office. In it, she read with delight that she should approach Surgeon-General Hayward R. Whitehead, the Director of Medical Services in Salonika, and also the surgeon Colonel English, with a view to finding employment with them. Without confirming the reality of any such appointment, she tendered her resignation to Louise McIlroy.

She had to deal with some ongoing practical issues: the design of inflatable cushions for positioning and an improvised frame for localisation of a foreign body in the eye. Some electrical items needed to be reordered because they had gone down with a transport ship that had been sunk by a submarine. She had been asked by the Equipment Committee to prepare a complete inventory of the equipment in her care. There was continuing concern in Edinburgh about the overlap between SWH equipment and her own and also that she was inclined to over-equip her unit in comparison with the others. The typed list she prepared suggests that she thought that the whole thing was a bit of a waste of her time [23]. It includes the items that might be expected, five X-ray tubes of various types, a couch (war office type), her old engine and a new one that had been bought to replace it, the interrupter and coil agreed to replace her own, screens, radiometers, meters and so on. Equipment to enable localisation includes a plumb bob arrangement, a lead ring on a wooden handle, a horizontal bar with ball joint and a slide rule. Batteries, accumulators, cables and fuses are all listed in detail and then all the spare parts, even down to two half inch nuts. The petrol and oil pump are listed with two copper pipes, one for each fluid. The second half of the inventory lists the equipment that she had bought from the French supplier Gaiffe. She thought it was a waste of her time to translate the delivery notes, so she listed most of these items in French.

Correspondence from this time with Mrs. Laurie records that she was now being paid on a par with the doctors. Her salary in February was £16-13-4, raised to £20 in May 'for all medical women'.

The long-anticipated arrival of the X-ray van happened at the end of May. By this time Edith had a well-deserved reputation with her medical colleagues outside the SWH as someone who set the highest standards in radiological practice. The most knowledgeable had seen X-ray vans elsewhere and were looking forward to seeing her design. Their disappointment matched her embarrassment. None of her recommended changes had been made. Glassware had been broken in transit, and

---

[2]Archibald Reid edited the English edition of Ombrédanne and Ledoux-Lebard, *Localisation and Extraction of Projectiles*. 1918 (published in French in 1917).

the engine needed attention. She felt the criticism deeply, seeing it as a slight on her own competence.

She finally wrote to General Whitehead on 1 May just after she had formally written to end her contract with SWH and immediately was invited for interview. The outcome was that that Whitehead gave her a verbal offer to lead the X-ray department in the Fourth Canadian General Hospital, the same hospital at which John Mackenzie had been based the previous spring. By 4 May she had received a letter through the Red Cross confirming the appointment. The appointment of a woman into such a position in an overseas military hospital would have been unique. However, Whitehead was surprised when he heard from the War Office on 18 May that it did not intend to proceed with the appointment, stating that Edith was still employed in Louise McIlroy's Unit. Edith pointed out that she had already resigned, information that was relayed back to the War Office in London by Whitehead, but this made no difference to the decision. As far as Florence could make out, her sister had indeed been offered a job, but only as a VAD orderly at a rate of £20 a year and reporting to the Matron.[3]

As a result, Edith was left without a job, neither with the SWH nor with the army. Edith and George trained a new orderly, Ida Moir, to carry out the routine radiography. A 'lame mechanic', Harold Bentley, was taken on, whom Edith scathingly reported had arrived with no tools. The photograph in Fig. 12.3 shows Edith Stoney, George Mallett and probably Harold Bentley, in the X-ray tent, in May 1917 just before George Mallett left. They are surrounded by some of the equipment that she had by this time assembled, both for radiography and electrotherapy. The high-frequency equipment that Edith bought in Paris before she departed for Serbia can be seen on the left: her brochure for it is shown in Fig. 12.4.

In managing her departure, Edith retained her demand that George Mallett should leave at the same time as she did. In doing so she was consistent with her declared position in December 1915, during the uncertain first days in Salonika. Mallett wanted to stay. Confused, he wrote 'I very much regret leaving my unit in Salonika by the request of Miss Stoney. I beg to state that I did not leave on my own accord or through bad conduct. I have from Dr. McIlroy a reference of appreciation of my services to the unit'. Conscription had been introduced for all men aged 18–40 in January 1916. Shortly after arriving back in England, he was called up, and on 1 August 1917 he was recruited as a private into the 19th Battalion Middlesex Regiment. He survived the war, however, and was discharged on 6 October 1919, returning to live with his mother and brothers in Cricklewood. His reluctance to return to Britain is easily understood. He knew that recruitment into the army would follow immediately on his return, and he had seen enough of the effects of bombs and bullets on human flesh to know what might follow.

Edith's intractable position needs to be explained. In the first place, she was not strictly in a position to decide on his future, however closely they had worked

---

[3] A Voluntary Aid Detachment (VAD) orderly was a volunteer civilian who provided medical aid to the military but was not under direct military command.

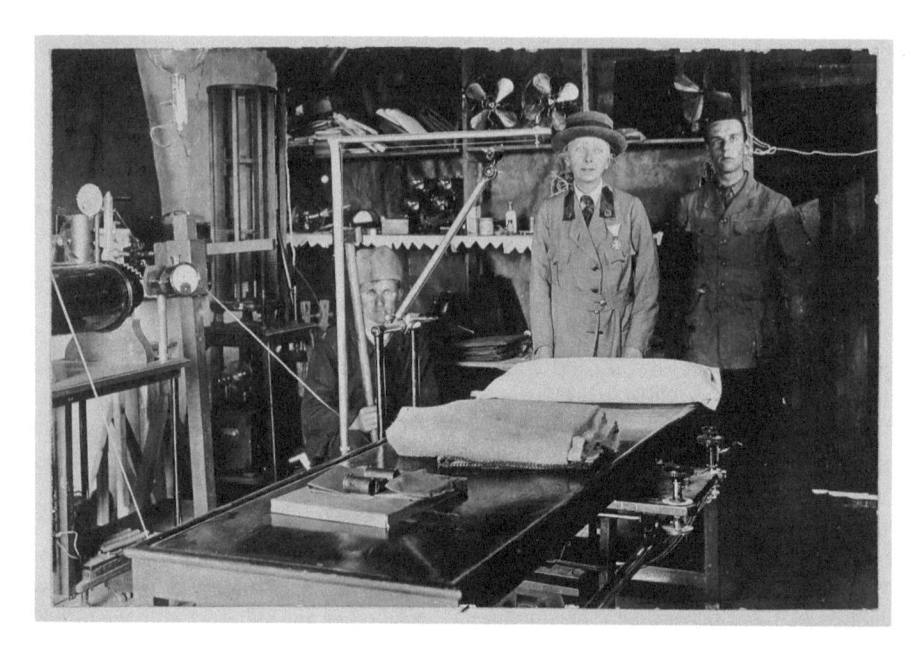

Fig. 12.3 Edith Stoney with George Mallett and Harold Bentley (seated) in the Salonica X-ray and electrotherapy department. The hot-air douche and diathermy coil are on the left, and spare X-ray tubes on the back wall. (London Metropolitan Archives H71/RF/R/02/02/008)

together during the previous 2 years. However much it might have irritated her, it was the personnel committee in Edinburgh, under Mrs. Russell, who recruited staff and who made decisions about the renewal of contracts. Locally, Louise McIlroy was in overall charge, and Mallett could have appealed to her over Edith's head had he wished to do so. However, he knew only too well that he was vulnerable to the argument that he should be in the army and that he could expect no official support from the SWH once Edith decided he should go.

Why, then, did Edith pull the plug in his continued employment with the SWH? Until this time she had been completely supportive and loyal to him. She knew quite well that by demanding his departure she sealed his fate. They both knew that he faced conscription on his return and might have avoided that fate by staying away. She knew, too, that Louise McIlroy had explored the suggestion that Mallett should take her place when she left. It was this suggestion that she opposed. She was consistently and vocally opposed to any circumstance where a man filled a job left vacant by the departure of a woman. Splitting hairs, she had accepted that a new position could be temporally filled by a man, in the way that George had become her technician 2 years before. Her more senior position, secured and retained with effort, should not be relinquished. Had George stayed, he would have taken her position, and he was a man. Therefore he had to leave. She was prepared to sacrifice him in the cause of women's advancement.

A. GAIFFE
à Paris

N° 7
HAUTE FRÉQUENCE

SELLETTES
CONDENSATEUR ET ÉCLATEUR AVEC RÉSONNATEUR

Effluves et Fulgurations.

Auto-Condensation.

Applications directes.

Electro-coagulation.

d'Arsonvalisation.

Thermo-pénétration.

like mine large one
EAS

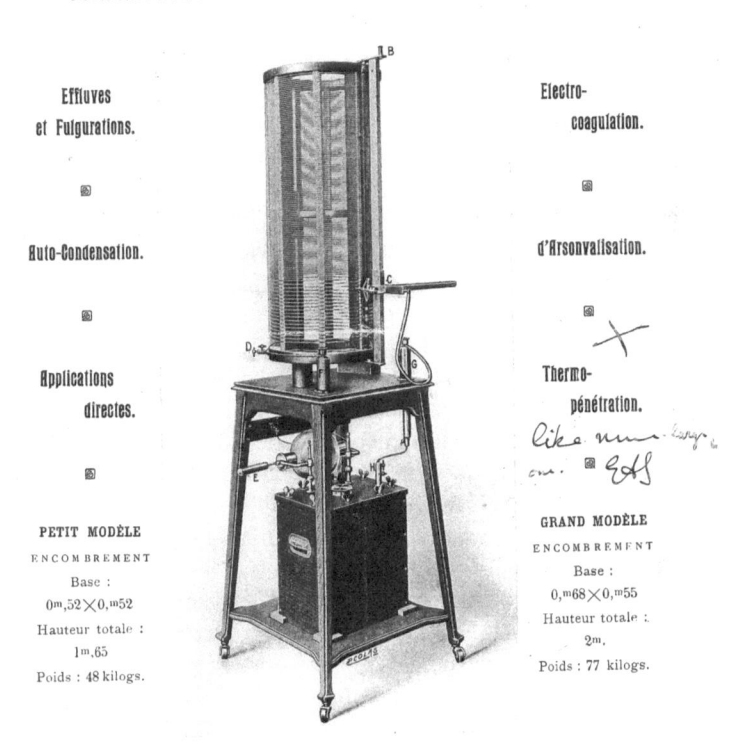

PETIT MODÈLE
ENCOMBREMENT
Base :
0^m,52 × 0,^{m}52
Hauteur totale :
1^m,65
Poids : 48 kilogs.

GRAND MODÈLE
ENCOMBREMENT
Base :
0,^{m}68 × 0,^{m}55
Hauteur totale :
2^m.
Poids : 77 kilogs.

Fig. 12.4 Edith's brochure for a Gaiffe high frequency unit she bought in Paris in October 1915 and shown in this figure. She has added 'like mine large one' and signed 'EAS'. (Glasgow City Archives)

The difficulty in recruiting skilled staff was emphasised after they had both returned to England, when the male radiographer appointed to Ostrovo, William Ross, only lasted a week. A further male assistant had been appointed in Salonika to help with the electrical work in her absence, a reliable ex-soldier John McAllan who had previously been at the SWH unit at Valjevo. Edith had found him to be 'very hard working', a characteristic she greatly admired. She was rather less enthusiastic when she learned that he was being groomed to replace her, which he did. Writing to Mrs. Laurie she said 'I fear that I do not see why you make a corps of women for women surgeons, and then place the most difficult department (under camp conditions) in the hands of a man. There are plenty of women can do the work'. Returning to a theme that she had raised when she was treasurer of the British Federation for Women Graduates, she added 'Are we trying to set men free for other work or are we not and why should we not want women to take up engineering work as well as other work' [24]. She understood that the fight to open medicine to women was already engaged and was being won, whilst that to open engineering to women had barely commenced.

Edith needed a break, and she eventually left Salonika on 22 July 1917. Much of the return journey was now overland, because the route through the Mediterranean had become too dangerous. At this stage she believed that she was still under contract to Salonika and that her resignation had tacitly been withdrawn once more. She left her equipment and some of her personal possessions behind [25]. A complete list is given in an Appendix to this chapter. Edith did not return directly to London. She stopped off first in Rome, where she saw the powerful Fiat vans that took Countess Gleichen's Red Cross mobile X-ray unit into the mountains of Italy [26], so much better than the inadequate X-ray van that she had left behind in Salonika.

Before she left, Louise McIlroy had approached Edith to ask if she would consider taking a new role with her in Salonika. She was in negotiation with Edinburgh about a new orthopaedic service and wondered if Edith might consider taking charge of the therapeutic services. This initiative was still in the planning stage, and it would not be until September that the Committee authorised it to go ahead, using money raised in Calcutta by Elizabeth Abbott. It would be called the Calcutta Orthopaedic Centre. However, Edith was by now much clearer about what she could do and conversely what was not appropriate for her skills. The Calcutta Centre would need a medically qualified person to lead it, and she was not the right person. However, she knew that she could assist in the identification and selection of the best equipment, a role that she was very competent to carry out. The question was left open during the ongoing negotiations between McIlroy and Edinburgh.

Continuing home, she made a week's stop in Paris. It is likely that she stayed in the Lyceum Club of France at 8 Rue de Penthièvre. She visited Gaiffe to establish a costed list of equipment for the physiotherapy facility in Louise McIlroy's planned orthopaedic department. Apparently on her own initiative, she submitted the list to Edinburgh for their consideration, with an estimate of £600 for the electrical equipment and £1500 for the mechanical exercise equipment. It was not well accepted, the committee giving several reasons for refusal. They pointed out that no decision has yet been made on the orthopaedic unit, that there was no extra space in Salonika and that the equipment costs were prohibitive [27]. Edith's enthusiasm had led her to be ahead of the game. By the autumn Louise McIlroy had gained agreement to establish a 300-bed orthopaedic department specifically for the treatment of Serbian soldiers on a new, healthier site in Salonika with a reliable mains supply of electricity [28].

Edith was still torn between her feelings of allegiance to the Newnham and Girton Unit, to which she had dedicated 2 years of her life, and the need to move on to a new venture. The war had 18 months of trauma and destruction still to run, and there was still much for her to do. Those colleagues who worked with Edith Stoney were the first to observe the emergence of a new professional role in medicine, that of the scientific and technical expert, and to respect its importance. Nowadays, medical physics departments are to be found in the majority of large hospitals, and graduate engineers manage the wide range of biomedical equipment that forms the bedrock on which modern medical diagnosis and surgery depend. Then, no such structure existed, and doctors largely took a do-it-yourself attitude to the use of modern technology and to learning the new skills associated with this equipment. The modern view of protected, medical specialisation had no place. Improvisation and rapid skill development were the orders of the day in most military hospitals and may be seen especially in the roles played in the SWH units. Louise McIlroy, a gynaecologist, became expert in extracting bullets and in orthopaedic surgery. The X-ray department at Royaumont, where Edith would go next, was run by a dermatologist and a journalist. In this context, asking Edith to play a hands-on clinical role becomes much less surprising. Greatly to her credit, and without any pathway defining her future, she chose a different career route. She started to demonstrate that future medical care would become multidisciplinary and that specialist scientists and engineers of the highest calibre would play roles that were essential and complementary to those of their medical colleagues. Very few could understand this to be the opening stages of the future for high-tech medicine.

Appendix

The following is a complete and exact transcription of the detailed financial agreement between Edith Stoney and Louise McIlroy for reimbursement for goods and equipment that Edith left in Salonika when she returned to England in July 1917 [25]. For completeness, Edith added at the end a summary of the costs, which gave a total of £231:17:0, noting again without comment the agreed price of £150.

LIST OF X_RAY GOODS

Agreed price £150—Agreed between Dr. McIlroy and Miss Edith Stoney—The Apparatus left with the S.W.H. at Salonique by special request from Dr. McIlvoy.

12" Spark coil in special portable box with condenser—(this was used for the corps from June 1915 - July 1916 when no other had been supplied; it is much better than the new one supplied with many of its fittings being of pre war German make)—£36:0:0

Spare parts - MacKenzie Davidson Interrupter - spare motor switch board - milliampere meter , ameter, on special baskets, oscillograph, 2 valve tubes - lead wires - sparkgap regulator etc.- special portable box for Interrupter & switch board.—£30:3:0

Upright Tube stand with special set of diaphragms and special portable base—The tube box specially protected also safe for treatment work etc. The stand made with graduated arms for accurate work—cost more than £10:18:6

Fluorescent screen, 12 × 15 with lead glass protection and special protecting handles—spare lead glass—(this is really a very special American pre-war screen & cost £15 originally). £9:3:0

2 fans, 3 tubes, stereoscopic apparatus—localising apparatus. £37:10:0

15 doz. whole plates, 8 doz. 10 × 12 plates, 12 doz. packages of developer - dark screen holder fluoroscope- developing dishes—£34:2:6

Other things I have supplied are now worn out or out of date and are not included here as 6 boxes of 6 cells each accumulators £36. —stretcher couch with underneath rail etc. £11. - Intensifying screens—chemicals—viewing box, etc. (£18 omitted from the text but indicated below)

Clothes, tools measuring instruments, resistances, switch boards, books, hand camera, plate glass viewing box, hand stereoscopic charging board for accumulators, small hand grind stone, stock of small Gaiffe switches & store of nails sirens etc. & other electrical fittings have to be returned to London. These are other than those measuring instruments etc. above mentioned, most of the tools, the charging board, switches etc. and grind stone etc have been replaced by things belonging to the corps. The list of corps things was left with Miss Moir—my own tools etc are in special packing cases as also my winter clothes—These boxes are open, or if locked Miss Baughan has the keys, so that they can be looked over if desired before being packed. Miss Moir knows about the resistances switch boards, and charging board having to be replaced. I left replacements for these ready, but my own were up, and better than those Dr. Erskine sent me in July 1916.

(Sgd) Edith Stoney 26/9/17

The Tent and Camp bed were −£18. This was not included in the £150.

References

1. 'F.A.S.' (Florence A Stoney). N.U.W.S.S. Scottish Women's Hospitals. Girton and Newnham Unit at Ghevgali. The Common Cause. 1916 May 19;78.
2. Louise McIlroy to Miss Mair. 1916 Jan 31. ML. TD1794.
3. Edith Stoney to Mrs Russell. 1916 Mar 10. ML. TD1734/2/6/9/21.
4. No 10 Mobile X-ray Unit. Mar–Dec 1918. March 18th. National Archives WO 95/4807.
5. Part of a letter from Edith Stoney. 1916 Feb 17. ML. TD1734/2/6/9/14. The letter is unaddressed.
6. 'F.A.S.' N.U.W.S.S. Scottish Women's Hospitals. Girton and Newnham Unit at Ghevgeli. The Common Cause. 1916 May 19;78.
7. Mackenzie KC. Number 4 Canadian Hospital. The letters of Professor J J Mackenzie from the Salonica Front. Toronto: Macmillan; 1933. p. 198, 229.
8. The Common Cause. 1915 Dec 10;477.
9. McIlroy AL. Hôpital Auxiliare Bénévole 301, L'Armée d'Orient, Salonica. 1916 Aug 8. ML. TD1734/2/6/9/39.
10. Letters from Dr Erskine. ML. TD1734/2/4/1/19.

References

11. Scottish Women's Hospitals. Personnel files. 1917 Feb 20. ML. TD1734/1/4/2/135.
12. Ellie Rendel to Ray Strachey. 1916 Oct 29. WL. LSE: 7/BSH/2/2/5.
13. The Common Cause. 1916 Oct 27;367.
14. Stoney EA. The Girton and Newnham Unit of the Scottish Women's Hospitals for foreign service. National Union of Women's suffrage societies. Newnham Lett. 1917;25–40.
15. Edith Stoney to Mrs Laurie. 1916 Dec 8. ML. TD1734/2/6/9/57.
16. Edith Stoney to Mrs Laurie. 1917 Jan 24. ML. TD/1734/2/6/9/58.
17. Edith Stoney to Mrs Laurie. 1917 Feb 10. ML. TD1734/2/6/9/61.
18. Mrs Russell to Mrs Laurie. 1916 May 16. ML. TD1734.
19. Louise McIlroy to Mrs Russell. 1917 Jan 28. ML. TD1734.
20. Edith Stoney to the Secretary to the Director General Army Medical Services, War Office. 1917 Aug 26. ML. TD1734/2/6/9/69.
21. Phillips CES. Bibliography of X-ray literature and research 1896–1897. London: The Electrician; 1897.
22. Stoney EA. Electrical &c Department Report XXVIII Week. 1917 Apr 14–21. ML. TD1734/2/6/9/65.
23. Salonika G&N Unit Inventory of X-ray outfit. 1917 Mar. ML. TD1734/6/2/3/9.
24. Edith Stoney to Mrs Laurie. 1917 Oct 1. ML. TD1734/2/6/9/79.
25. Memoranda between Edith Stoney and Dr McIlroy. 1917 Sept 26. ML. TD1734/2/6/9/77.
26. Gleichen H. A mobile X-ray section on the Italian front. Blackwood's Mag. 1918;24:145–77.
27. Edith Stoney to Mrs Erskine. 1917 Aug 30. ML. TD1734/2/6/9/71.
28. McLaren ES. A history of the Scottish Women's Hospitals. London: Hodder and Stoughton; 1919. p. 384–92.
29. The Zander Institute London. Mechanical exercise a means of cure. London: Churchill; 1883.

Chapter 13
Mobile Radiography

When Florence left work in the afternoon of Friday 30 July 1915, she did not go directly back home to Hampstead. Instead, she made her way to Regent's Park and to the grounds of Bedford College for Women. Her purpose was to view the new X-ray ambulance that had been bought by the Scottish Women's Hospitals and was on display there. It would have been better had Edith accompanied her, so they could have discussed the advantages and disadvantages of this new vehicle, but her sister was by then in France, setting up the radiology department at Troyes with George Mallett.

Mobile X-ray units were not new at the outbreak of war in August 1914. There had been numerous prototype examples of X-ray equipment mounted in a variety of vehicles for use in the battlefield. Nevertheless, although the idea had currency, army medical corps had yet to include X-ray vans as a necessary part of medical planning. Nations, and their armies, had different official views on the value of such vehicles. The French were enthusiastic. By 1915, a French guide to war radiology devoted a whole chapter to *Les voitures radiologiques* [1]. Conversely, the *United States Army X-ray Manual* contained not a single reference to X-ray vans, reflecting the lack of interest by the US Army Medical Corps in such vehicles [2]. When the United States entered the war in 1917, any interest was limited to small vehicles equipped only for fluoroscopy, intended simply for brief visits to support rapid medical decisions in the evacuation areas [3]. Similarly the British War Office showed only muted interest in X-ray vans. Only 14 mobile X-ray units were deployed by the RAMC over the whole period of the war, 10 in France, 2 in Salonika and 2 in Mesopotamia [4].

The public were more enthusiastic. As Marie Curie had discovered, donations became more generous when attracted by the purchase of a piece of exciting new medical technology. Using her celebrity status as woman Nobel Prize winner, she helped to raise funds to purchase, eventually, 20 of her X-ray vans, nicknamed 'little Curies'. The Scottish Women's Hospitals' X-ray van project had a precedent in Britain too. As early as November 1914, a War Fund had been started by the Guild of Cheltenham Ladies' College. The subscribers were so generous that by 8 December there had been sufficient donations for the College to cover the estimated cost, £500, to fund a mobile X-ray unit to go to the front. There was a very strong network of contacts between Cheltenham and London, including Louisa Aldrich-Blake, Sir Alfred Keogh, the Director of the General Army Medical Services, and Archibald Reid, who later became the Chair of the War Office X-ray Committee.[1] By January 1915 it had been agreed to fund a Cheltenham unit with a design that had 'evolved after long and careful consultation between the English and French authorities' [5].

Keogh and Reid may have had an ulterior motive in accepting the donation, which probably anyway was insufficient to cover the whole cost of a vehicle plus equipment. Stimulated by the Cheltenham Ladies' initiative, they decided to commission not one but two mobile X-ray units. These were almost certainly both built on an Austin ambulance chassis. The 'Cheltenham College' unit was in France by the first week in June, initially under the command of Dr. Basil Lang FRCS (1880–1928), a surgeon from Bart's who specialised in ophthalmic surgery [6]. It was quickly followed by its companion, the 'No. 1 Mobile X-ray Unit' under Captain S. H. Gibson RAMC, which reported to General Headquarters 2 on 9 July and left Paris for its first assignment on 16 July [7].

Whilst the Cheltenham Ladies' College vehicle was first to reach the front line, it was only subsequently that it was included in the numerical listing of RAMC mobile units, becoming officially No. 2 (Cheltenham College) X-ray unit, losing the word 'Ladies" somewhere along the way [8]. It carried the label 'Presented by the Ladies' College Cheltenham, for use of the Wounded in the war 1914–'. The Cheltenham Guild also gained agreement from Dr. Reid that once there was no further need for the vehicle in war service, it would be donated to the New Hospital for Women in London. At the time this was agreed, in the first months of 1915, Florence was still nominally the person in charge of the X-ray service there. The plan would have made sense, making available X-ray services in poorer, smaller urban hospitals that lacked such facilities, operating as an outreach service from a centre of excellence. This certainly did happen after the war. However, if the Cheltenham vehicle was indeed used in this way, no record remains of its activities.

The Royaumont X-Ray Ambulance

The procurement and deployment of the SWH X-ray ambulance happened more or less at the same time as that of the Cheltenham College and No. 1 Units for the RAMC. There is much to suggest that the War Office took a strong interest in the SWH project, but they did not manage it. Indeed there were differences in purpose between the vehicles, which may have been reflected in their designs. In particular, the Army's purpose was to create peripatetic radiology units that would provide

---

[1]The War Office X-ray Committee was formally set up in late 1915 with responsibility for the planning, equipping and organising of X-ray services at home and on the battlefield, although it operated informally before that.

emergency radiology at the Casualty Clearing Stations, very close to the front line, fully staffed with a radiographer, technician and driver. On the other hand, the SWH hospital at Royaumont had no mandate to work in this way, and the intention was to work out from the main hospital and visit local hospitals in the area that lacked radiology, without the luxury of extra staff dedicated to the mobile unit.

No one in the SWH had procured a mobile X-ray unit before. It was the responsibility of Dr. Agnes Savill, the Royaumont radiologist, to lead the project, and she was invited by the London unit to return from France to do so [9]. She would have been happy to accept any experienced advice which might be available, especially if it could be drawn from the extensive network of professional contacts between women that had by now been established.

The offer of help, when it came, could not have come from a higher authority [10]. Hertha Ayrton (1854–1923) was a unique and pioneering woman engineer who stood alone in a profession that was otherwise exclusively male. Like Edith, she was educated at Cambridge and helped to form the first mathematical club at her own College, Girton. She completed the Maths Tripos in 1880, although she was not an academic high-flyer, as Edith would become a decade later. Her career began to mature when she joined her husband, William Ayrton, in his physics laboratory at Finsbury Technical College. Amongst other achievements, she became an acknowledged expert on the electric arc [11]. More importantly, she was hammering on the doors of the male bastions of professional science and engineering. She became the first female member of the Institution of Electrical Engineers in 1899, two decades before the next woman was admitted. In 1902 she was nominated to be a Fellow of the Royal Society. In this she was unsuccessful. Legal council advised this to be against its charter, because she was married, advice that was not reversed until 1923. Edith was well acquainted with her through their mutual involvement in national women's activities: Ayrton served as a vice president of the British Federation of University Women when Edith was its treasurer, and she also served as vice president of the National Union of Women's Suffrage Societies.

It was not that Hertha Ayrton herself could bring expertise in the design of a mobile X-ray car. She had no personal experience in medical radiology. But her close friend, Marie Curie, who she had known since 1903, did. They had first met when Pierre Curie had addressed the Royal Society on the subject of radium, when the Ayrtons had invited the Curies to dinner, remaining lifelong friends thereafter. Hertha Ayrton had been particularly caring for her widowed friend when, during 1912, she was suffering from a life-threatening illness that had required renal surgery and from continuing gossip resulting from the scandal of her affair with Paul Langevin [12]. In the summer, convalescing in Thonon-les-Bains, Marie Curie was worried that the press would discover where she was. Hertha invited her to escape to England. At the end of July, travelling under the name Madame Sklodowska, she found refuge with her old friend in an old mill house at Highcliffe-on-Sea, Hampshire, to be joined by her daughters Eve and Irène after a few days. Described briefly in her biography of her mother, Eve reported that 'her friend, Mrs. Ayrton, received her and her daughters in a peaceful home on the English coast. There she found care and protection' [13]. Before leaving England,

Marie Curie met Hertha's daughter Barbara at her house in Norfolk Square, learning more of her experience as a prisoner in Holloway Prison, convicted of suffragist activities earlier that year. At that time, Hertha Ayrton had written to Marie Curie, asking her to support a petition protesting the imprisonment of the leaders of the suffrage movement. Hertha Ayton had explained that she was a 'member of the association whose leaders are now in prison, and I know those leaders personally and look on them as persons of the utmost nobility of mind and greatness of purpose'. Marie Curie, who normally was very cautious about attaching her name to causes, agreed because the request came from her friend. 'I accept your using my name for the petition of which you tell me, because I have great confidence in your judgement.... I am very touched by all that you have told me of the struggle of English women for their rights; I admire them very much and I wish for their success'.

Hertha understood that she was in the ideal position to learn from her friend's experience and to ask for her advice in the design of the new mobile X-ray unit. She was well aware that Marie Curie had, very early in the war, focussed her efforts on supporting medical radiology in France. In the first weeks of the war, she had procured her first vehicle and X-ray equipment so that, in September 1914, she was able to provide radiological support for the flood of wounded who were arriving in Paris from the battle of the Marne.

Mari Curie's advice gave careful details of the specification she had used for her own X-ray vans [14]. She said:

> The bodywork of the car is from a larger model, and the power of the motor should be 15–20 HP. It needs to be strong but robust in motion, carrying 100 kg of useful load in addition to the bodywork, with pneumatic tyres to cushion the shocks that might damage the equipment. The size of the superstructure we have used is: height 1.60 or 1.65 m: length 1.9 m: width 1.4 m. But these dimensions may be altered a bit. The frame is light, from wood or steel. It has a glass door at the back. The frame holds the furniture and the photographic equipment.

She went on to describe how her vans were being used. 'The car goes into the hospitals at the front line and the doctor directs the examination of the wounded. I very often have carried them out myself, and they have been very successful, and saved many lives or prevented illness'. This matched with the aspirations of SWH, which similarly expected to support the work of smaller French hospitals near to Royaumont, lacking their own X-ray facilities. Intended to be entirely independent, power for the Curie vans was supplied by a dynamo driven from the van engine itself. Marie Curie described a couple of alternative means by which this was achieved:

> I fixed a dynamo on the running board on the side of the chassis at the front. The dynamo is driven by a drive-belt passing over a pulley on the motor axis, so that when the car is stationary, the motor drives the dynamo. If the car is of the type of construction that has a free end of the axis under the feet of the driver, it is also possible to mount the dynamo at the front of the car, with a pulley 30 cm in diameter. The dynamo generates 2 kW or a bit less (15 A at 110 V).

On 31 May 1915, a two-page quotation for the X-ray equipment arrived at the headquarters of the London Branch of the SWH from Fred R Butt & Co,

Manufacturers of X-ray, High Frequency and Electrotherapeutic Apparatus, 147 Wardour Street, London, at a total cost of £185 4s 9d. The most expensive items were the coil (£34-15-0), the accumulators (£27–14-0), the 4 X-ray tubes (total £18-18-0), the control panel (£15-10-0) and the interrupter (£11-3-8).

Much of the equipment was standard for the time. The imported Macalister-Wiggin gas tubes had a reputation for reliability and high output and with the 12″ coil should have been sufficient for most abdominal as well as peripheral radiology. Both screening and film radiography were catered for. Safety had been considered, and one operator could have been protected using the lead gloves and lead apron. The order added that 'The above Apparatus would have to be suitably arranged in the Ambulance Van for ease in taking down and erecting'.

Both Agnes Savill and Florence were familiar with radiological equipment. What was of greater interest to both women was the practical matter of fitting this into a vehicle. A separate quotation from the Austin Motor Company offered a 20 HP ambulance 'built to War Office requirements' to house the equipment. The stretchers and fittings were to be removed to make room for the X-ray equipment and darkroom facilities. The superstructure was to be made of aluminium to be fully lighttight. Austin informed the client that there was no permanent roof over the driving seat, perhaps being aware that it would be women and not men driving the vehicle. There was, however, to be a folding waterproof cover that could be used to protect the driver [15]. The quoted cost was £600. The specification that was received from the Austin Motor Company did not include an integral generator. A freestanding 15 A generator was included at delivery, loaded into the back with the other equipment. Generators designed for X-ray work were widely available from several suppliers by this time (Fig. 13.1).

The SWH vehicle was designed to provide two functions, to transport the X-ray equipment and to serve as a darkroom. In transit, the X-ray equipment was carried in the back. On arrival, some equipment, such as the couch, would be unpacked and set up in a tent for the examination, with the main van used as the darkroom with its own water supply. The 10-foot spring rheophores (cables) linked the electrical supply from van to the couch and tube in the tent. The heavier equipment, such as the control panel, coil and generator, would have usually stayed inside the van, to be operated from outside.

By the end of July, the ambulance was sufficiently complete to be shown off. There was a private viewing on Wednesday, 28 July, at the headquarters of the *Croix Rouge* in Knightsbridge, where M. Paul Cambon, the French Ambassador, and his daughter-in-law, Madame de la Panouse, President of the *Croix Rouge* in London and wife of the French Military Attaché at the Embassy, were present. They were accompanied by Miss Kathleen Burke and Miss Beatrix Hunter from the London Unit of the SWH [16]. On the same day, notices appeared in the press that the SWH X-ray ambulance would be on view to the public in the Bedford College Grounds in Regent's Park during the next two days, during the afternoon and early evening. Tickets were free: this was not to be a separate fundraising event. Photos appeared in Thursday's papers. The ambulance was draped in the Italian colours for the visit of the Marchesa Imperiali, the wife of the Italian Ambassador. The press described the ambulance as 'the finest and most up to date ever constructed', and that 'many

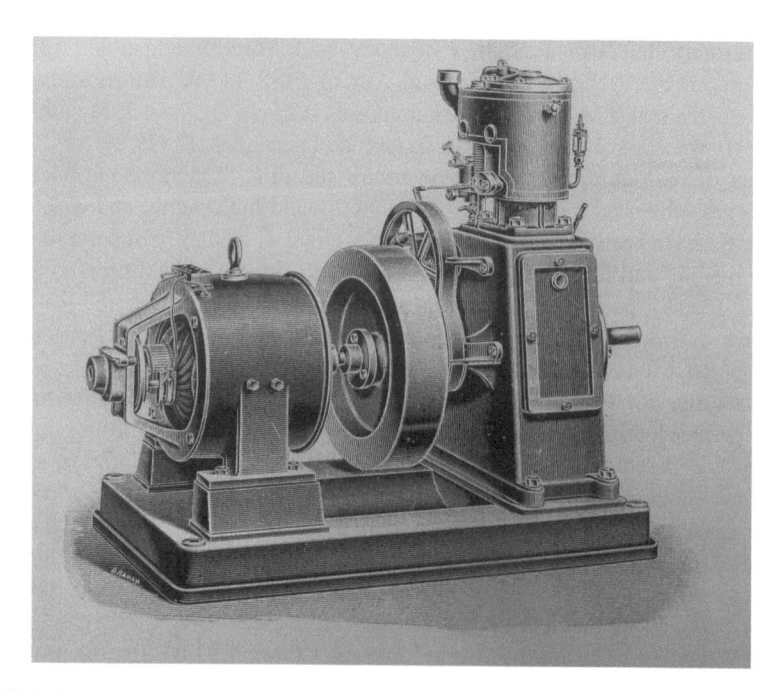

Fig. 13.1 A generator for X-ray work, from the Cavendish Electrical Company catalogue of X-ray and Electromedical Apparatus, 1914

prominent advocates of the women's movement' visited. The X-ray van was variously referred to as an *Ambulance Flottante*, or an *Ambulance Volante*. The final cost had risen to more than £1000, to cover the additional cost of the generator and the tent. The publicity value of this high-tech unit, run entirely by women, was exploited to the full.

The War Office was monitoring this initiative of the SWH with considerable interest, even though the purchasers were nominally a civilian organisation. This included the specification of the 'War Office Field Service Pattern' for equipment, and three of the items in the SWH van, the folding couch, the induction coil and the folding stereoscope, were identified by the supplier as conforming to this standard. This suggests both a close liaison between Fred Butt and the War Office and also that Savill and the SWH purchasers were being guided by the supplier. Following close on the heels of the Cheltenham College and No. 1 Units, Austin could declare that its ambulance conformed to War Office requirements. The embryonic War Office X-ray Committee would have been particularly interested in comparing the design of the SWH unit with that of their own two X-ray vehicles.

Florence was probably the only visitor with any first-hand knowledge of military radiology and was there not only through her personal interest but also in an official capacity. The reporter for the Scotsman described her as the 'Chief Radiographer to the War Office', which suggests an official position by which she reported back to Reid and his Committee [17].

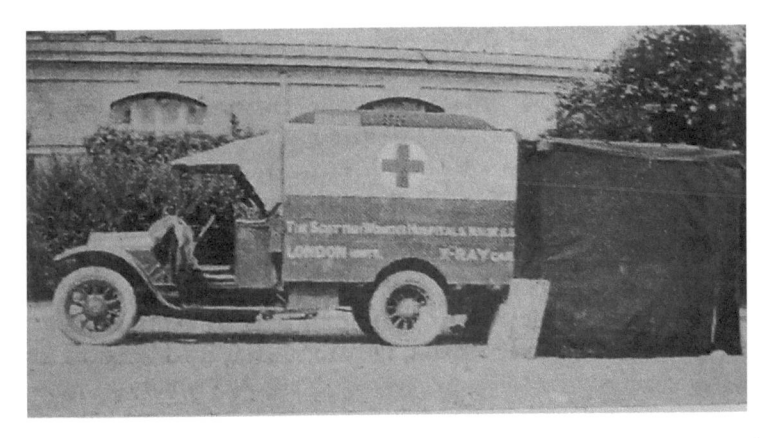

Fig. 13.2 The Scottish Women's Hospital London Unit X-ray ambulance at Royaumont showing the radiographic tent erected. (Abbeye de Royaumont archive and elsewhere)

The ambulance was now apparently ready for dispatch to France. There was a short hitch for which the War Office got the blame [18]. Perhaps the War Office and Austin wished to carry out further tests on this prototype vehicle to assist in the design of future X-ray vans for the Army. The Army were sufficiently interested that military radiological personnel, Major Barratt and Captain Humphries, were assigned to advise the Royaumont staff on setting up and using the van and quite likely to assess its potential in the army's own plans. Eventually, Agnes Savill was able to report on 11 September that the X-ray ambulance had arrived in France and that it was 'simply a perfect thing' (Fig. 13.2). It was soon put to use supporting the smaller hospitals in the neighbouring villages of Chantilly, Chambly, Laversine and Louvieux, where there was still no electrical supply [19]. The ambulance continued to be used intermittently up to the early part of 1918. However, by end of the war, there was a greater need to provide transport than mobile X-rays, and the Royaumont mobile X-ray unit was stripped of its equipment and adapted as an ambulance to carry four stretchers [20].

Towards the end of the war, in a paper on the design of mobile X-ray vans, Howard Head described the design of a van using an Austin ambulance chassis. He said 'One of the first equipments produced with this type of chassis was built in July 1915, and has since been in use near Paris'. This presumably referred to the RAMC No. 1 Mobile X-ray unit, although it is clear that the SWH ambulance was also in the vanguard of design, and much was learned from its use that was of value in designing later vans [21].

Head identified those design aspects that particularly resulted in its success. He noted specifically the loading line which, being quite low, made it easy to load and unload the back of the van. He also noted that the low loading line made it possible to reach the induction coil and control equipment from outside the vehicle, so only the X-ray stand and couch needed to be moved into the tented X-ray area. He remarked that the low centre of gravity helped with stability. By the time Head was reporting, his later van was considerably larger than that purchased for the London Unit of the

SWH. It included a lead-lined internal wall to separate the darkroom from the X-ray equipment and a specially designed dynamo driven by a chain from the ambulance engine. By 1918, much had been learned about the effective design of a vehicle to bring X-rays to remote medical facilities under war conditions.

The Edith Cavell X-Ray Van

During these heady early days of 1915, when the Austin X-ray ambulance was being arranged for the London Unit, it was discussed in the committees of the SWH whether more than one van might be procured, either for Royaumont or perhaps to support the Girton and Newnham Unit. Edith shared Florence's enthusiasm for the value of an X-ray van. Nevertheless, as early as May 1915, Edith was told that these plans would not be carried forward and that it was deemed unnecessary to include the X-ray van for the hospital at Troyes. When the Girton and Newnham Unit was posted to Serbia and then to Salonika, Edith returned to the question of mobile radiology with renewed interest. It was probably true that an X-ray vehicle would have been of marginal utility in Troyes. On the other hand, the conditions Edith had experienced in Gevgheli were much more challenging and more chaotic than in France. The terrain, too, was much more difficult, the roads unmade and the mountainous tracks often impassable. Outside Salonika, closer to the fighting in Serbia, it seemed to Edith that there was a real need for a rugged mobile X-ray unit that could negotiate the difficult travelling conditions to reach remote hospitals where there were few or no modern facilities. It would be a risk, but with the right equipment and planning, she knew that radiology could reach otherwise unsupported hospitals and was excited to try.

On 12 October 1915, shortly after the Girton and Newnham Unit left Troyes, the nurse Edith Cavell was executed for treason by a German firing squad, convicted of aiding allied soldiers to escape from German-occupied Belgium. This event caused a huge outcry of rage throughout Britain. In Scotland, public grief was turned to good purpose. Not long after the death was reported in the press, a 'Scottish Edith Cavell Fund' was set up by a tireless supporter of the SWH, Miss Etta Shankland of Greenock. Funds were quickly raised, soon enough to support eight 'Edith Cavell' beds in hospitals at the front [22].

By the beginning of 1916, soon after Edith had arrived in Salonika, Florence began lobbying the SWH head office on her behalf that they should provide another X-ray van, this one for the Girton and Newnham Unit [23]. At first this was not met with much support in Scotland. Then, in May 1916, new fundraising advertisements appeared in Scottish newspapers, independently from the SWH, stating that the Scottish Branch of the British Red Cross were raising money for an 'X-ray car for the Russians':

> The great distances to be covered between the Russian Front and the hospitals render it necessary that an accurate diagnosis of the injuries should be made before the wounded are dispatched to the base. The Scottish X-ray car will relieve the suffering of our gallant allies,

and will form a fitting addition to the Scottish hospital ward at Petrograd, and motor ambulances. [24]

Anything that the Red Cross were doing in Scotland must of course be matched or bettered by the Scottish Women's Hospitals. It was clear that the name Edith Cavell had strong emotional power, and soon the Glasgow Branch set about further fundraising for the Edith Cavell Fund. The Red Cross were already referring to their vehicle as 'The Scottish X-ray car', so another title was required to distinguish the two efforts. Miss Shankland wrote to Mrs. Cavell, who replied that nothing would please her better than that the SWH car be named after her daughter. This vehicle soon became known as the 'Edith Cavell X-ray van'. Nearly all the £900 required to pay for the fully equipped van was gathered by a single Flag Day in Glasgow [25]. The contract was awarded to Mr. Prosser, 68 Hope St, who was the Glasgow Wolseley Agent. Prosser knew nothing about radiology, of course, and the supply and installation of the X-ray equipment was subcontracted to D. B. Selkirk, Scientific Instrument Makers of 100 Bath Street, who procured the actual equipment from a number of other suppliers.

There remained a question about the ultimate destination of this new car. At the beginning of July, Florence heard from Mrs. Laurie that the X-ray car could not be secured for Salonika [26]. This was partly because of the new hospital unit that was being planned at this time to go to Serbia, and there was uncertainty whether the X-ray van might be placed there instead. On 14 July Elsie Inglis, who was particularly interested in Serbia, promised to consult Edith, whilst it was left to Miss Kemp, a committee member, to talk to Dr. Erskine [27].

It was soon realised that the purchase of an X-ray van would provide an extremely effective focus for further fundraising. As early as the end of July, the treasurer wrote to Elsie Inglis that, once the van was completed, 'we propose to show it to make a little money' [28]. The publicity value of a high-tech item designed and built north of the border was too good to miss. The Glasgow donors believed they had the local engineering expertise to execute the project. Marian Erskine knew about X-rays: she was honorary physician at Bruntsfield Hospital and in charge of the X-ray and electrical department there. Her committee colleagues would have considered her as an expert in radiology. What could go wrong?

It is at this point that the initiative, sadly, started to unravel. The design brief given to Prossers appears to have been unclear, and, in the absence of any clarity or actual expert advice, the garage interpreted the brief in its own way, within the budget it was given. As a result, the requirement was interpreted in a rather narrow way. Edith and Louise McIlroy were too far away to make clear what was their actual operational need, and anyway there was a muddle whether the van was to be placed in Salonika or in the new 'America' unit in Ostrovo, Serbia, which would be opened in September. What is fairly clear is that the initial idea was for a fluoroscopic X-ray van more aligned with the US Army design than that of the Royaumont ambulance. Film radiology would not be required, and so no darkroom was planned. The fluoroscopic imaging would be carried out in the lighttight back of the van, which itself would be entirely self-sufficient in electrical power, with its own engine and dynamo. It was a neat, simple package. Quite early it was realised that, one way or another, a tent would be required, either to allow examinations outside the vehicle or to make a darkroom for film processing, so that was added to the specification, for an additional £50.

By the time Edith got back from Salonika to London at the end of September, the X-ray van was complete, as Prosser had understood the specification. When Edith met Marian Erskine in London on 6 October, she was invited to travel to Scotland to inspect the vehicle in Glasgow and report to the Committee in Edinburgh. She had hoped to inspect the car before the meeting on the 11 October, but in fact she was invited to meet them first, only then travelling on to Glasgow. Probably everyone was hoping that this inspection would be a formality so that the van could quickly be dispatched. But even before she travelled to Scotland on the overnight train, Edith had learned enough from talking to Erskine, who had not yet seen the van, to raise serious concerns in her mind.

Edith had very firm views of what she expected, and this included a sufficiently powerful X-ray set installed in a sufficiently rugged lorry with a ready supply of spare parts [29]. Furthermore, she anticipated that most of the studies would be carried out using film radiography, not fluoroscopy. She may have known of the Fiat X-ray vans used by the radiographic units of the British Red Cross in Italy, under the command of the aristocratic Countess Helena Gleichen, cousin of George V. Her vehicle with its 14½-inch clearance and double wheels allowed access over the worst of rough mountain roads. Edith knew that the widespread use of Fords in Salonika meant that their spares were easy to come by. Having such standards, she was shocked and embarrassed when she first saw the small low-slung Wolseley lorry when she arrived at Prosser's garage to inspect the vehicle. The letters she wrote during the next year or so exhibit the complete range of emotions she experienced as she battled to come to terms with what had happened: confusion, frustration, disbelief, irritation, anger, disappointment, embarrassment and ultimately profound sadness [30–37]. These letters have allowed the following detailed description to be set out, avoiding, as far as possible, her own repetition of unresolved criticisms, and in some cases altering the chronology of her comments slightly in order to clarify the themes. The letters certainly included a large degree of rational self-justification, which at times would have come over as irritating. Nevertheless, she consistently argued that surgeons would have been able to save more soldiers' lives had an effective mobile radiology unit been available earlier and genuinely wished for the van to be placed where it was most needed.

When she returned home to London from Scotland, she immediately prepared a formal written critique, giving her initial views both on design problems with the vehicle and also the design problems with the X-ray equipment.

Her critique opened with a polite paragraph expressing her very great appreciation for the trouble and care that has been taken to provide this car. She then sets out her criticisms. Her main concern was undoubtedly the size of the vehicle. Accepting that it was not going to be a van as robust as the Fiat she had seen in Italy, she had hoped that at least it could have been the Wolseley Colonial van with its higher clearance, and not the smallest van in the Wolseley range. She proposed that, for a little extra money taken from the available maintenance budget, the X-ray equipment could be refitted into a higher specification vehicle. 'It is a beautiful car—but the clearage (5½ inches) is very small for Serbian roads'. The vehicle might be useful in the Serbian towns, but only if it could be transported there from Salonika by rail.

Edith had other concerns, not critical, but worrying nevertheless. The power available from the mounted dynamo was low, and the novel method of coupling to the engine was of concern. Indeed, she knew that smaller lighter generators now made it possible to be independent of the vehicle's engine, as was done in the SWH X-ray van. There was a further practical issue. Unlike the Royaumont Austin van, the Wolseley had no electric self-starter. Edith knew that women drivers would find it difficult to operate this vehicle in the absence of such a facility, especially during the cold Serbian winter. Furthermore, she felt that the 20 HP van was underpowered, carrying about 4 tons even without passengers, driver, water, petrol and plates. She also anticipated problems with the availability of Wolseley spare parts in Salonika.

She was only able to test the X-ray equipment on fluoroscopy, there being no means to carry out film radiography. She was broadly positive about the X-ray equipment, which she thought was well constructed and of good quality. But she only managed to reach a maximum tube current of 2.5 mA and was disappointed to be unable to image anything thicker than a hand. The time was insufficient to determine why the performance was so poor, and she was of the opinion that this was because the equipment was not all from one maker. Edith would have preferred the larger water-cooled Macalister-Wiggin tubes, capable of operating with a higher tube current, as were included both in her own X-ray system and that in the London Unit ambulance. Nor could she properly test the lighttightness of the van within the subdued lighting of the garage workshop, and the tent was not yet available to evaluate. An important omission was the plumb line, essential for foreign body localisation: no one in Glasgow seemed to have had understood that foreign body localisation was the most important wartime use of X-rays. And, finally, in a detail that reveals her complete knowledge of the technology, she was fairly certain that she would not be able to find a source of coal gas in the villages of Serbia: the mercury jet-break interrupter supplied was designed to work with a coal gas dielectric instead of the more practical paraffin or alcohol. Betraying her sensitivities, she observed that 'the X Ray expert would not have asked a *man* X Ray specialist to pass it in the way it worked' and suggested that Florence might be asked to try out the X-ray system once it was fully up to specification, in order to pass it for clinical use.

Later, in a pointed criticism of the parochialism that caused the poor specification, she asked rhetorically, 'What could be said of a policy which decided that Glasgow soldiers might only use guns made by some eminent Glasgow firm, eminent in other ways, but which had never made this kind of gun before? If added to this no expert tested the guns before the gallant men risked their lives with them, you have a parallel to your committee insisting that a Glasgow firm must fit the car as the money was raised in Glasgow'. Such barbed comments were guaranteed to further alienate her from the committee members in Edinburgh.

Edith knew that the car would have little relevance in Salonika, with its several well-equipped hospitals, and expressed her provisional support for its deployment to support the work of the more remote SWH hospitals in Serbia, such as the America Unit in Ostrovo. Assuming that the technical details she had identified would be rectified, possibly including a more appropriate vehicle, she hoped that it could be dispatched by January, in preparation for the expected spring offensive.

The Glasgow team did not allow Edith's concerns to interfere with the publicity value of the new X-ray van, even if they were made aware of them. On Tuesday, 17 October 1916, the 'magnificently equipped X-ray motor ambulance' was formally presented to Mrs. Mair, the President of the SWH, by the Lord Provost of Glasgow and his wife, Sir Thomas and Lady Dunlop, in the quadrangle of Glasgow City Chambers [38]. The proceedings were presided over by Lieutenant Colonel Dalziel. They were in no hurry to ship it on. The newspaper reported that 'Prior to proceeding to the Front the car will be placed on exhibition in various Scottish towns, and demonstrations of the working of the X-ray apparatus will be given.' The vehicle set off the following Monday, and by the time the tour ended in Carlisle on 18 November, it had travelled as far north as Elgin and as far east as Aberdeen and Dundee, including stops at 32 towns along the way. It was estimated that 9000 people visited the car. Fourteen thousand postcards of Edith Cavell were sold. The tour resulted in over £650 more in donations, substantially greater than was needed to cover the extra cost of the tent [39, 40] (Figs. 13.3 and 13.4). The surplus was banked to provide support and maintenance. The tour gave plenty of opportunity for press photography [41] (Fig. 13.5).

A month later the 'Edith Cavell X-ray Wagon' was still in Glasgow, where the general public were invited to inspect it at Prosser's Garage, for an admission fee of 1 shilling during the day and sixpence in the evening [42]. 'This X-ray Wagon, built and fitted by Glasgow firms, is the first of its kind to be equipped in Scotland, and in its recent tour throughout England and Scotland created unflagging interest'. Edith was of course irritated by the delay this caused in shipping the vehicle and made her feelings known, writing to a committee member later that she 'had urged you to send the car last Autumn instead of taking it round on show to raise money'.

During the next few months, Dr. Erskine seems to have made little attempt to respond to Edith's criticisms. She argued that no tent 'is absolutely light-proof in the brilliant light of Macedonia' and that they had a similar problem with a tent she chose for Ostrovo. The best suggestion she could offer was that they should find a lighttight hut at each hospital they visited, or, failing that, the plates could be taken home to be developed [43]. The van was still in Glasgow in February, but set to be in the next consignment, by which time Prosser, having been paid, was not very interested in dealing with any of the technical criticisms, saying that he was not an X-ray expert [44].

The X-ray van finally arrived in Salonika in late May 1917. Edith was appalled to find that none of her recommended changes had been made. Further problems became apparent. Tubes and lamps had been poorly packed and arrived broken. The 'light-proof' tent, not seen in Glasgow, was made of canvas that was so thick and was so large that it was too heavy to erect. Furthermore, there was a severe practical problem. The way in which the dynamo had been coupled to the engine caused considerable vibration of the whole van. This meant that film radiography

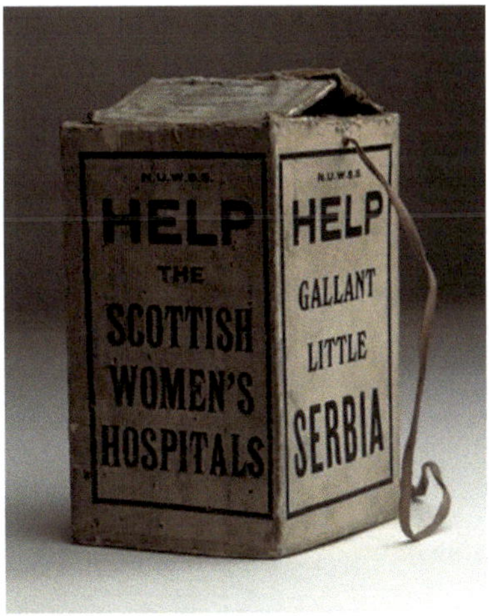

Fig. 13.3 A Scottish Women's Hospitals collecting box. (National Museum of Scotland)

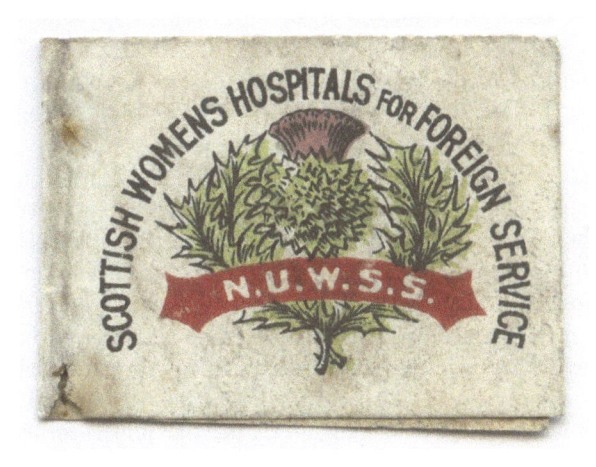

Fig. 13.4 A Scottish Women's Hospitals fundraising flag

was impossible because the movement blurred the image, and even fluoroscopy was compromised. Finally, the sunny Mediterranean conditions were always a challenge, but the small Wolseley became almost unbearably hot during use. It was clear that she had received a grossly inferior van, and Edith was embarrassed to demonstrate it to her more experienced visitors. She took the view that the van would have so little operational value that the equipment should be stripped out and used elsewhere and that the van itself should be used as a general-purpose ambulance.

She was late producing her final report and later wrote to her friend Mrs. Laurie, 'Dr. Erskine is very angry with me over my report and treats me as Major Carter was treated in Mesopotamia' [45]. Major Carter, of the Indian Medical Service, had

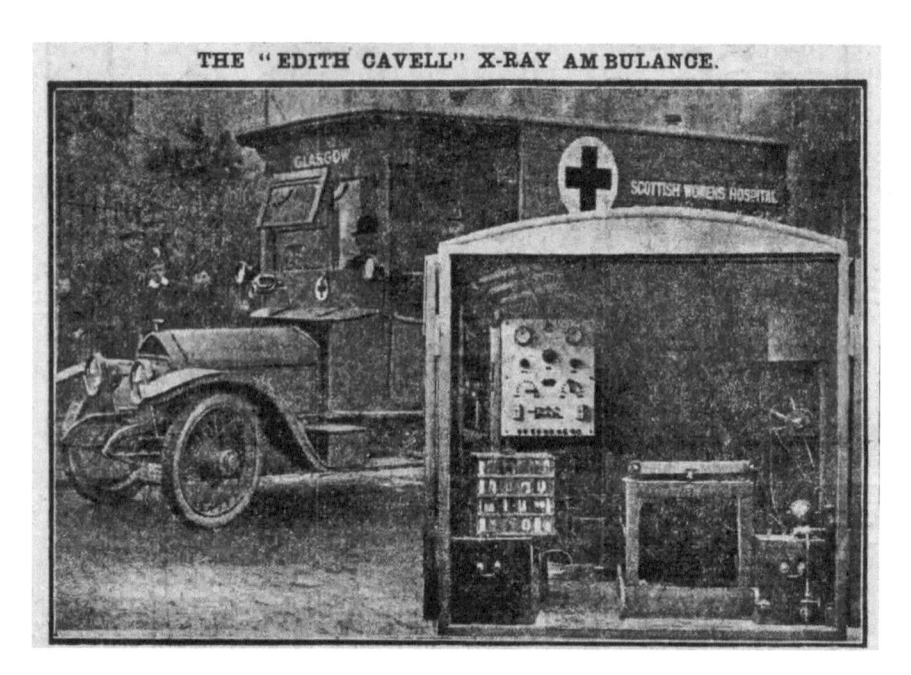

Fig. 13.5 The 'Edith Cavell X-ray Ambulance' exhibited at St Roque's Garage, Dundee. Inset is a view of the interior. Dundee People's Journal 4 Nov 1916. (British Library Newspaper archive/DC Thompson)

written an official letter to describe the sufferings of 600 sick and wounded people crowded into a small river steamer in the Mesopotamian battles of late 1915 and 'was treated with great rudeness... General Cowper... threatened to put him under arrest and said that he could get his hospital ship taken away from him for a meddlesome, interfering faddist.' [46]. Clearly there were times when Edith got a bit carried away by her own self-righteousness, although it had actually occurred to her to make the issue public [47]. It is easy to understand why Dr. Erskine was angry. The X-ray van was a costly, public, high-tech, prestige project for the SWH. What she wanted from Edith was a glowing report that demonstrated how their women were at the vanguard of medical care for casualties in the mountains of Serbia, if possible supported by photographs with grand scenery and grateful wounded. What she had received was a scathing criticism of a mismanaged project, which supplied badly conceived and constructed equipment, too late, to an inappropriate location.

Even now, Edith lived in the hope that something could be recovered from the wreck of the project. By now she understood that it all started with Etta Shankland, the enthusiastic fundraiser who had been so naively influential in setting the scene at the early stages of the project. So, on 30 August 1917, Edith wrote a long letter to her, which starts 'My Dear Miss Shankland, I do not know how to tell you how very sorry I am over this business of the X-ray car you gave so much time and thought and labour getting the funds for.'

She reiterated the need:

> I had several requests for the use of the car—and knew it would be most useful at the small forward surgical outpost (of about 30 beds) of the Ostrovo Unit of the Scottish Women's Hospitals. This had no X-rays tho' a surgical unit!. Much good work could have been done up where it was also in neighbouring Serb and Russian Clearing Stations, there being no X-rays and much need of them. But this was at Dobravenij—some 50 miles further over the mountains than Ostrovo—and only a car high off the ground ... could have got there with the heavy X-ray outfit.

On the whole, Edith places the greatest blame on the Wolseley agent Prosser and the equipment supplier Selkirk. She felt very sore that the men who designed and manufactured the X-ray van had paid no attention to the critical points that she, a woman, had made. 'It was disastrous mistake I fear putting the outfit of the car and the choice of the chassis, in the hands of a Glasgow firm who had not made a very special study of the very special subject of X-ray *car* outfits'. She expressed the hope that even now there was a possibility of replacing the chassis with one more suited to the mountains of Serbia. 'I do very greatly trust that you may be able to induce the Scottish Women's Hospitals Committee to make such sacrifice and additions as will make this Edith Cavell car of great use and success in skilled hands—they have taken the matter out of mine'.

She ended the letter 'Some day when you are in London it would give great pleasure to my sister and to me if you would come to see us—With very great regret for disappointing you—I am heartbroken over it all. Yours sincerely, Edith A Stoney'.

Edith recognised that it was not easy to design a mobile X-ray van. Both the technology and the operational requirements were changing rapidly, with no general consensus on the specific medical needs for X-ray vans close to the battle. If the US Medical Corps was correct, all that was needed to support the casualty clearing stations was a simple fluoroscopic system, similar in concept to the original SWH specification. As it happens, Edith herself did not believe this approach was correct, noting reports that numerous American vehicles lay unused in French ports, but it was an approach that certainly had its place, especially as high casualty numbers led to increased use of fluoroscopy over film radiography throughout all military hospitals. As the front stabilised in France and the military hospitals were better established and better equipped, even the argument that a van might help to support the smaller hospitals became weaker. Writing as early as March 1917 of the London Unit's experience, Florence observed that 'it is pity the (X-ray ambulance) at Royaumont was not made more use of—the difficulty is to get things just where they are wanted' [48]. As Edith pointed out, the strongest argument for mobile radiology arose not in France, but from the more remote areas of conflict, where field hospitals were more primitive, and radiology could indeed support surgeons trying their best in very difficult conditions. But this could only have worked with a high-specification van with a rugged design and by having high performing, reliable X-ray equipment installed in it. Sadly, the SWH van supplied for work in Salonika and Serbia simply did not meet this need. About 6 months after Edith left, the RAMC finally deployed two mobile units in Salonika and the surrounding district, built to a more suitable design for the conditions there [49].

References

1. Massiot G. Biquard. La manuel practique du manipulateur radiologiste. Paris: Maloine; 1915. p. 140–80.
2. United States Army X-ray Manual. London: Lewis; 1919.
3. Christie AC. Mobile Roentgen ray apparatus. Am J Roentegenol. 1919:358–67.
4. MacPherson WG. Official History of the War. Medical services general history, vol 1. Appendix E. London: HMSO; 1921. p. 401.
5. Cheltenham Ladies' College War Fund. Interim Report Jan 1915. Cheltenham Ladies' College Magazine. 1915 Spring.
6. Lang BT. A Day's work with the mobile x ray unit. Cheltenham Ladies College Guild Leaflet. 1916:63;22–24.
7. Army Troops No 1 Mobile X-ray Unit. National Archives Kew. WO 95/259/5.
8. Army Troops. No 2 (Cheltenham College) X-ray Unit. National Archives, Kew. WO 95 503/1&2.
9. de Navarro A. The Scottish Womens Hospital at the French Abbey of Royaumont. London: Allen & Unwin; 1917. p. p161.
10. Perthshire Advertiser. 1915 Aug 4.
11. Ayrton H. The electric arc. London: The Electrician; 1903.
12. Quinn S. Marie Curie a life. London: Heinemann; 1995.
13. Curie E. Madame Curie. Tr. Vincent Sheean. New York: Doubleday Doran; 1938. p. p281.
14. Scottish Women's Hospital archive. WL. 2SWH.
15. Van Tiggelen R. Radiology in a Trench Coat. Brussels: Academia; 2013. p. p158.
16. M. Cambon and Scottish Women's Hospital Equipment. The Scotsman. 1915 Jul 29.
17. X-ray Motor Ambulance. The Scotsman. 1915 Jul 30.
18. Crofton E. The women of Royaumont. East Lothian: Tuckwell Press; 1997. p. 49.
19. de Navarro A. The Scottish Womens Hospital at the French Abbey of Royaumont. London: Allen & Unwin; 1917. p. 162.
20. Crofton E. The women of Royaumont. East Lothian: Tuckwell Press; 1997. p. 182.
21. Head HC. Mobile X-ray wagon unit. J Rönt Soc. 1918;93–99.
22. The Scotsman. 1916 Oct 18.
23. Guy JM. Edith (1869–1938) and Florence (1870–1932) Stoney, two Irish sisters and their contribution to radiology during World War I. J Med Biog. 2013;21:100–7.
24. Aberdeen Daily Journal. 1915 May 9.
25. Edith Cavell X-ray Car. Peoples Journal. 1916 Nov 4.
26. Florence Stoney to Mrs Laurie. 1916 July 6. ML. TD/1734/2/6/9.
27. Inglis to Kemp. 1916 July 14. ML. TD1734/2/6/4/2/43.
28. Mrs Laurie to Inglis. 1916 July 20. ML. TD1734/2/6/4/2/45.
29. Edith Stoney to Mrs Laurie. 1916 Oct 6. ML. TD/1734/2/6/9/44.
30. Edith Stoney to Mrs Laurie. 1916 Oct 16. ML. TD1734/2/6/9/47.
31. Edith Stoney to Mrs Laurie. 1916 Oct 17. ML. TD1734/2/6/9/48.
32. Edith Stoney to Mrs Laurie. 1916 Dec 8. ML. TD1734/2/6/9/57.
33. Edith Stoney to Mrs Laurie. 1917 Jan 24. ML. TD1734/2/6/9/58.
34. Edith Stoney to Dr Erskine. 1917 Aug 30. ML. TD1734/2/6/9/71.
35. Edith Stoney Miss Shankland. 1917 Aug 30. ML. TD1734/2/6/9/72.
36. Edith Stoney. 1917 Aug 31. Lord Northcliffe speaking of the Italian Front August 1916. ML. TD/1734/2/6/9/73.

References

37. Edith Stoney to Mrs Laurie. 1917 Oct 14. ML. TD1734/2/6/9/81.
38. Edith Cavell memorial. Presentation of X-ray Motor Ambulance. Daily Record. 1916 Oct 18.
39. Report on the tour of the Edith Cavell X Ray Car. 1916 Nov 14. ML. TD1734/1/11/6.
40. Care of the Wounded – "Edith Cavell" X-ray car. The Scotsman. 1916 Dec 9.
41. Dundee People's Journal. 1916 Nov 4;8.
42. Daily Record. 1916 Dec 18.
43. Dr Erskine to Mrs Laurie. 1917 Feb 19. ML. TD1734/2/4/1/19.
44. Mrs Laurie to Dr Erskine. 1917 Feb 16. ML. TD1743/2/4/1/19.
45. Edith Stoney to Mrs Laurie. 1917 Sept 20. ML. TD1734/2/6/9/74.
46. Mesopotamia Commission. Hansard. 1917 Jul 4.
47. Edith Stoney to Mrs Laurie. 1917 Nov 10. ML. TD1734/2/6/9/86.
48. Florence Stoney to Mrs Laurie. 1917 Mar 1. ML. TD1734/2/6/9/63.
49. No 9 and No 10 Mobile X-ray unit. National Archives, Kew. WO 95/4807.

Chapter 14
Villers-Cotterêts

Edith arrived home in Hampstead on 16 August 1917. She now had the loosest of formal relationships with the Scottish Women's Hospitals. Mrs. Russell thought so too and wished this to come to an end. Before she went away on holiday in August, she arranged for a letter to be sent to Edith, telling her that her resignation was now 'taken to be final'. Mrs. Russell must have gone away a happy woman, having finally got rid of this difficult troublemaker. She could not have been more wrong.

Edith was in a quandary. She needed a job, an income. She had sent off her passport to be stamped with a Greek visa, under the unwarranted expectation that she would be returning to Salonika, only to learn from Mrs. Russell that her contract with SWH had been terminated. Both her heart and some of her possessions were still in Greece and she retained a belief that she might be given a new contract to return there to assist with the technical support of McIlroy's planned orthopaedic unit. The rest in London was certainly welcome, but she needed to sort out what she could do next. Florence was financially secure in her position as radiologist at the Fulham Military Hospital so could cover her expenses for a while, but Edith had no pension and had no intention of being dependent permanently on her sister for financial support. She needed to explore other options that would match her unique skills and experience. She learnt that Countess Gleichen, who had been running one of the X-ray vans in Italy, was returning home on sick leave, suffering from the major occupational hazard of war radiography, radiation burns to her hand [1]. Countess Gleichen's misfortune (or bad radiological safety practice) generated a vacancy in the British Red Cross Unit in Italy, and Edith was approached to determine if she was available. She initially refused the offer, claiming a commitment to the Salonika Unit. Without a radiological expert to lead the Italian Red Cross Unit, it closed during October.

Back to France

It was not until 27 September that her future was decided. Louise McIlroy had been in Edinburgh where she had at last gained permission to go ahead with her orthopaedic unit. She put in a request that she should be allowed to recruit Edith for a few months to set up the electrotherapy equipment. However, there was another more pressing SWH initiative in France that needed Edith's expertise, and it took priority.

During her brief stay in Paris on her way home in July, she had visited the SWH London Unit hospital in Royaumont Abbey, to find out how the X-ray and electrotherapy work was progressing there under the leadership of Agnes Savill. Royaumont was the flagship hospital of the Scottish Women's Hospitals. It had been established in the old Abbey of Royaumont when it was offered by its owner Edouard Goüin to the *Société de secours aux blessés militaires* in December 1914 to be used as a hospital to care for the wounded.[1] The main drive brought incoming ambulances to the main door, from where the wounded were moved towards set up in the high-vaulted rooms. When they overflowed and the weather was good, they set up beds in the cloisters on the four sides of an enclosed garden. Staff were accommodated in rooms upstairs. Electricity was supplied from a water-driven dynamo. Senior doctors and politicians from London and Paris were regular visitors, admiring the smooth efficiency with which the Chief Medical Officer, Frances Ivens, conducted operations. Agnes Savill wrote 'Royaumont placed a spell upon all who saw it; on those who dwelt within its walls the spell was so mysterious and so potent that it inevitably drew them back from all other interests and occupations. . . . Custom never dulled ones appreciation of its beauty, nor did long familiarity during the passage of the years ever blur the sense of satisfied delight aroused by the peaceful proportions of its cloisters, its arches, its great grey pillars and groined roofs' [2] (Fig. 14.1). At the time of Edith's visit, the fighting had moved away, the wounded being largely shipped to other hospitals served by a different railway, and the hospital had become a bit of a backwater. Savill wrote 'During these peaceful interludes there were musical and other entertainments of a wide variety in the wards'. For recreation, staff could walk in the surrounding parkland and woods. To Edith, the contrast with the tented hospital in the swamp in Salonika that she had just left could not have been greater.[2]

During her brief visit, she was able to offer advice on the equipment both at Royaumont and at the new SWH hospital at Villers-Cotterêts that was being set up at the time [3]. She suggested in particular that Frances Ivens should request a different

---

[1]At the same time, the SWH set up a typhoid annex for Belgian children in Calais under the leadership of Dr. Alice Hutchison (1874–1953). This hospital closed in March 1915. It continued to Valjevo in Serbia, where it was overrun in November 1915. After release from confinement as a prisoner of war, Hutchison worked in other SWH hospitals, returning to London at the end of the war.

[2]A French-language film clip showing contemporary and wartime sequences at Royaumont may be found at https://www.youtube.com/watch?v=DMKwr3p7U6E

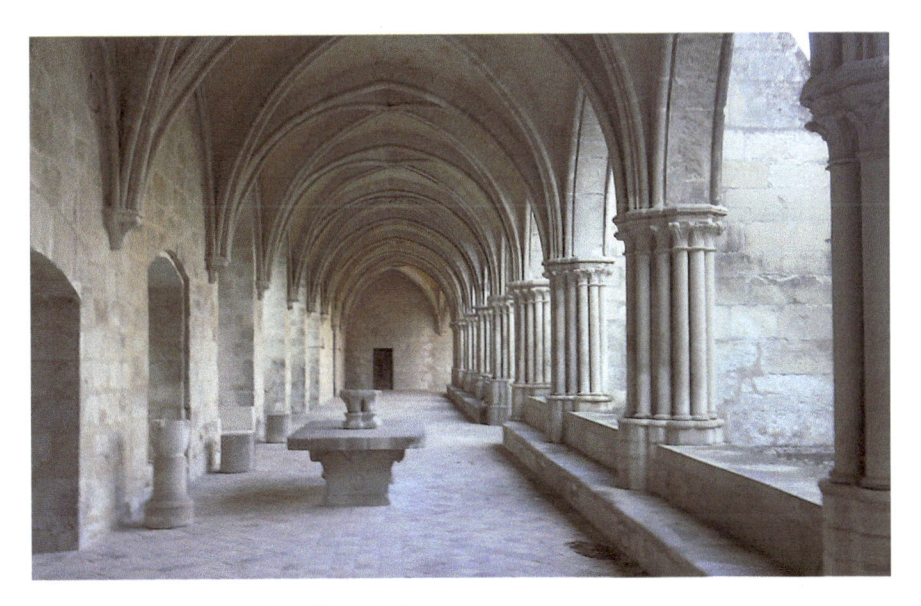

Fig. 14.1 The Cloister of the Abbaye de Royaumont

generator to operate the X-ray equipment at Villers-Cotterêts, the one that had already been installed being of insufficient power.

Edith was pleased to renew her acquaintanceship with Frances Ivens (Fig. 14.2). The two women, whilst not close friends, were well known to one another. Edith had first come across her as high-flying student who had graduated MBBS from the London School of Medicine for Women in 1902. When Ivens became surgical registrar at the Royal Free Hospital in 1904, she took on Florence's responsibility for the X-ray equipment for a couple of years, no doubt being advised by Edith in its technical aspects. The two women had worked together again as officers of the Federation for University Women after Frances Ivens had been appointed as gynaecological surgeon to a new unit in the Liverpool Stanley Hospital. These experiences had resulted in a high mutual respect for one another's complementary skills and dedication to hard work. Miss Ivens had a clear understanding that the technical aspects of radiography must be looked after, otherwise the service would be inadequate at best and absent at worst. Agnes Savill wanted to return soon to look after her medical practice in Harley Street during the winter, and Ivens needed someone to take on responsibility for running the X-ray unit at Villers-Cotterêts. She was increasingly aware that successful X-ray departments demanded active technical support. Equipment went wrong, got broken and needed adjustment. Agnes Savill knew Florence well and was aware that the Fulham Military Hospital was fortunate to have engineers for this technical support, allowing Florence to concentrate fully on her clinical work. Frances Ivens proposed that Edith should be posted to France to fill a similar role in her unit. The initial cautious appointment was for a temporary stay of 4 months. She appreciated Edith's talents and was willing to

Fig. 14.2 Frances Ivens, Chief Medical Officer of the Scottish Women's Hospitals London Unit, Royaumont Abbey

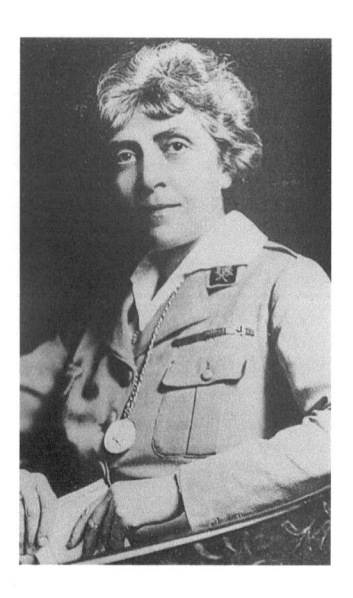

risk the reputation that she had gained in Edinburgh for being difficult to work with. She must have been very persuasive, because the Chairman of the Committee, Nellie Hunter, noted her regret that 'the Personnel Committee had re-appointed Miss Stoney, as she considered Dr. McIlroy's reports, and Miss Stoney's letters, showed that she was too difficult to be a member of a unit' [4].

On 27 September Edith received a letter from Mrs. Russell offering her a post at Royaumont. Given all the history between these two women, one can only imagine Mrs. Russell's gritted teeth and Edith's wry satisfaction. Rather perversely she decided to play hard to get, claiming that she had not heard back from the Red Cross about the Italian job but stating that she would be glad to go to Royaumont if she were now free to accept. She also protested about being posted to France rather than Salonika claiming that she had been tied to her post in Salonika and had lost several posts as a result, though this seems a little disingenuous in retrospect [5]. She also wished to recover her own tent from Salonika before setting off, having heard from Agnes Savill's sister of the 'discomfort and unhealthiness' at Villers-Cotterêts [6]. This request was rejected and she was given a room in one of the huts. She could never have stayed in a tent in the depths of the winter anyway.

As Florence and her colleagues in London were swamped with casualties from the battles around the small village of Passchendaele, Edith waited for her papers to move to France with increasing frustration. Lack of communication, as she saw it, allowed her to place the blame for the delay firmly on SWH bureaucracy, which she did with considerable fury and much underlining in yet another letter, sent once she had safely arrived in Royaumont en route to Villers-Cotterêts [7]. She finally left the comfort of their Hampstead Garden Suburb home for France at the end of October, arriving at Royaumont on 3 November, nervous about what lay ahead. She wrote to her friend Mrs. Laurie 'one always is frightened over a new job', allowing her usual uncompromising facade to slip for a moment, although she knew that the initial posting was only a temporary one. The last time she had set off for France she had George Mallett to help. This time she was on her own.

The SWH hospital at Villers-Cotterêts had been authorised by the French Ministry of War on 11 July 1917. Its purpose was to provide additional casualty clearing beds in the area, anticipating another offensive with its further surge of casualties. This was not the first time that war had reached this part of France. When the SWH hospital had first been established at Royaumont Abbey, it was only 25 miles behind the front line, but now the trenches were too far away for it to be usefully placed for casualty clearance. Anticipating this, the French military authorities had made a request to Frances Ivens for a new advance casualty clearing station to be set up close to the new front line. Ivens was fully aware of the French strategy and wholeheartedly agreed. Detailed accounts of the establishment of this hospital at Villers-Cotterêts have been given by Eileen Crofton in her complete account of *Abbaye Royaumont* [8] and by Leah Leneman in her biography of Elsie Inglis [9] from which much of the following account has been drawn.

After several false starts, a team from Royaumont came across a deserted wooden-hutted evacuation centre beside the railway at Villers-Cotterêts, which was about 40 miles nearer to the front line, which suited their requirements. Vera Collum recorded that 'nothing could have been more different than this ultra-modern barraque hospital from our own ancient Abbaye. Rows of wooden huts with oil-papered windows and composition roofs, on either side a new road sweeping through the camp to the railway line at the back'. There were two rows of derelict huts, one for most of the wards and the second housing the operating theatre, X-ray and laboratory facilities, other offices and staff accommodation. Much work had to be done, using a workforce of German prisoners and *infirmiers* (soldiers unfit for military duty), overseen by General Descoings.

Agnes Savill

Over 2 years previously, Agnes Savill had been appointed as the senior doctor in the X-ray department of Royaumont Abbey and had the responsibility for setting up the X-ray equipment there. Before the war she had practised as a dermatologist, using X-rays mostly for treatment rather than diagnosis and would have had little practical experience in X-ray imaging and certainly none relating to the diagnosis of wartime casualties. Nevertheless, she knew something about X-ray equipment, how it was assembled and operated. She had none of Edith's practicality, however, writing that 'The mystery embodied in every marvellous invention makes a strange appeal: the affection I have for my X-ray tubes and other electrical apparatus, and that some feel for their bicycles and motor-cars, is a real, not a feigned emotion'.

The X-ray room had been set up on the first floor, close to the operating theatre. The suite could be easily reached from an upstairs ward through the gallery at the end of the huge refectory, looking down on its nine great stone pillars. However, all new stretcher cases had to be carried up and down a flight of stairs, both to and from the X-ray room and the operating theatre. The developing room was downstairs. The electrical power came, at first, from the water-powered dynamo intended for lighting.

The equipment itself was functional but simple, a 'little Army pattern mule-back Butt installation'. At that time it was the only X-ray installation in this area [10]. When the boxes were delivered to Royaumont in December 1914, she had opened the 69-page 'Field Service X-ray Outfit Instructions, with numerous illustrations and diagrams' with a mixture of determination and awe:

> The purchase of the X-ray apparatus was confined to what was indispensable, and at lowest possible prices. The arrival of all the complicated and delicate instruments at Royaumont without a single breakage was not only a welcome surprise to the Staff, but a credit to the British packers. When the strong young orderlies had emptied the voluminous cases, their contents presented an accumulation bewildering even to the professional eye. Fortunately, the radiologist was equal to the occasion, and promptly coaxed the heterogeneous collection into a harmonious combination, putting up couch, coil, switchboard, and tubes in a single morning. A tour de force. An arrangement having been planned the previous afternoon, after careful examination of the many parts, all fitted magically in their appointed places. [11]

Somehow, the account makes it sound as though she was erecting a piece of IKEA furniture (Figs. 14.3, 14.4, 14.5 and 14.6).

In contrast to Edith's ability to provide immediate on-site technical maintenance when faults inevitably developed with her equipment, here in Royaumont the Gaiffe X-ray engineers would have been brought in from Paris, about 35 miles away, when things went wrong.

Dr. Savill still had needed a crash course in the practice of military radiography before she could start to contribute to the work at Royaumont. It was Florence who visited there in order to give this training, even before she returned to London in March 1915 from the Women's Imperial Service League Unit in Cherbourg. Florence was in a position not only to give Savill general guidance in radiological technique but also to pass on her experience of radiography of wounded soldiers.

Fig. 14.3 The War Office Pattern Field Service Couch, folded. (Women's Library, 2SWH)

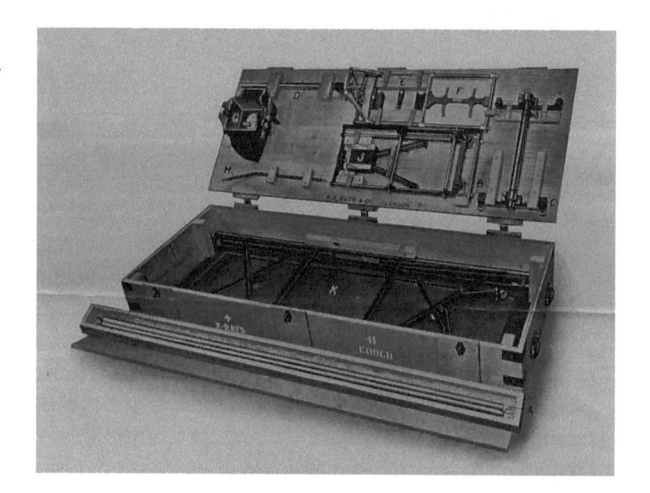

Fig. 14.4 The War Office Pattern Field Service Couch, erected. (Women's Library, 2SWH)

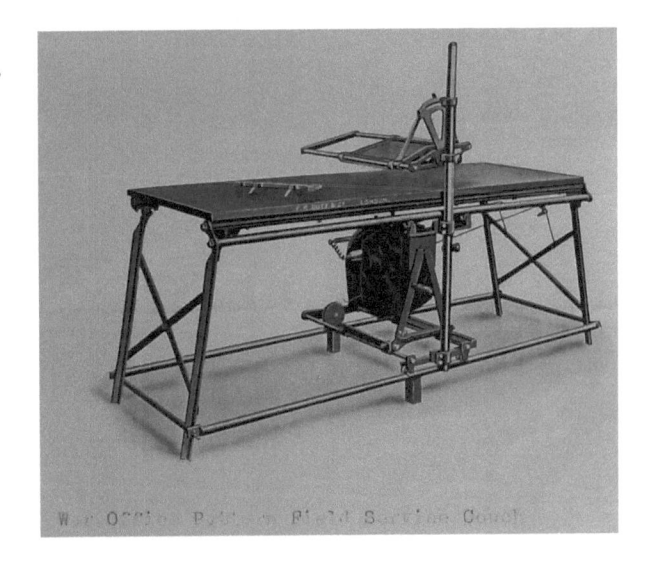

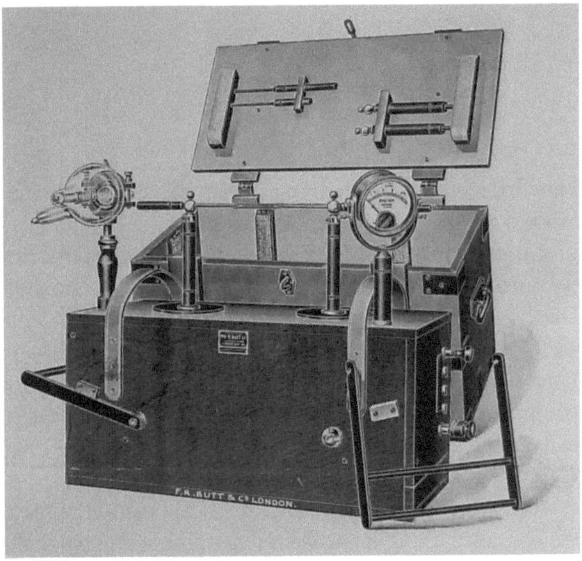

Fig. 14.5 Boxed X-ray equipment, including the induction coil, for war radiography as specified by the War Office and supplied by Fred Butt and Co. (Women's Library, 2SWH)

She also took on the supervision of the SWH X-ray van. Edith later credited Savill with its design, but her limited background in X-ray imaging implies that she had gained expert advice from others.

Savill described working with this equipment. In the absence of a mains supply, it was run from 'one set of 36 ampére-hour accumulators', recharged using an adjacent charging-board, and Savill noted that 'this was so much more convenient than taking the accumulators to be charged elsewhere'. In her London practice, she would have operated her X-ray equipment from the mains, and she admits to having no

Fig. 14.6 The illustration supplied by Butt for the controller, labelled 'Control similar to above suggested'. (Women's Library, 2SWH)

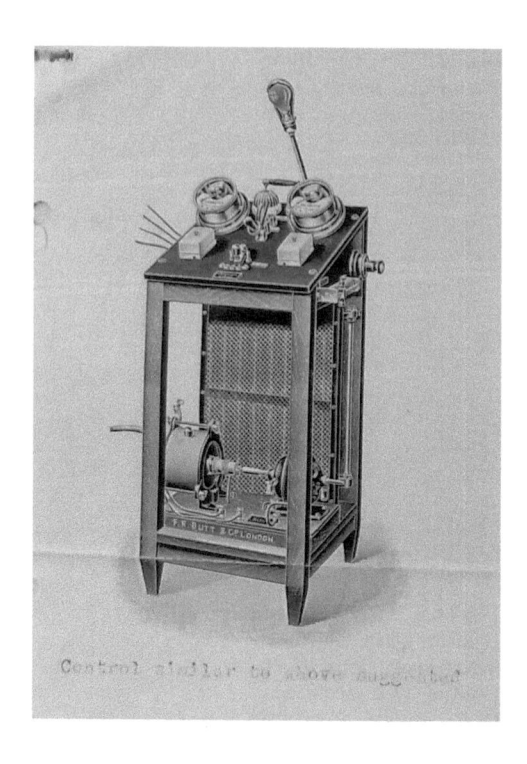

knowledge about maintaining rechargeable accumulator batteries and seems to have learned on the job. She included in her report the advice that 'a daily charge was given until hissing of the acid was audible'. At first the exposures used only 0.33 mA, requiring lengthy exposures, but eventually she settled on using small cheap hard tubes operated with a current of 1.75 mA, claiming that the screening was as clear as could be achieved with other tubes at 3–4 mA and that her tubes lasted longer than the more expensive Macalister-Wiggin tube. Savill admitted that the equipment was not sufficiently powerful to obtain radiographs through the shoulder and upper thorax, limiting her ability to localise of embedded fragments in that region, prior to surgical removal [12].

Agnes Savill maintained her medical position as the senior radiologist throughout the war, even though she shared her time with responsibilities in London, where she ran her own medical practice and remained head of the skin clinic at the South London Hospital for Women. During her periods of absence from France in the winter months, other doctors took over formal medical responsibility. She was in France during the summer of 1917 at the time that the hospital was being established at Villers-Cotterêts and so had taken the lead in setting up the X-ray room there. She was soon able to report that 'our X-ray hut is huge, magnificent, all provided by the military genie'. She wrote privately to Mrs. Russell that she had 'installed a lovely X-ray room here with the aid of a very smart mechanicien (possibly Mr. George Day, mechanic with the London Unit between November 1916 and November 1917). I have made such charming accessories at a few shillings cost', no doubt being aware of the view from Edinburgh that X-ray equipment could be costly. On her own admission, Savill prided herself on limiting expenditure, previously describing herself as 'a canny Scot who can run things cheaply' [13].

The field Butt equipment was transferred from Royaumont, leaving one X-ray room operating there, which had been installed immediately prior to the Battle of the Somme in the summer of 1916. Since that time the workload had diminished, and two rooms were barely needed. It would have been an easy and cheap decision to release the older equipment for use in Villers-Cotterêts. All that was needed otherwise was a source of electricity, for which a cheap second-hand engine had been found.

By the beginning of August, 211 beds were prepared with space for another 60, comprising about 13% of the military hospital capacity in the area. The hospital was called *Hôpital Bénevole 1 bis 6ième région (SWH)*. But the summer of 1917 had been quiet. They waited for casualties. None came. They were inspected and approved with enthusiasm. French attacks were muted, partly from mutinies within the French army. The first wounded were admitted on 27 August, but very few followed. Only about ten patients came through the X-ray department each week [14]. There was a slight increase in October during the French attack on Chemin des Dames, but the sporadic ebb and flow of the French battles at Verdun were too far away to affect them. 1917 proved to be the only year during the war when the summer offensive resulted in no significant surge in casualties for the London Unit of the SWH.

When Edith arrived at Royaumont, many of the staff had experienced well over 2 years dealing with military casualties. Agnes Savill had gained the respect of her colleagues as a caring member of staff, with a broad concern for their welfare. Her interest in music had led her to hire a pianola from Paris almost as soon as Royaumont had opened, for both staff and soldiers to play. She and several of her assistants had as much clinical experience as had Edith in wartime radiology, so Edith had every reason to be confident that she was moving into a much more competent environment than she had previously experienced. For the first couple of weeks, she covered for Dr. Savill at Royaumont whilst she dealt with a sudden rush of work at Villers-Cotterêts. Then, when Savill went home on leave, Edith took her place (Fig. 14.7). Savill was slightly in awe of Edith, once remarking in a letter 'what an amount of abstruse knowledge she possesses'.

Radiology at Villers-Cotterêts

Edith's arrival at Villers-Cotterêts on 14 November enabled both Agnes Savill and the senior radiographer Vera Collum to return to London. Savill was not well, and this was nearly the end of her association with Royaumont, though she did return, looking 'absolutely cadaverous', to help during the end of the major offensive the following summer. Collum intended to return home permanently after nearly 3 years' service, not knowing that the following March would find her back at

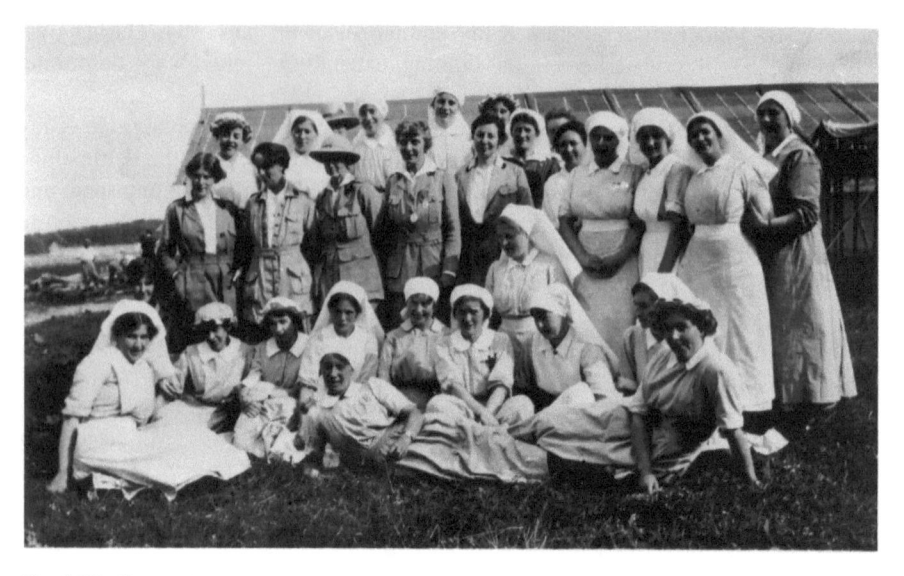

Fig. 14.7 Group photograph of some of the Villers-Cotterêts staff including, in the second row, Agnes Savill, Edith Stoney (in the wide-brimmed hat) and Frances Ivens

Royaumont, helping with another surge in casualties. The radiographer Phylis Berry was left in charge of the Royaumont department.

Dr. Helen McDougall, the physician who was temporarily in charge of X-rays at Villers-Cotterêts, was also away, in Paris. McDougal had been originally recruited to join the SWH Serbian unit at Kragujevac in July 1915, only to have an uncomfortable time as a prisoner of war when the hospital was overrun in December by the Austrian advance. By the time Edith arrived she had been working at Royaumont for a year. It had been so difficult to find competent staff that Marie Curie had been approached to ask for the assistance of one of her assistants, a Miss Brock being appointed for a few weeks before Edith arrived.

Edith described the location of the hospital to be in a lovely forest clearing at an elevation of 400 ft. The area had been explored by Vera Collum who wrote 'I had the opportunity for long walks in the forest of Villers-Cotterets, visits to Corcy, Longpont and the war-scarred little hamlet that sits on the crest of a hill, on the doorstep as it were, of Cœvres. . ... It was the agony of 1914 that was brought home to me in the forest, with its shell-torn trees, its little scattered graves of the Scottish Highlanders and English Guardsmen. Nothing was further from our thoughts, in 1917, than a second agony of anxiety for Paris in the forest of Villers-Cotterets, a second great victory of the Marne'.

Perhaps Edith had similar thoughts during the next few months, in the quiet times. Unfortunately, she had little opportunity to explore the area when she arrived. The weather had broken, and the rain that was causing the trenches of Passchendaele to become seas of mud and that drowned wounded soldiers in the shell holes of Ypres also fell on Villers-Cotterêts. Everything was soaked. Dampness caused the high-voltage leads to spark and discharge, making it difficult or impossible to operate the X-ray equipment. Such conditions, she knew, could cause catastrophic failure.[3] Soon after her arrival, Edith wrote:

> Here it is very wet—drifting mist everywhere and I have not yet got the X Rays into working order—The damp running down the walls and through the roof of the X Ray baraque last night flooded the floor and put out the stove. . ... Wet leaking on to electrical apparatus is not good for its longevity [15].

At least the clinical workload was modest during her first months: 89 in December, 78 in January and 67 in February [16]. Winter was always quieter on the front. Edith took the opportunity to find her bearings, settle in to her new accommodation and to sort out the equipment. Before long she had set up the electric lighting, as she had done in each of her previous hospitals. She realised that the X-ray ambulance was sitting idle at Royaumont and arranged with Frances Ivens to have it driven over to Villers-Cotterêts so she could have two X-ray sets in operation [17].

During the first months of 1918, they experienced what was reportedly the coldest winter since 1870; 'It was cold—colder even in its way than December 1915 in Serbia' with no heating in the personal barracks and temperatures as low as −22 °C. All the toiletries, sponge, toothbrushes and soap were all frozen hard. An auxiliary nurse, Etta Inglis, described how 'our breath froze to the sheets, our hair to the pillows, our rubber boots to the floor. . ... The camp was under snow for three months and huge icicles hung from the roofs of the huts' [18]. Edith often had to start up the 'very crazy old' engine at 5.00 a.m., to give enough light so that the wards could be washed and the patients given breakfast, only to return to bed to warm up once everything was in hand. She admitted, though, that 'it was nice in that glorious bracing forest air!'

She was pleased to find that one of the two X-ray rooms had been equipped with new, French equipment from Gaiffe shortly before her arrival, quite probably on her recommendation. It had always been Frances Ivens' plan to ensure that Villers-Cotterêts was equipped to a level that would enable it to withstand the anticipated influx of casualties from a now offensive and remembered the pressure on the surgical and X-ray capacity at Royaumont during the summer of 1916. Edith Procter, an orderly, wrote to her mother at the end of October that the X-ray department was now 'very smart and beautifully equipped, with 2 X-ray apparatus' taking the view that the SWH was 'an enormously wealthy society and they don't mind how much they spend' [19].

Edith had by now worked out a strategy for dealing with the Edinburgh bureaucracy. First and foremost she had Frances Ivens' full support in building a robust X-ray facility. Secondly, she had learned from bitter experience that she had to curb her natural inclination to purchase equipment without authority. The SWH now had a more formal purchasing policy, requisitions having to be signed off by those

---

[3]RAMC No 4 Mobile X-ray unit diary twice noted X-ray tubes being perforated due to damp. National Archives Kew: WO 95/503/1,2.

authorised to do so, Frances Ivens in France and Marian Erskine in Scotland. Finally, she knew that Florence could help through her good relationship with Mrs. Laurie in Edinburgh. Florence wrote to Mrs. Laurie on Edith's departure, with a not-so-hidden message that she could soon expect further requests for expenditure from France:

> It is most disheartening for her (Edith) to feel that those in authority do not care for the quality of the work, but only for the quantity—and resent any attempt to improve the quality. It is impossible to have the best work without both efficient apparatus and an efficient person to work it—the one without the other is not much use. You have no idea how she has been worn out trying to fill the deficiencies of incompetent materials and assistants. Forgive the explosion but we feel you are her only friend on the Committee. With kind regards, Florence Stoney. [20]

Edith was careful not to offend. Marian Erskine came on an official inspection soon after she arrived and wrote 'Miss Stoney is sweeter than honey. Long may it last!' [21]. So far so good.

Edith was soon writing to Mrs. Laurie herself:

> very aghast at present at the makeshift way the apparatus has been put up here . . . The engine was old and out of work constantly—and there always seemed to be burst pipes to be soldered—kitchen drains to be seen to—broken windows in the men's barraques to be mended etc. . . . I only hope that I can secure enough apparatus to make the work efficient. [22]

Edith quickly realised why there had been such insistence that she was posted here to France, rather than back to Salonika. The need was not simply that they needed a skilled working radiographer with experience in handling military casualties. Edith could, and did, carry out that clinical role with total competence. The main requirement was to bring the Villers-Cotterêts X-ray department up to a standard that could cope with the anticipated next major offensive. By the beginning of 1918, Edith was becoming more confident that she could make a difference. Unlike some in Edinburgh, Dr. Ivens understood the value of employing a person who possessed a detailed understanding of X-ray technology to be part of the professional team of a modern hospital, complementary to the medical role played by the doctors. Ivens would not be browbeaten by the officials in Edinburgh either and had already got into trouble for authorising 300 beds for Villers-Cotterêts, a number that the committee members in Edinburgh had not authorised and that they stated that they could not be held responsible for. This was Edith's kind of woman. It was not difficult for Edith to persuade her that penny-pinching on X-ray equipment was not for the best. In early January she ordered four large tubes to replace the smaller ones she found on arrival, deliberately placing a requisition for 'the expensive French ones and not the cheap £3 ones' [23]. Once she found her feet, further equipment was added to bring the unit up to a high standard, including two more X-ray tubes, these with tungsten targets. The selection of more robust tubes was for a purpose. They were preparing to accept a similar influx of casualties to that they had arrived during the Battle of the Somme in 1916. Edith knew that meant that the X-ray tubes would be driven all day, every day for several weeks, and that they must have confidence that could be done without overheating them. This required either tungsten-anode tubes or water-cooled tubes, both of which she added to her shopping lists as she developed the department.

She ordered X-ray plates of several sizes, including some for dental examinations, and accelerating screens for most plate sizes. A total of 2000 X-ray plates were bought during the first 5 months of 1918, an average of about four per patient. She also started to use daylight printing paper, to be used with cassettes with an inbuilt intensifying screen. Film made with a photographic emulsion coated on to a base of cellulose nitrate had been available since the earliest days of X-rays, but it had been little used, partly because it was highly inflammable. In 1917 Eastman-Kodak introduced double-coated film that was widely introduced into military hospitals. This may have been the film that Edith ordered although, knowing that she was always at the cutting edge of technology and highly conscious of safety, she may have procured some of the nitrate-based X-ray film produced by Kodak at Harrow before the end of the war.

Other equipment started to bring the X-ray department at Villers-Cotterêts up to the level that she had established in Salonika: a stereoscope; two cooling fans to work off different voltage supplies; an exposure slide rule; an oscilloscope tube for testing the discharge duration and magnitude; three valve tubes, probably as spares; a gas bag for the coal gas used in the interrupter; and a ring localiser. The 'crazy old engine' was replaced. Villers-Cotterêts soon became better equipped than Royaumont.

Edith's role in upgrading and maintaining her X-ray facility was one that was a requirement not only for the SWH but also for the War Office as a whole. It was of sufficient logistical importance to be subsequently mentioned in the formal military history of the war [24]. A total of 528 X-ray outfits were issued during the war, and their maintenance involved the supply of a very large number of X-ray tubes and X-ray plates, over 4100 of the former having been issued during the last 2 years of the war. In total, the requisitioned spares amounted to a large number of complete outfits. Furthermore, processing required supplies of equipment and chemicals, estimated to have cost the War Office £52,000 in 1 year alone. Radiology did not come without significant expenditure.

Frances Ivens was more than satisfied with Edith's performance and requested her retention in France, which was granted. Edith was assigned three radiographic assistants, Patricia Raymond, Marian Butler and Florence Anderson, a chauffeur Hilda Smeal, and Monsieur Defarge, a French male orderly and mechanic, who she rather disparagingly described as being only half-trained and often ill and who used to flee to the fields whenever there was danger. Finally, after over 2 years of intermittent acrimony, Edith felt fully supported by her senior medical colleague and the central place that radiology held in military medicine. For example, such was the value given to X-rays in the diagnosis of gas gangrene that Frances Ivens encouraged all surgical staff to spend some time in the X-ray department to learn to recognise the radiological appearance of the disease (Fig. 14.8).

Edith set about organising the requests to the radiology department. She designed a form for each request, requiring the patient's name, the diagnosis of the injury and the name of the surgeon in charge. Gone were the rather casual arrangements allowing any doctor to bring a patient to the X-ray room, hoping that a radiograph might help. Edith was building a tightly professional department with clear structural

Fig. 14.8 Radiograph showing striations diagnostic of severe gas gangrene

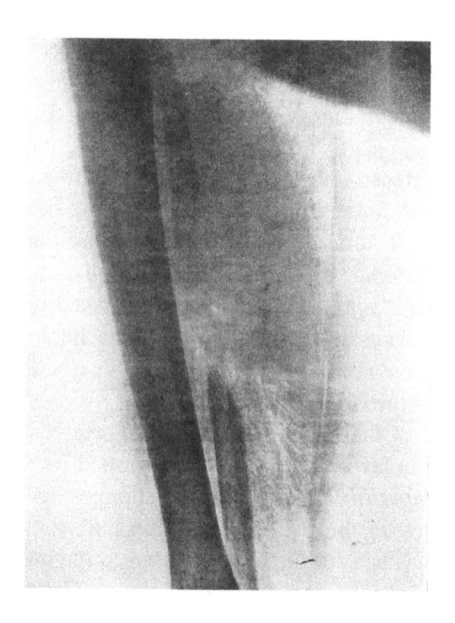

procedures and internal organisation. Referring surgeons were expected to have a clear purpose for each referral. There were four categories of request. Only two were radiological, for either a radiograph or a localisation. The other two were for electrical treatment and for nerve testing. Each form had a space for the report to be written and signed off by the radiologist. Casual verbal reporting was a thing of the past.

Edith had yet another reason to be content, which had nothing to do with the events in France. On 6 February 1918, the British parliament finally passed the Representation of the People Act giving some women a vote in national elections for the first time. The long-anticipated news must have given a great boost to all those at Royaumont and Villers-Cotterêts, many of whom had been active participants in the campaign for women's suffrage before the war. Yet the record is muted about their response. It could well be that they felt no particular enthusiasm for a law that established full male suffrage without its full extension to women. If there were any celebrations amongst the SWH women, they remained unremarked in the letters and reports that passed between France and Britain at the time.

There was a sudden influx of wounded from 21 to 25 March, British Fifth Army casualties from the German attack known as Operation Michael, when the German forces moved on a broad front along the Somme from St. Quentin, advancing some 40 miles into Allied-held territory. Whilst Villers-Cotterêts was some way south of this battle, the hospital played an important role in taking many of the wounded. Edith and her team carried out 60 radiographs and 46 fluoroscopies in 1 week. The hospital had been located, deliberately, alongside the main railway route, and as the battle intensified, they were increasingly subjected to aerial bombardment aimed at disrupting the rail transport. Nevertheless, April was quiet again, and she was happy to remember the 'delicious long lazy spring days in that beautiful forest clearing'. It would not stay quiet for long.

27–31 May 1918

At 01.00 on Monday, 27 May, a major offensive was launched by the German forces over the River Aisne (Fig. 14.9). The weather was calm, and so, from her bunk some 30 miles to the southeast, Edith could have become aware of the sound of the distant bombardment as, for over an hour, Allied targets were attacked with explosives and

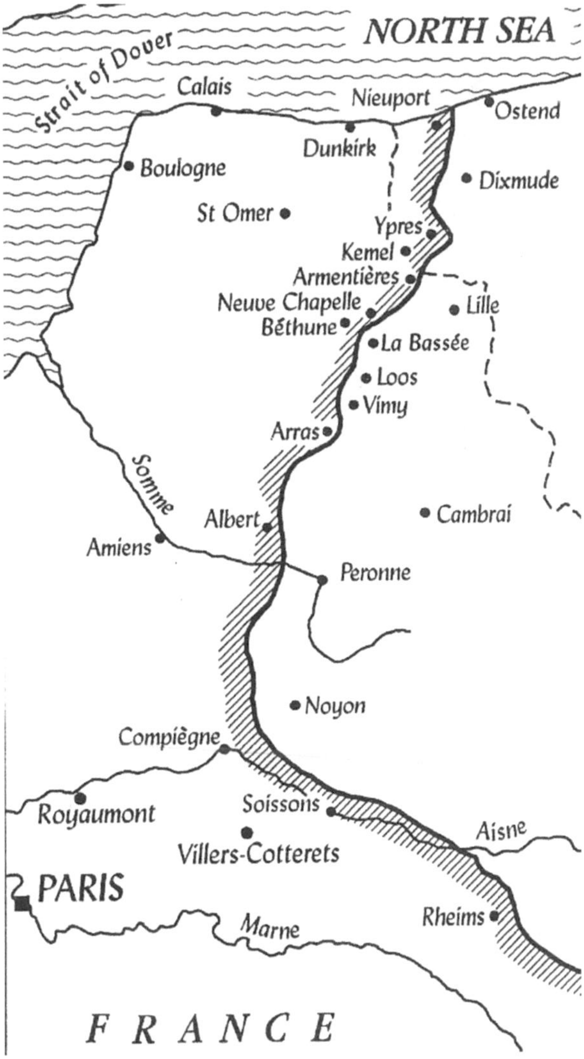

Fig. 14.9 The front line before the German attack over the Aisne on 27 May 1918

mustard gas. The slight easterly breeze drifted the gas towards and beyond the trenches. The Allied front collapsed. By the evening, casualties started arriving, growing from a stream to a torrent during the next 4 days. The SWH unit at Villers-Cotterêts came under direct Army control as the only Casualty Clearing Station in the district. Young Dr. Leila Henry recalled this as 4 days 'when time did not exist'. Even Edith, usually scrupulously accurate, was a day adrift when reporting her recollection of these few traumatic days.

Florence learned about the attack from *The Times* on Tuesday morning, and she would have immediately appreciated the threat to her sister and the whole hospital at Villers-Cotterêts. She would have also understood that they were in exactly the right position to provide maximum assistance as the casualties started to come out from the front-line fighting. Under a headline 'New German Offensive. Great Battle on the Aisne' under which was the reminder 'The War: 4th Year: 298th Day', Florence read 'Germany reopened her offensive on a big scale against the Allied Armies in the West early yesterday. The main attack was made on a wide front between Soissons and Reims'. She would not have needed expert analysis to realise that this attack had Paris in its sights and that her sister was exactly on the intended route. If she was in any doubt, *The Times* also printed telegraphic dispatches received from GHQ in France from the day before. '10.42 a.m.—Strong hostile attacks, preceded by bombardment of great intensity, developed early this morning, on wide fronts, against the British and French Troops between Reims and Soissons'. And '9.8 p.m.—On our left the enemy succeeded, after heavy fighting, in pressing our troops back to a second line of prepared positions. Severe fighting has taken place all along the front and is continuing'.

By the time Florence learned of what was happening, the casualties had started to arrive at Villers-Cotterêts. During the following 3 days, more than 300 of the most severely wounded cases passed through the hospital many with wounds already infected with gas gangrene. 'Their wounds were terrible, and in most cases they arrived at the hospital minus even a field dressing. For four nights and three days they (the staff) worked without ceasing except for meals. We began to lose all sense of time and worked like machines' [25].

Edith's recollections are contained in a letter to her friend James Mackenzie-Davidson [26] and in another to Mrs. Walker [27]. She improvised to provide a few 50 candlepower lights shaded in cocoa tins, but the surgeons, Frances Ivens, Edith Martland and Jessie Berry, still often had to work by candlelight. She kept the engine going to provide power for the X-rays.[4]

Collum reported the words of a theatre orderly:

> A hell and a shambles. Nine thigh amputations running; men literally shot to pieces; the crashing of bombs and the thunder of ever-approaching guns; ..... the operating hut with its plank floor and the tables on them literally dancing to the explosions; the flickering candles,

---

[4] All these three women, Frances Ivens, Jessie Berry and Edith Marjorie Martland, were former students at the London School of Medicine for Women.

the anxiety lest the operated cases might haemorrhage and die in the dark; the knowledge that the next bomb might get them. [28]

Then, on 'Wednesday (29 May) we had orders to pack—and we got both X-ray installations down and packed, and all the wiring down' in preparation to evacuate Villers-Cotterêts and retreat to Royaumont, about 50 miles away. By then, the German advance had crossed the Aisne at Soissons, only 15 miles up the main road to the northeast.

Early in the evening the decision to withdraw was abruptly reversed. The wounded were continuing to arrive, and all the neighbouring hospitals had closed their X-ray and operating facilities. By 11.00 p.m. Edith and her staff had re-erected one of the X-ray rooms, and the wiring was all in place again.

The X-ray orderly, Florence Anderson, recalled:

The ward next to the X-ray department was a nightmare. Black blankets on the beds. On each men were dying, screaming, unconscious and delirious, the sisters doing their work the best way they could with lanterns—Miss Ivens was operating, operating, operating by candle light. Six amputations of the leg, and all the time the horrible bang bang of the bombs and the munition train, and shrapnel falling sometimes on the roof. [29]

Edith recalled being sent to bed at 4.00 a.m. and finding her X-ray technician Marian Butler still working with the surgeon Jessie Berry when she came back on duty again 3 hours later.

The staff remaining at Royaumont had no clear news about what was happening at Villers-Cotterêts, and at one point on Thursday, 30 May, the communiqué was so bad that they felt justified in feeling that Villers-Cotterêts had already fallen into German hands. Then, about mid-morning on the same day, the final decision was made to accept no more wounded and to evacuate the remaining casualties. Although the aerial bombardment during the past few days had not been aimed at the hospital, they were lucky to avoid being collateral damage, and that it suffered no direct hits and no staff were injured. The immediate area suffered damage and casualties, however; 'the village a mile off was blazing—a woman and children were killed at the corner of our hospital grounds' and a bomb destroyed a cottage at the level crossing close by their sidings.

The proximity to the railway should have made it relatively easy to arrange the evacuation. Unfortunately, a train loaded with ammunition had suffered a direct hit during the bombardment. The resulting disruption to rail transport, together with the large numbers of other troops being moved away from the front, left Frances Ivens with 50 casualties and the remaining staff to travel by road. Some were taken in their own cars, once they had arrived from Royaumont (Fig. 14.10). Some went with American car drivers who told them that the front line had already reached Longpont, only 3 miles away, and was still advancing. Some younger staff set off to walk, joining the civilian refugees, hitching a ride from any road or rail transport when this was possible. There was no space or time to bring anything, except for their handbags and packed knapsacks that all staff members had been told to prepare in case rapid evacuation was required. Other baggage, including the trunks containing personal possessions, was stacked by the hospital railway sidings, an

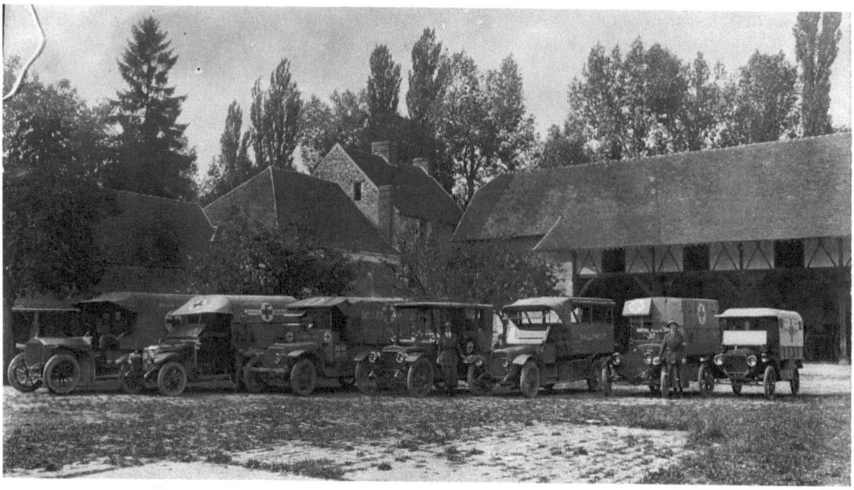

Fig. 14.10 The vehicles of the Scottish Women's Hospitals London Unit at Royaumont Abbey, with two women and two men drivers. (Archives of the Fondation Royaumont)

invitation to looters. One lorry, carrying eight of the staff, had enough room to include the theatre equipment and a few X-ray tubes, but no room to carry the rest of the X-ray equipment. The last evacuation car finally got back to Royaumont at 5.00 the following morning.

Edith's own report encapsulates the drama:

> We worked till 4.00 p.m. Thursday seeing X-ray cases. Then the order came to pack up finally. At 1.30 p.m. Miss Ivens sent off the younger doctors and orderlies walking, and hoping for odd lifts—this included my three assistants Anderson, Butler and Raymond. Then my last helper, the X-ray *infirmière* was needed to carry the *blessés* (casualties)—and help with the wounded—the doctors and nurses remaining were desperately busy with patients. The whole of the X-ray equipment was however repacked by 6 p.m. and we went for supper. During supper the shelling began, and the splendid American ambulance men came along for the last of our *blessés* whom we had not yet been able to evacuate in our own cars. And this left our returning cars free for the last of us to luxuriously drive to Royaumont. We were heavily bombed on the way—as indeed we were the night after when a few of us had gone up for the apparatus.

Edith was determined not to abandon her equipment, as Florence had been forced to do when she left Antwerp. Her return visit to Villers-Cotterêts on Friday morning was foolhardy and almost certainly not authorised. She would have had difficulty anyway in finding Frances Ivens, who had set off early to Senlis to discuss the changing situation with the medical authorities there, as the French hospital at Creil, too, was threatened. It is quite in keeping with Edith's character that she made the decision independently of any authority, which would almost certainly resulted in her being denied permission. In retrospect it was a highly dangerous act because, as far as they were aware, the hospital could have been overrun by the advancing front by then, and, in any event, it was so close to the advancing lines that it was under constant bombardment. In fact, the German advance finally stalled at the far edge of the Forest of Villers-Cotterêts, in what was the climax of this Second Battle of the Marne.

The first part of the route back was fairly well protected as they drove out of the Oise valley through Gouvieux and past the Chateau of Chantilly, which the German army had reached, briefly, in September 1914. Beyond Senlis, with its damaged houses from 3 years earlier, the next part of the journey was very exposed, the straight road running across open fields for mile after mile, any vehicles an open invitation to attack by enemy aircraft. Even after they had passed through Crépy, there were more open fields for several miles before they finally reached Villers-Cotterêts, a total journey of at least 2 hours. In Edith's own words:

> Friday I went up early with Ramsay Smith (Madge Ramsay-Smith, administrator) Graham (Margaret Graham, chauffeur) and Tollit (Florence Tollit, storekeeper)—but shelling began again before we were at the hospital more than 20 minutes. Our things had not yet been looted—We loaded up the car and sent it on—waiting for another promised one ourselves. The shelling got worse and the car did not come (Miss Ivens had to use it for blessés), so after leaving—it seems that we should also go. We had seats in cars part of the way and walked when these were needed for blessés overtaken en route. We could therefore carry no apparatus. Finally when nearly back we met two cars from Royaumont sent out to look for us. I returned with them to Villers Cott. for more apparatus, splints, drugs etc. as we heard that the shelling had ceased for a while. It started again before we were at Villers Cotterets more than 10 minutes. I broke open boxes and repacked as hastily and as well as I could the more essentials to make up one complete (X-ray) set.

As they finally returned retraced the dangerous journey back to Royaumont in the evening, 'the roads were heavily bombed—so much so that the French stopped our second car and made the 2 girls in it fly to the fields for the night. A great red light was let down over Crêpy, one could have read by, on some sort of parachute—which hovered for about 15 min and gave light to bomb.—We had only got a couple of hundred yards through at the time, and could have read easily by the light'.

Returning one more time, they found that:

> our boxes had been broken open—and much damage done even when things were not taken—as for instance the X-ray plates were mostly spoilt. The personal luggage was looted—I had not had time to pack my own trunk—but my loss is only the same as others as all trunks were broken open.

In her official report, Edith made a statement that revealed, at least in part, why she made this desperate journey to recover the X-ray equipment. 'The Butt coil has come back and works well' she wrote, but 'the Butt break (i.e. interrupter) is broken—The Butt table has not come back—most of the photographic material—plates and developer is lost—the intensifying screens are lost—part of the overhead tube stand of the Gaiffe is lost... I trust the Committee will realise the difficulties before blaming me too much for the heavy loss of apparatus entrusted to my care. Our cars were all needed for the blessés at Creil—and the whole X-ray apparatus had had to be twice hastily packed so that much of the original order attempted in the original packing was lost'. It may also explain why she asked Ramsey-Smith to accompany her, to corroborate her subsequent report that she did her best to recover as much of the expensive X-ray equipment as possible. She was only too well aware of the conflict between her view of a well-equipped department and that of Marian Erskine, who was always liable to exert financial and hence managerial control. She knew that, during the last few months, she had been able to set up an extremely well-equipped two-room X-ray department in a hospital that officially was only a forward annex to the main centre at Royaumont. The fact she had been encouraged by Frances Ivens, who knew that it would be Villers-Cotterêts and not Royaumont that would be, literally, in the firing line when the German army advanced, was no great comfort to her. She felt personally responsible.

In London, Florence learned what she could from the pages of *The Times*. On Thursday, 30 May, she read, to her undoubted concern, that 'The enemy are now on the high-road which passes through Villers-Cotterets'. Briefly, it would have seemed quite possible that her sister was about to become a prisoner of war. News at the end of the week was more reassuring, with reports that the attack had stalled and especially that American troops had been brought in to reinforce the French. Nevertheless, the map that appeared on 3 June, with the front line placed immediately to the east of Villers-Cotterêts Forest, showed how close it had been.

By that time Edith had done what she could at Villers-Cotterêts and was now embedded in the work of Royaumont. In spite of the fact that she had endangered the lives not only of herself but also of three other members of staff, she seems to have suffered no criticism for her action. Indeed, her efforts throughout the week to maintain the necessary X-ray support for the surgeons, during a time of extraordinary stress, earned her a new position of respect.

Edith's action was not heroic. That word is reserved for saving people, not things. Yet Edith contributed no less to the saving of lives by saving her equipment. It was essential for the continued effective operation of the hospital in Royaumont, where the X-ray facilities were already stretched to the limit. But it also points to a much deeper change in the practice of medicine, which Edith sensed perhaps more strongly than any of her colleagues. It was becoming increasingly dependent on technology and instrumentation. Even at this stage in the development of medical care, the removal of new technologies would diminish the ability of doctors to diagnose and treat their patients. This change, which would continue to accelerate throughout the twentieth century, has utterly transformed medicine. If a modern hospital were to be forced to evacuate and relocate, it would have to bring anaesthetic trolleys, diathermy and laparoscopes from the operating theatre, ECG and pulse monitors from intensive care, ultrasound scanners and portable X-ray units from the imaging department and auto-analysers and spectroscopy from the laboratory. Some imaging installations, magnetic resonance and X-ray computed tomography, could only be moved by major engineering. At least Edith's X-ray equipment, in her skilled and knowledgeable hands, could still be dismantled and reconfigured. Warfare was forcing the pace of technological change that would transform medical and surgical care out of all recognition during the century to come.

References

1. Edith Stoney to Mrs Laurie. 1917 Oct 1. ML. TD1734/2/6/9/79.
2. Music SA. Health and character, vol. 17. London: Bodley Head; 1923. p. 49–50.
3. Edith Stoney to Mrs Laurie. 1917 Sept 2. ML. TD1734/2/6/9/74.
4. Scottish Women's Hospitals. Hospitals Committee minutes. 1917 Sept 28. ML. TD1734.
5. Scottish Women's hospitals. Minutes of the personnel committee. 1917 Oct 23. ML. TD1734/1/4/3.
6. Edith Stoney to Mrs Laurie. 1917 Oct 14. ML. TD1734/2/6/9/81.
7. Edith Stoney to Mrs Laurie. 1917 Nov 10. ML. TD1734/2/6/9/86.
8. Crofton E. The women of Royaumont. East Lothian: Tuckwell Press; 1997. p. 133–47.
9. Leneman L. In the service of life. The story of Elsie Inglis. Edinburgh: Mercat Press; 1994.
10. Crofton E. The women of Royaumont. East Lothian: Tuckwell Press; 1997. p. 24.
11. de Navarro A. The Scottish Women's hospital at the French Abbey of Royaumont. London: Allen & Unwin; 1917. p. 159.
12. Savill A. Some notes on the X-ray department of the Scottish Women's hospital. Royaumont, France. Arch Radiol Electrother. 1916;20(12):401–10.
13. Letters from Agnes Savill. 1916 May 10. ML. TD1734/8/1/2/17.
14. X-rays at Royaumont and Villers Cotterets. Jan 1919. ML. TD1734.
15. Edith Stoney to Mrs Laurie. 21 Nov 1917. ML. TD/1734/2/6/9/89.
16. Villers Cotterets work-load. ML. TD1734/8/4/1/2.
17. Les annales de la guerre No 44. Documents officiels de la section cinematographic de l'armee Francaise. 14.18 A44. www.ecpad.fr/janvier-1918-les-annales-de-la-guerre-44. The X-ray van can be seen in this short documentary film of Villers Cotterets dated 4 January 1918.
18. Crofton E. The women of Royaumont. East Lothian: Tuckwell Press; 1997. p. 152.
19. E M Procter to her Mother. 1917 Oct 30. Imperial War Museum.
20. Florence Stoney to Mrs Laurie. 1917 Nov 6. ML. TD1734/2/6/9/85.
21. Crofton. Quoting Dr Erskine to Miss Kemp. 1917 Nov 22. p. 138.
22. Crofton E. The women of Royaumont. East Lothian: Tuckwell Press; 1997. p. 169.
23. Letters from Agnes Savill. 1916 Jan 10. ML. TD1734/8/1/2/17.
24. MacPherson WG. Official history of the war. Medical services general history, vol. 1. London: HMSO; 1921. p. 169.
25. Crofton E. The women of Royaumont. East Lothian: Tuckwell Press; 1997. p. 158–67.
26. Edith A Stoney to Sir James Mackenzie Davidson. 1918 July 7. Mackenzie Davidson papers 40. Royal Society archives.
27. Edith Stoney to Mrs Walker. 1918 June 30. ML. TD1734/2/6/9/102.
28. Skia (VCC Collum) Blackwood's Magazine. 1918 Nov;629.
29. Crofton E. The women of Royaumont. East Lothian: Tuckwell Press; 1997. p. 164.

Chapter 15
Royaumont Abbey

Florence, in London, waited anxiously to hear news of her sister. She would have known from newspaper reports that the hospital at Villers-Cotterêts had remained, just, in French hands, and so it was unlikely that Edith and the others had been taken prisoner. It is quite possible that she had been able to obtain an outline of what was occurring at the front through her military and medical contacts. It must have come as a huge relief, nevertheless, when Edith's first letter after the evacuation reached her on 17 June, 3 weeks after the attack had commenced. Edith had written the letter at the end of a 30-hour marathon session that had started at 8.00 a.m. the previous day. Normally the sessions were only 18 hours, but she had been needed to cover for a sick colleague. Florence immediately wrote from work at the Fulham Military Hospital to Mrs. Laurie in Edinburgh to let her know that she had heard from Edith. She passed on the news:

> The last 48 hours at V.C. she had to pack and unpack the x Rays twice over, as fresh wounded came in, and within 24 hours of being at Royaumont she had her X-rays all set up and actually working. I don't know how she managed with all the wiring and getting electricity. It is a marvelous performance. [1]

The pressure did not let up once the evacuation of Villers-Cotterêts was completed: far from it. The beds at Royaumont had been largely emptied during the week, anticipating the new influx of wounded. The flood of injured soldiers started on Saturday. The radiographer Vera Collum wrote 'On the 31st of May began for us at the Abbaye the period of greatest stress and strain our staff had ever known'. Amalgamating the two hospitals expanded the number of beds to 480 and then to 600, stretching the accommodation for wounded to the limits. Space had to be found for the extra staff, too, some of whom had to sleep in chairs or share beds between day and night staff. The hospital was transformed into an emergency front line hospital operating under the direct control of the Army. They opened three operating theatres, two of them working 24-hour days (Fig. 15.1). Fleets of ambulances ferried the wounded from Senlis, the closest Casualty Clearing Station because Creil, near the railway junction, was now under threat of bombardment. Ramsay-Smith, the

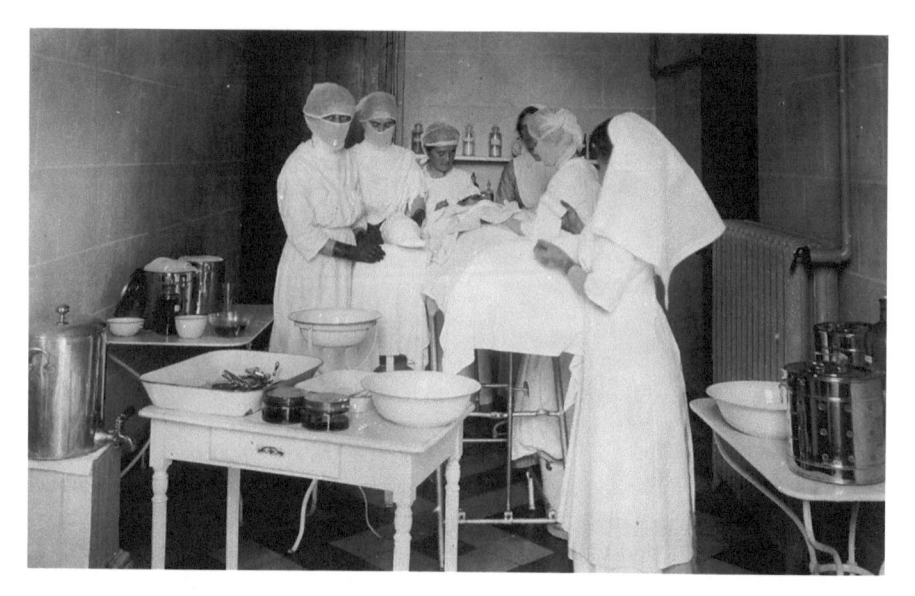

Fig. 15.1 The Royaumont Abbey operating theatre (Archives of the Fondation Royaumont)

administrator who had helped Edith to recover the equipment from Villers-Cotterêts, reported 'We have received over 400 in 3 days and we evacuate as quickly as we can and there is hardly ever an empty bed' [2].

Vera Collum

The senior radiographer at Royaumont, Vera Collum, was one of the longest serving staff there, originally offering her help as a driver for the SWH in September 1914, the first woman to do so. She had been appointed in November 1914 and joined Royaumont as an orderly in February 1915. Much of what is now known of Royaumont, apart from the official archives, comes from her article in *Blackwood's Magazine*, under the pseudonym 'Skia', and her contributions to *The Common Cause for Humanity*, the magazine of the National Union of Women's Suffrage Societies (NUWSS) [3]. At the outbreak of war, she had been working as a freelance journalist also employed in the Press Department of the London Office of the NUWSS. She was a woman of considerable personal initiative, and the ethos established by Frances Ivens at Royaumont encouraged anyone, like her, who wished to learn new skills and take on greater responsibility. She remained convinced that it was the women orderlies, even more than the women doctors and nurses, who were responsible for the working success of the hospital and found the informal, non-hierarchical environment in the early times motivating. She soon outgrew her position in charge of the *Vestiaire* (cloakroom) and expressed interest in radiography.

She wrote:

> I had the luck, helped by photographic knowledge, to get in to the only medical department in which a lay person could rise to full charge ... I was helped in every possible way to develop what originally was nothing more that some amateur skill in photography into a practical working knowledge of radiography, so that, for the last months of my life at the hospital, I was in charge of the department I had entered as an orderly more than 2 years before.

At first she worked in the darkroom, processing the X-ray plates. Dr. Jane Hawthorne, covering for Agnes Savill during her leave in summer of 1915, saw her talent and interest and trained her in the practice of radiography. She was joined by two others, Phylis Berry and, for a while, Gladys Buckley, a medical student who later specialised as a radiologist. They learned on the job, developing their skills, with Collum especially earning a reputation for care and compassion for the injured soldiers during radiographic procedures.

Vera Collum had her own dice with death when, returning from leave in March 1916 on the *Sussex*, the boat was torpedoed in mid-channel. She sustained severe injuries including a smashed foot, a damaged back, strained muscles and internal injuries and was in considerable pain. Eventually she was picked up by the British Navy and spent 3 months recovering in 'one of the great London Hospitals' where she was able to compare the standard of her own radiography, favourably she felt, with the X-ray images she saw there.

This was the experienced colleague who Edith joined on her arrival at Royaumont. Very different in background, the two women respected one another's competence and skill and willingness to rise to any challenge. By any standards, Edith's recovery of the Gaiffe equipment from Villers-Cotterêts was remarkable. Even more impressive was the re-establishment of the equipment in an anteroom in Royaumont, in full working order, within 24 hours. Edith knew exactly what she was doing and had equipped herself with the necessary measuring instruments and means to repair the damage that had inevitably occurred in transit [4]. It meant that two working X-ray rooms were now again available at Royaumont. The new Gaiffe room was fully working by 4 June. There was no way that the hospital could have coped without it. Edith and Vera Collum worked both rooms simultaneously. Collum reported 'I do not know how many men were brought in during that first 24 hours of 31st May—but I know that I personally made 85 X-ray examinations, and that neither my assistant nor developer got to bed till dawn'. As the wounded continued to flood in from Senlis, they carried out 1000 X-ray studies in 16 days and over 1200 radiographs, fluoroscopies and operations under X-rays during the first 3 weeks of June. Edith's workload statistics showed the dramatic increase that occurred during this time (Fig. 15.2). Even though things slowed down towards the end of the month, Edith's still recorded 1379 X-rays during the month of June, twice the number that had swamped those who had been working the two X-ray rooms during the peak influx from the Battle of the Somme 2 years before. To set the work in a peacetime context, Collum's 85 examinations in a single night was about the same as Florence's monthly total of diagnostic radiographs that she performed in the London Women's Hospital before the war.

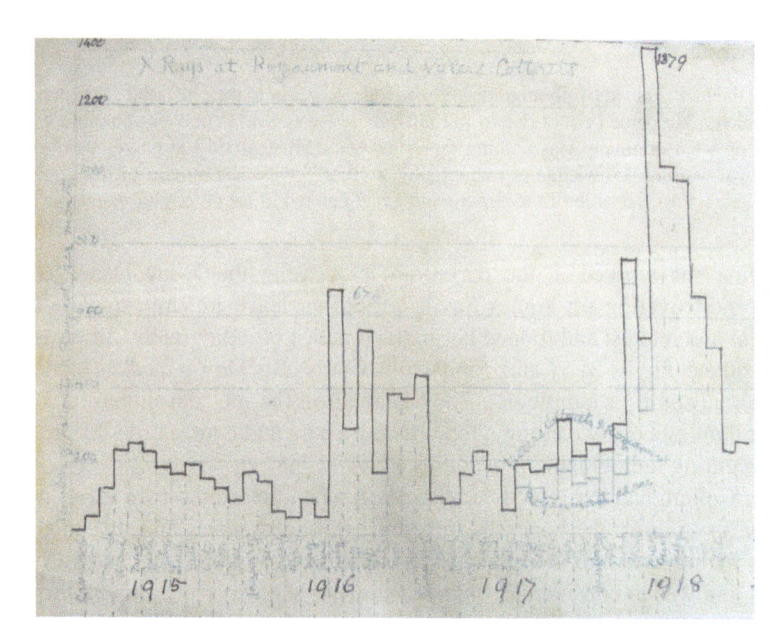

Fig. 15.2 Edith's record of the numbers of X-ray studies carried out at Royaumont and Villers-Cotterêts during the period December 1914–December 1918. (Glasgow City Archives)

In order to manage the workload, the X-ray and theatre staff roughly organised themselves into shifts, working 18 hours and resting 6. They were desperate for help, and Edith even drafted in one of the cooks, Eva Ashton, who 'most gallantly and most ably helped us in the worst of the rush when we had night work with the lights not able to be shown because of the raids overhead' [5]. 5 June came and went. For the first time in 7 years, dealing with the immediate crisis gave her no time to dwell on the anniversary of her father's death.

The basic Butt X-ray equipment was the only X-ray equipment that Collum ever used and was partly responsible for her later radiation-induced sickness. Whilst she recognised that the newer Gaiffe equipment that Edith had recovered from Villers-Cotterêts was a considerable improvement over her more basic system, it was unfamiliar to her, and she was more comfortable using her simple equipment with its 'reliable foolproof functioning', which 'never let the radiologist down'. This, written many years after the event in a tribute to Frederick Butt, may have been slightly through rose-tinted glasses [6].

Collum gives a vivid description of what it was like working as a radiographer during the periods of extreme pressure, experiences that would have been very familiar to Edith:

> We were fighting gas gangrene, and time was the factor that counted most. We dared not stop work in the theatre until it became physically impossible to continue. For us who worked, and for these patient suffering men, lying all along the corridor outside the X-ray rooms and theatre, on stretchers, waiting their turn, it was a nightmare of glaring lights, of appalling stenches of ether and chloroform, and the violent sparking of tired, rapidly-hardening X-ray

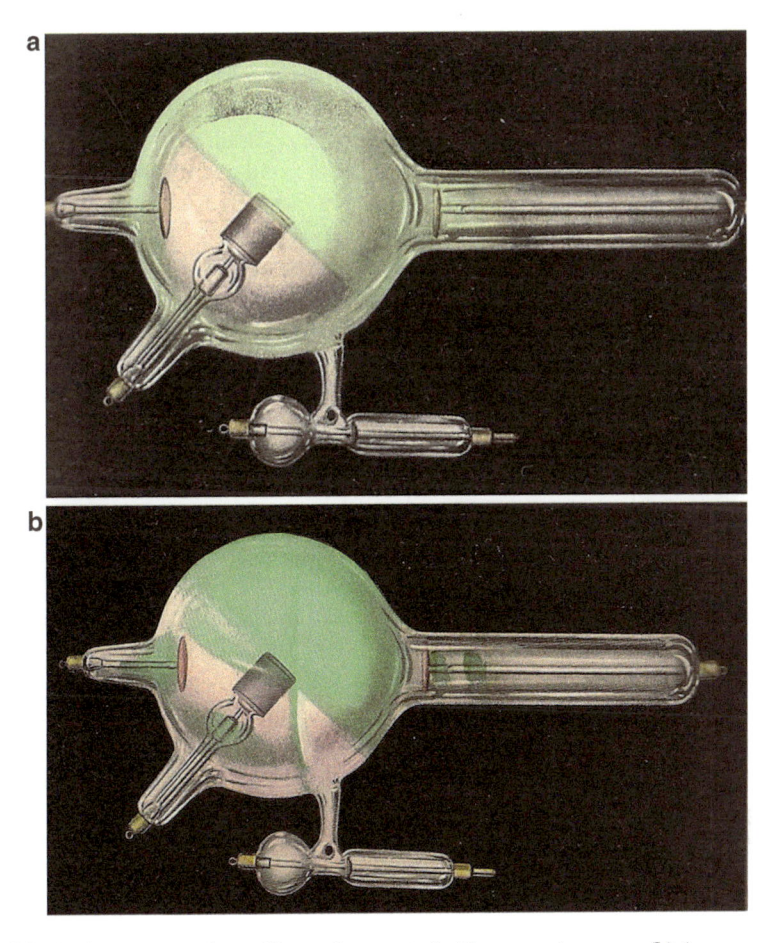

Fig. 15.3 (**a**) Appearance of a gas X-ray tube operated with a correct vacuum. (**b**) Appearance of a gas X-ray tube after it had hardened to a high vacuum

tubes, (Fig. 15.3a, b) of scores of wet negatives that were seized upon by their respective surgeons and taken in to the hot theatre before they had even had time to be rinsed in the dark room ….. and with us it was anxiety for the life of our hard-worked overheated tubes, anxiety to get the gas gangrene plates developed first, to persuade them to dry, to keep the cases of the six surgeons separate, to see that they did not walk off with the wrong plates—for we had pictures that were almost identical.

This had been Collum's experience during the Battle of the Somme in July 1916. The experience of dealing with casualties at that time led the French authorities to reorganise the way of dealing with the wounded. Instead of being transferred as soon as possible out of the danger zone, to hospitals such as Royaumont, they were initially dealt with in Casualty Clearing Stations near the front line, where first-line wound treatment was carried out. As a result, Royaumont during 1917 was a much quieter place, 'a sort of depot for the surgical cases that merely required skilled dressing or small secondary operations and good care'. Edith's graph shows the result of this changed strategy on the X-ray workload. The German attack of May 1918 abruptly returned the function of Royaumont from a back-up hospital to one that was responsible for dealing with casualties brought directly from the front line.

By the end of June, the tide had turned on the front, and the torrent of casualties arriving at Royaumont had slowed to a steady flow. Exhausted, Edith's assistant Patricia Raymond went off on well-deserved leave, having earlier taken over from Collum in the Butt room. The cook, Ashton, was needed back in the kitchen. Katherine Grandage, another Royaumont orderly, who had returned at the beginning of March, continued in the darkroom.

Radiation Safety

There were more serious reasons why staff had to leave.

Radiation injury was an ever-present hazard for these early radiographers. Ever since the earliest work with X-rays and radioactivity 20 years before, it had been realised that radiation could be dangerous. In the immediate pre-war years, anyone who entered radiography for the first time ran a risk of death due to radiation exposure that has been estimated at about 1–2%. For novice workers who started at the beginning of the war, the risk was higher, about 3%, reducing again as the war went on [7]. In the review from which these data are drawn, 71% of all the victims died from metastasized skin cancer. The other deaths were either from electrocution or from a wide range of radiation-induced blood disorders. Thus, whilst the radiographers who worked at Villers-Cotterêts and Royaumont certainly suffered from radiation-induced medical problems that will be detailed below, their risk of death from such reactions, though finite, was relatively low.

Furthermore, the principles that could limit a worker's exposure to radiation were also understood. It was known that radiation effects were dependent on the integrated radiation dose that built up over time. This meant that the longer a radiographer worked, the higher was the chance that she would develop symptoms. The effects were worse from more intense beams, closer to the tube, so that those not actually needed at the bedside should step back. However, the conditions under which radiography was carried out in hospitals such as Royaumont and Villers-Cotterêts, especially when overrun by casualties, could easily mean that radiation safety was not a high priority.

The radiation dose depended on, first, the design of the equipment and, second, how it was used. The design of the Butt Field systems paid scant attention to radiation safety. This was a general concern that was identified in the official report on the history of the WW1 medical services, where it was noted that the early equipment 'did not sufficiently protect the operator when working under war conditions'. The report added that, in due course, means to improve the protection afforded by the equipment was added and special radiation monitors were developed to survey the safety of the equipment already supplied [8]. These additions included protective metal screens partially surrounding the X-ray tube, limiting diaphragms to restrict the main beam of X-rays to only the region under investigation and thicker couch-tops and aluminium filters to prevent the low-energy X-rays reaching the skin. Some of these improvements were included in the new Gaiffe equipment that Edith had rescued from Villers-Cotterêts and Edith was clear that 'without the Gaiffe table .... the wreckage amongst the X-ray staff would have been greater for burns' [9].

Early in the war, the British military were not too concerned with such matters. Reviews of wartime X-ray equipment show a wide variety of tube protection [10]. Neither, sadly, was Frederick Butt himself, whose name is now inscribed on the Martyr's Memorial in Hamburg. F R Butt (1877–1937) started work as works manager for Harry Cox (1870–1931), an engineer who had commenced manufacturing induction coils and vacuum tubes shortly after Rontgen's discovery was announced. These included an early mobile X-ray apparatus for military use [11]. In 1908 he established Frederick R Butt and Co Ltd. at 147 Wardour St, and the Butt military field sets became standard issue during WWI. Butt's radiation injuries were sufficient to result in the surgical amputation of his left arm, and he finally died of disseminated cancer in 1937.

Lead-lined gloves were supplied, but were often not worn, because they were too bulky to allow any delicate mechanical or surgical manipulations to be carried out. Florence, who completely understood the risks she was taking, never used protective gloves when carrying out her fluoroscopic procedures.

What were the reported symptoms for the X-ray staff of the Scottish Women's Hospitals? First we will deal with Edith. In a letter to Mrs. Laurie from Royaumont in which she speaks of the previous winter in Villers-Cotterêts, she includes the casual comment 'my hands gave out—and it is not easy to write with one's hands bandaged up' [4]. She should not have allowed that to happen. She knew enough about the dangers of X-rays for her to take sufficient care to avoid overexposure. Skin reddening to the hands similar to sunburn was the first evidence to a radiographer that she might have received a high radiation dose.[1] Edith had not worked with X-rays since she left Salonika in July, and she had made no earlier comments on radiation-induced reactions from her previous posts. How was it that, after being in Villers-Cotterêts for only a few months, she had developed problems with her hands? Initially she was working on her own, and this may have been a contributory factor. In addition, it may have been that she was not sufficiently careful when working with the unfamiliar and poorly designed Butt equipment, perhaps making multiple exposures in an attempt to achieve the radiographic quality that she had reached with her equipment in Troyes and Salonika. Whatever was the cause, she continued to have problems, noting in a letter to Sir James Mackenzie-Davidson from Royaumont early in July 1918 that she had a septic hand [12]. If this means that her radiation burns had ulcerated, she would have received by then a dose of about 24 Gy. She was only too aware of what might happen. In the same letter she remarks

---

[1] Skin reddening may occur once the radiation dose to the skin reaches 2 gray (Gy) and will occur once the dose is 5 Gy.

'do not hurt your hands answering this', anticipating the surgery he would need later in the year for his radiation-induced malignancy.

During 1918, Edith required that the Royaumont radiographers had blood tests in Paris to test for any cellular changes that were by then known to arise from excessive exposure to radiation. At the end of June 1918, Vera Collum was advised to stop all X-ray work for at least 10 years, following her blood test. By then, on her own testimony, she had burns not only on her hands but also on her neck. Edith reported that 'Collum has been so badly burned with the old Butt Table's want of adequate protection that she could do no X-ray work. I am very thankful—very thankful indeed—that those working the Butt coil have now a better protected table in this new Gaiffe table' [5]. Florence Anderson took over Collum's role in the X-ray room whilst she continued to assist Miss Grandage in the darkroom until finally leaving France for the last time at the end of July [13]. Marion Butler, the radiographer who had worked for so long with Vera Collum, was also suffering from radiation burns after the influx of wounded at Royaumont in March and April 1918. She, too, had evidence of haematological effects from radiation in her blood test and returned to England.

That was not all. There was a change in practice that considerably increased the radiation dose, which was the increased use of fluoroscopy. From the earliest days of X-rays, there had been two ways in which the X-ray image could be viewed. The first was to create an image on film that was processed and examined later. The second used a screen of a material, usually barium platinocyanide, which glowed faintly when exposed to X-rays. Particularly during the busy periods, the surgeons wanted to learn as quickly as possible about the fractures and embedded fragments, and did not want to wait until the X-ray plates were processed. During these times, the proportion of studies using fluoroscopy increased from 20% to about 40% [14]. The X-ray tube was operated continuously, whilst the surgeons, radiographers and radiologists explored the wound for embedded metal under X-ray guidance. With gas tubes it was not possible to turn the output down, so the intensity was about the same whether the tube was used for fluoroscopy or for taking films, but for fluoroscopic screening it continuing for many minutes. As a result the total dose to the hands of the operator after many such examinations could eventually reach hazardous levels.

The radiation burns to the neck may have arisen when the radiographer helped the surgeon during an operation. The glow on the fluoroscopic screen was too weak to see under the bright lights of the operating theatre. So the radiographer used a closed hood with the screen mounted in front of her eyes, looking straight at the main beam of X-rays. The beam was then much larger, and any X-rays that passed by the hood and screen struck the skin of the radiographer, typically on her neck.

Some radiographers used their hands to test the X-ray settings. Edith knew that there was a safer and more accurate way of setting and testing the tubes. The equipment that she took to Troyes and Salonika included a Wehnelt radiometer. This simple device consisted of an aluminium 'step wedge', a small staircase of aluminium layers of progressively increasing thickness. This was usually placed over a small fluorescent screen, giving a standard target with which to judge how penetrating the X-ray beam was. It could also be used with film. Novice radiographers undoubtedly spurned the radiometer as being not the real thing. Equally certainly, it would have been the tool that Edith, the physicist, would have used to set her tubes, saving her own hands from unnecessary exposure.

Apart from the effects of radiation, there was another important reason why some staff had to take time off from their work. Back in London, Florence understood the stress that Edith and her colleagues were under. 'We may indeed be proud of them all but I fear there will be a heavy aftermath to pay for the great overwork they are undergoing. Here, in London, we think we are busy, but it is a backwater compared with Royaumont' [15].

Florence was right to be concerned. By the autumn, the unit had lost three of their doctors who had broken down under the strain, Berry, Martland and Walters. Mrs. Berry suffered a complete nervous breakdown. 'Perhaps it was ….. her highly-strung and sensitive nature and the terrific pressures of the spring and summer of 1918 which became an increasing and ultimately intolerable strain upon her, leading to her collapse'. Her husband believed that the chief cause of her depression was the feeling that she had been of no use to Royaumont [16]. Much later, Dr. Henry confided to her daughter that she still had recurrent nightmares about the evacuation from Villers-Cotterêts [17]. One is left wondering how many others suffered silently from post-traumatic stress following their ordeal. By contrast, Edith was damaged physically but not mentally. Those best able to cope were probably those who focussed firmly on the task in hand and were not naturally inclined to feel empathy with the wounded.

During the extreme pressure on the two X-ray rooms that summer, Edith had bought a mobile X-ray system, using funds donated directly to the hospital [4]. This equipment could be taken into the wards, making it unnecessary for some casualties to be taken to the X-ray room for examination. A mobile set was a simple but innovative development, only very recently available. The US army had developed a standard bedside design during the war, and a similar system had been devised by Ledoux-Lebard in France at about the same time [18, 19] (Fig. 15.4). In the French system, all the electrical equipment was mounted within a wheeled cabinet divided into four separate compartments, two large ones back-to-back at the top and two smaller ones at the bottom. The larger compartments carried the coil and the milliammeter in one and the interrupter, designed to operate on either DC or AC electrical supply, in the other. The accessories, screen, gloves and so on were carried in the lower compartments. The tube was mounted on a separate, wheeled stand. Some parts may have been salvaged from the X-ray ambulance [20], and it was well within Edith's capability to create a bedside system using some new and some old parts. Edith appreciated the need for further ambulance capacity, but still harboured the idea that it could be possible to transport the new portable equipment in the back, so reinstating the X-ray van if this became necessary.

Other changes in the X-ray team occurred. Marion Butler, who had been at Villers-Cotterêts with Edith, went home after her 6-month appointment. Agnes Savill came back from London in July, even though she herself was ill, bringing her own X-ray assistant, Ruby Large, to help. She was pleased to find that the

Fig. 15.4 The Ledoux-Lebard portable X-ray system c. 1920. front view

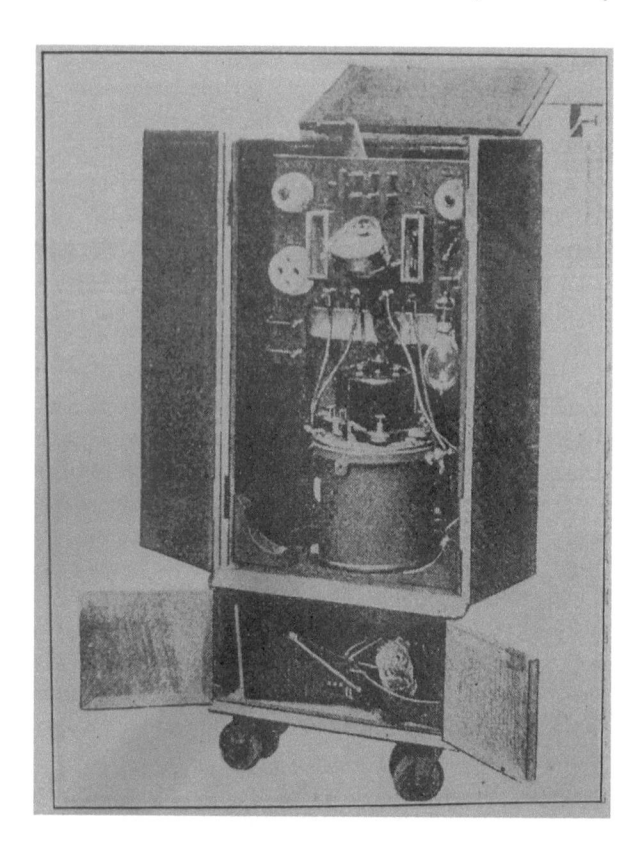

department was working well, even though still under considerable pressure. This allowed Edith to go home for a couple of weeks on leave. She had developed a ruptured varicose vein in her leg, which she believed was the result of the many hours she had spent standing. She allowed Florence to treat it with ionisation therapy, a technique that she herself had used in Salonika. Florence was very pleased with the result, and Edith confirmed, cautiously, that 'it is wonderful when properly done, sometimes', although adding that 'this electric treatment is so often quackery', and was concerned that 2 weeks was rather too short a time for her leg to fully recover. Florence had apparently decided that the high-frequency electrical therapy that she had advocated for the treatment of varicose veins a decade earlier was not as successful as she had hoped [21].

Planning Ahead

Edith continued to log the numbers of X-ray investigations being carried out. It was not until September that the total dropped to below the April peak. The team continued to operate the two rooms side by side, getting though about

500 examinations each summer month in each room. As the pressure released, they could relax a bit. In an undated letter, Edith told Mrs. Laurie that they were having a welcome rest, with only three of the wards 'full of fractured legs and femurs, otherwise the hospital is not full'. The weather was 'delicious'. The brief respite gave an opportunity for a fancy dress party and concert when:

> one of the men dressed as Miss Ivens in white overall—with an attendant 'sister' in blue cotton and white service cap—and an attendant orderly—one without a leg and one without an arm . . . . We laughed and laughed and they laughed and laughed.

Edith was thinking about what she was going to do next, following the expiry of her current contract in November. She was genuinely concerned about finding appropriate employment when she left the SWH. At home on sick leave in Reynolds Close at the end of July, she confided to Mrs. Laurie that 'one's inside (most of us who are not medical) is so eaten up these days with dread of not getting useful enough work'.

Florence and Edith had been in touch with their friend and radiological colleague Sir James Mackenzie-Davidson, exploring whether he could suggest any of his contacts who might have a vacancy that would suit Edith's skills and experience [12]. In her letter to Mackenzie-Davidson, Edith cogently and openly summarised the problem she faced in finding employment as an older woman scientist, 'It is very hard to get work when one is (1) a woman (2) not strong (3) 48 years of age (4) and not with a medical or nursing qualification'. On Mackenzie-Davidson's advice, Florence had approached a Captain Cooper on Edith's behalf, who was looking for radiologists for France. He had written back a friendly letter saying that the British War Office would not employ women radiologists abroad in War Office hospitals but that he would look out for an opening for an X-ray assistant in a Red Cross Hospital. Edith pointed out that she was not in a position to fund herself: she needed a paid job. She still hoped that she might secure an appointment on a hospital ship as a radiologist and that Mackenzie-Davidson might be in a position to help.

It was all impossible, of course. In the letter, she explains her frustration over the barrier to finding a senior position in a department of radiology as a result of her lack of a medical qualification. She speculates whether the prejudice was not only because of the lack of qualification:

> Is it because women are generally not good on the side of care of apparatus—on the engineering side? That is the side I am some good on—at least I imagine myself to be less bad on than on the other sides. I have not the huge good fortune these days to be medically trained—but I have now done war work for 3¼ years –and often without a mechanic—or with only occasional and half trained help.

By now, Edith had come to understand her true value to the hospitals in which she worked and was frustrated by a system that obstructed, as she saw it, the provision of the necessary expert scientific and technical support that she knew was necessary to the performance of an effective radiological service. She was very critical about the failure to provide such a service in some other SWH units. For example, she was disappointed to learn that, after she had left Salonika, no properly trained person was appointed to look after the X-ray equipment in Ostrovo, leaving it in the care only of a radiologist. She claimed that the X-ray equipment shipped to the SWH unit in Russia had never once worked because the doctor in charge did not have the technical knowledge to set it up. Furthermore, she asserted:

> The X-rays of the Elsie Inglis corps in Macedonia does not work—and is in the hands of a junior doctor who asked Florence to teach her all about X-rays in 3 days! The apparatus was that which had gone out and come back from Russia—and when Florence offered to look over it,—or urged them to get it properly looked over—before taking it out to Macedonia—this small (!) precaution was refused as too much trouble! [4]

When Edith had offered her services to the SWH 3 years before, she had naively assumed that her academic qualifications and experience, Cambridge educated and then lecturer in physics at the London School of Medicine for Women, would place her on a par with her medical colleagues, to whom she was bringing complementary but equivalently senior skills. She had been happy to do battle with the Edinburgh managers when she felt their judgements were incorrect, having no understanding of a hierarchy that placed her on a lower status. After a very successful year working with Frances Ivens, where she felt respected and valued, she was now clearer about the difficulty she faced. It was not that she had any inferior place in the medical hierarchy: as a technical expert she had no agreed place in it at all. Collum had noticed how, 'as our hospital grew in size and numbers, it grew, too, in rigidity and convention. Where tradition had served as an ample guide for the few who had watched over its birth and infancy, regulation and restrictions, rules and maxims, had to be introduced' [22]. Since arriving back in France, Edith had worked effectively within rules she now understood to her own advantage and that of the X-ray department. Up to now, having the support and understanding of her local medical colleagues, especially Frances Ivens, it had only mattered up in Edinburgh that she was not medically qualified, not here in France. As rules and structures crystallised, however, and as new staff arrived, her position became progressively more difficult.

Edith returned from Hampstead to Royaumont in August to find Agnes Savill 'quite unable to do more than an hour or so of work—She is very plucky over her want of strength' [9]. Finally Savill returned to London at the end of September. By this time the X-ray workload was beginning to reduce, though it was still three times the level they had experienced during 1917. The biggest challenge to Edith was that there had been an almost complete turnover of staff whilst she was away. Catherine Lowe had arrived on 22 August and was quickly trained. Nevertheless, with both Agnes Savill and Edith ill, with the departure of experienced staff and with new faces in the surgical team who didn't seem very interested, it had not been possible to maintain the excellent methods they had established for X-ray-guided localisation. For someone who had been admired for the precision of her localisation, this must have been a huge disappointment.

Unfortunately, in the middle of October, and at the point she was beginning to train the new staff, she went down a respiratory problem that Frances Ivens diagnosed as influenza and Edith described as asthma. Feeling very low, she gave in when the X-ray Sister, Marion Macalister, unclear about Edith's status in the medical hierarchy, challenged her authority. When Agnes Savill left at the end of September, she was not prepared to accept instructions from Edith, who wanted Macalister to become competent to use the Gaiffe equipment for localisation. The nurse reacted badly:

> she used language I could not have passed over when I tried to shew her the Gaiffe apparatus and other French things we have—things new to her—which she therefore naturally could not work without getting it out of order. As I was likely to have to go on account of my own health, I thought it easier to go rather than complain and so force her to go.

It was all about the medical hierarchy. The Sister knew her place. This was to do the bidding of all medical staff, and that would have applied whether they were women or men. She could instruct the junior nurses, orderlies and VADs, who were all below her in status and would do as they were told. As far as she was concerned, Edith was not a doctor nor was she a nurse, so she was an orderly, in no position to give her instructions. As Edith wrote to Mrs. Laurie, 'It's a funny world—That I have 4 university degrees would count nothing to her—even if she knew it'.[2]

Irritated, Edith raised the matter with Frances Ivens who advised her not to press the issue and suggested sensibly that, for her own health, she should go on sick leave. So Edith, feeling tired, ill and disillusioned, left Royaumont on 24 October for Cannes where she gratefully relaxed. Frances Ivens, wisely concerned for Edith's welfare, and apparently less bothered than Edith by any argument there may have been, ensured that she could take a proper holiday by providing her with a travel pass. Edith left the recently trained but competent Catherine Lowe to look after the steadily reducing X-ray workload. Lowe stayed until the end of the year, when she moved on to Salonika to work in the X-ray department there. Three weeks after Edith left Royaumont, the war was over.

Frances Ivens may have been right in her original diagnosis of influenza. Edith's sick leave had to be extended by what she described at the time as bronchitis. It could have been more serious. Outbreaks of so-called Spanish flu had started in the spring of 1918, an epidemic that would finally cause the deaths of over 50 million people before it was over. It was noticed that those who died were predominantly aged between 20 and 40, an effect that has been explained as arising from an acquired immunity amongst older people from an earlier strain of flu virus. Possibly Edith was one of the lucky older ones. At the same time, Florence, exhausted and in need of rest, was 'indefinitely away, sent on a long holiday in Ireland' [9].

The Closure of Royaumont

Edith returned to Royaumont before the hospital finally closed its doors to casualties on 31 December 1918. A small number of patients still needed X-rays, and, even during December, Edith logged over 200 cases. She still had enough time to visit

---

[2]Edith was counting two examination results from Cambridge Part I and Part II in the Maths Tripos and her BA and MA from Trinity College Dublin. Strictly the Cambridge qualifications were not degrees, but women were increasingly ignoring that detail as a relic from some other age.

Paris on 29 November, to see the visit by King George V, where she was quite moved by the reception he was given writing that 'one felt many in the crowd were more like crying than cheering—with thankfulness' [23].

On her return to Royaumont, she found that work had already started sorting the mountain of X-ray plates and records that had accumulated over the past 4 years. This was a huge job, which eventually kept her in Royaumont until February 1919. They had also received a specific request from the College of Surgeons in London, which was to supply copies of all their pairs of stereo X-ray photographs, an important request that recognised the quality of radiography in Edith's department at Royaumont. Frances Ivens had asked Sister Macalister to commence this task, knowing that the Sister would refuse to be instructed by Edith, who kept her distance. When she came to review Sister Macalister's work before dispatch, she discovered that the nurse had assumed that one of each stereo pair was a duplicate and had destroyed it [24]. Later commentary improperly placed the blame on Edith for this error [25].[3]

Nearly 1000 people crammed in to the main hall for the Christmas pantomime, which included Widow Twankey collapsing in a heap, pirates and the wicked baron being killed by a prince, a wandering minstrel playing the violin, minuets and Scottish reels. The grand finale was a tableau titled 'Victory' 'A very good-looking sister, all draped in white, with green palms in her hair and holding a shining sword which scintillated and looked dramatic' [26].

One last ceremony occurred before the hospital closed: the award of the *Croix de Guerre* to 23 of the staff, including Edith. The presentations were made in the lofty main hall, the beds of the Canada Ward cleared to one side (Fig. 15.5). The 'citations' were read out for each group in turn, the medal pinned on each breast, in the name of the President of the French Republic, and the accolade given. The ceremony ended with the 'Marseillaise' followed by 'God Save the King'. Frances Ivens received the *Croix de Guerre avec Palme.* Edith was amongst the group who received the *Croix de Guerre avec Etoile,* for whom the citation read '*Ont prodigué a l'hopital des dames ecosses, tant a Villers Cotterets qu'a Royaumont, leur Science et leur dévouement aux blessés français et Allies, sous des bombardements repétés*' (For dedicating their science and their devotion to the French and Allied wounded at the Scottish Women's Hospital, both at Villers Cotterets and at Royaumont, under repeated bombardments) [27]. The emphasis on Edith's contribution through science was especially important in the eyes of the French authorities, as was her bravery under fire.

On the last day of the year, the final 200 men left, leaving only 7 who were too ill to be moved. All qualified nurses were dismissed, and the staff was reduced to a team of 20 orderlies. A once thriving hospital went quiet. They had shown, without a

---

[3] A moment's thought reveals how incorrect it was to cast the blame onto Edith. She had been specifically excluded from authority over the X-ray sister, and it was Frances Ivens who had instructed her to sort out the photographs. Ivens was fully experienced in radiography and knew the importance of keeping both photographs in each stereo pair.

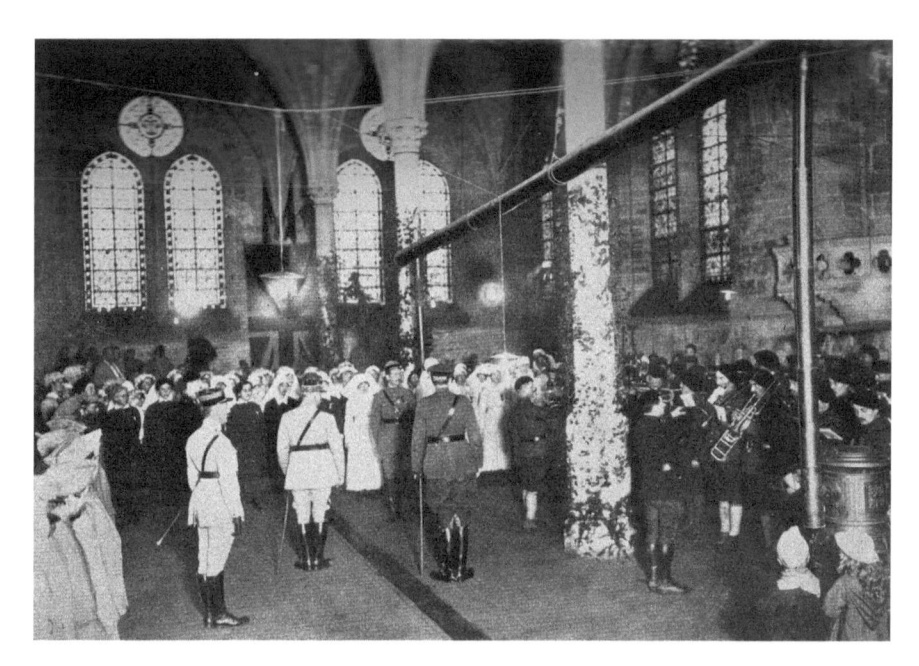

Fig. 15.5 The Croix de Guerre award ceremony in the hall at Royaumont Abbey on 12 December 1918. Edith was amongst the doctors in their dark uniforms on the left. The band of *12e Bataillon de Chasseurs Alpins* is on the right, with village children in the foreground. The awards were presented by General Nourrisson

shadow of doubt, the falsity of Isobel Emslie's friend who had assured her that 'the show won't last very long; these shows run by women never do'.

Edith's 50th birthday on 6 January was not a memorable occasion. The winter cold fatigued her limbs and numbed her mind. The excitement and challenge of military radiography had gone, its departure removing a major source of satisfaction that Edith gained from her job. The electricity supply, for which Edith felt responsible, periodically failed: it came from a dynamo driven by a water wheel, which froze. The men who had broken the ice to keep the water and electricity flowing in previous years were no longer available. It was cold inside the Abbey too, and there were no longer any soldiers to help bring logs in to feed the open fires. During the next couple of months, Edith slowly worked her way through the mountain of X-ray records and plates, doing her best to impress some order on the otherwise disorganised piles of results. She recognised that the X-rays formed an important part of the medical record, often central to any decision about the military pension to which a soldier would be entitled on discharge from the army.

Finally, Edith crated all the X-ray equipment. It left Royaumont as part of the load in 20 railway wagons full of equipment donated to *l'Hôpital Saveur* in Lille. On 10 February 1919, Edith eventually left Royaumont for the last time, returning to England to an uncertain future once more.

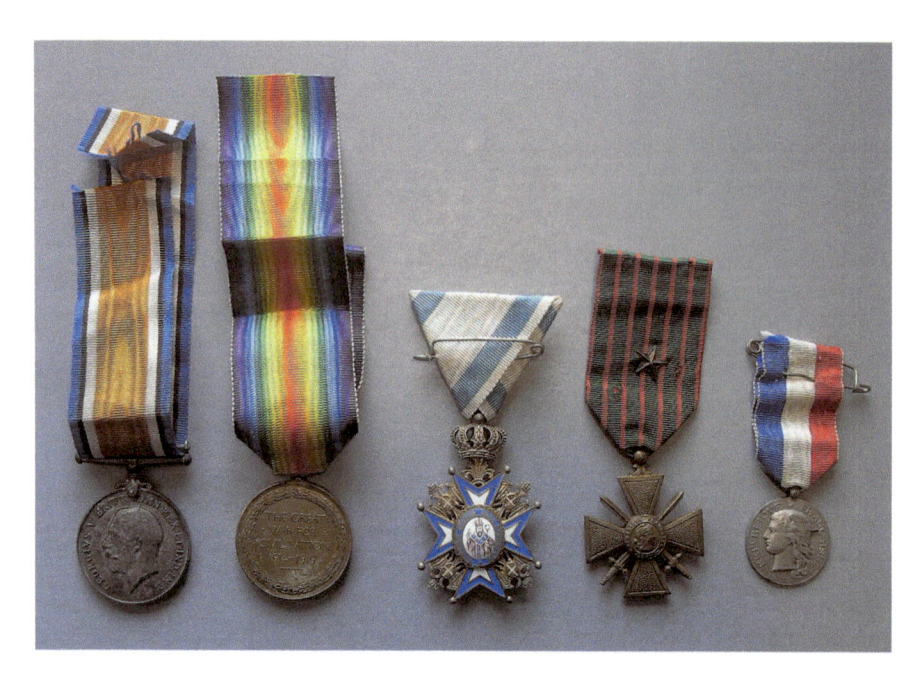

Fig. 15.6 Edith's medals. L to R. British War Medal, Victory Medal, Order of St Sava of Serbia, *Croix de Guerre avec Etoile. Medaille des Epidemies.* (Author's photograph from Newnham College, Cambridge archive)

Edith's war service was recognised by the British authorities by the awards of the Victory and British War Medals, given to all those who gave service during the war (Fig. 15.6). Shortly after she arrived home, Florence wrote once more to Mrs. Laurie:

> She (Edith) is not at all well—it is the price she has to pay for the help she has given during the war. Few people realise what the constant strain of X-ray work in the dark and stuffy atmosphere and with the X-rays about—mean to the worker—If she had been in the Army she would have had a pension, but that is one of the things where it is hard to be a woman. [28]

Edith went to Bournemouth to rest.

Edith's year at Royaumont and Villers-Cotterêts was the best time of her war. She was settled, confident and respected. This was noticed. When Marian Erskine came to Villers-Cotterêts on an official inspection soon after Edith arrived, she wrote 'Miss Stoney is sweeter than honey. Long may it last!' [29]. Mrs. Jessie Berry, acting Chief Medical Officer there during the winter of 1917–1918, later remembered her as a saint [30]. Agnes Savill, writing to Mrs. Russell in July 1918, when she returned to help during Edith's brief sick leave, was equally complementary about her, reporting that 'We are a very harmonious and congenial X-ray department now' [31]. After the unit was all but overwhelmed by the workload in the summer of 1918, Edith noted her own deep satisfaction to have been tested and to have risen to the challenge, writing that it was 'of the deepest pleasure to me to be on the Western Front in these days—and where such very excellent help was given when so desperately needed'

[4]. Florence wrote of Edith that 'she says what a privilege it is to be able to help in such work'.

In spite of this evidence, some later descriptions of the work of the Scottish Women's Hospitals singled out Edith as being a particularly difficult woman, and moreover that the difficulties that she had with her colleagues, especially her medical colleagues, were of her own making. An index even included a separate entry 'Edith Stoney; difficult woman', so the reader could easily look up the evidence for this opinion [32]. This somewhat negative view has since been accepted and propagated by others [33]. Edith was certainly tough, technically outstanding and uncompromising when she felt that her analysis of a situation was correct. In current parlance, being a 'difficult woman' is not infrequently used as a badge to be worn with pride [34], but at the time it was used as a critical comment on Edith's ability to engage with her women peers.[4]

In many ways she was closer in personality to her brother Gerald than to Florence. In his obituary, Gerald was described as being 'kindly, sympathetic and humorous', words similarly used on occasions to describe Edith when she was not under stress. But 'at times his Irish temperament showed itself. In controversy or under criticism, he was inclined to be scornful but did not seem to realize the irritation that this caused, even in ordinary conversation'. Furthermore, whilst Gerald was an outstanding engineer, he was poor at staff management, a failing that led to his acrimonious departure from Charles Parsons' employment in June 1912. Much of Edith's character could be described in these terms [35].

Edith herself was not indifferent to the tensions and conflicts that existed in the organisation, not only between herself and others but also between her strong-minded and independent colleagues. She also understood the role that Jessie Laurie had in the SWH played during the war and expressed this very clearly in a letter written to her after it was all over.

> May I thank you very warmly now for ... endless other warm-hearted courtesies. I do not suppose you have the least idea how much your constant cordiality has kept the Scottish Women's corps together and oiled many a temporarily grumbling wheel! [36]

Edith did indeed suffer from friction with some of her senior colleagues during her time with the Girton and Newnham Unit under Louise McIlroy. The fact that she worked well under Frances Ivens says as much about the two CMOs as it does about Edith. The record is clear, however, that Edith irritated Marian Erskine and Beatrice Russell beyond bounds by her complaining and critical letters. It is also true that, at a time of polite social interchange, some of Edith's letters exceeded the limits of acceptability, much as a modern email sent in haste might be later regretted. This did not mean, however, that she was wrong or that her position was unjustified. She just sometimes had a rather irritating way of making her point.

---

[4]Edith still retained an ability to irritate. Crofton reports Mrs. Berry begging a colleague to take Edith for a walk in the forest. 'If you do, I shall get you an egg for breakfast, and if you take her and lose her I'll give you two. And that was when eggs were scarce'.

Images are important too. The only photograph of Edith included in Crofton's book about Royaumont, taken during her time in Salonika and not in France, is an unnecessarily cropped and enlarged version of Fig. 12.3, tie askew, lower button undone and strangely pale eyes, presented as a stereotypical mad scientist. Looks are important, and this photograph is in strong contrast to the well-presented, posed pictures of her senior medical colleagues included elsewhere in the book.

Edith's colleagues were doctors first and women second. They were members of the first phalanx of women who had broken down the historic barriers that had prevented women from entering medicine, and they were deeply proud of that achievement. They were strongly bonded through this common experience. When recording their recollections of their war experiences, it is unsurprising that they speak warmly of those colleagues who had travelled the same path to professional status. The ties to other women who had chosen different life paths were not so strong.

In all this, Edith was an outsider. She was respected, but had no professional position or support from this clan of lady doctors. Her constituency lay outside it, the wider community of women who were still challenged to engage fully with the world. After the war, Edith left medicine behind, and there was not one to recall, and possibly not one who was bothered to understand, who she was and what she had achieved. It was a convenient fiction to give her a niche role during wartime as the difficult, unsocial scientist. Such portrayals are hard to dilute, to reverse. It is to be hoped that the present account may serve as a reminder that complex personalities cannot be so easily pigeonholed.

References

1. Florence Stoney to Mrs Laurie. 17 June 1918. ML. TD1734/2/6/9/100.
2. Crofton E. The women of Royaumont. East Lothian: Tuckwell Press; 1997. p. 285–91.
3. Skia (VCC Collum) A hospital in France. Blackwood's Magazine. 1918 Nov. pp. 613–40.
4. Edith Stoney to Mrs Laurie. 28 July 1918. ML. TD1734/2/6/9/104.
5. Edith Stoney to Mrs Walker. 30 June 1918. ML. TD1734/2/6/9/102.
6. Crofton E. The women of Royaumont. East Lothian: Tuckwell Press; 1997. p. 175. Quoting Collum.
7. Kemerink GJ, van Engelshoven JMA, Simon KJ, Kutterer G, Wildberger JE. Early X-ray workers: an effort to assess their numbers, risk, and most common (skin) affliction. Insights Imaging. 2016;7:275–82.
8. MacPherson WG. Official history of the war. Medical services general history, vol. 1. London: HMSO; 1921. p. 170.
9. Edith Stoney to Mrs Laurie. 27 October 1918. ML. TD1734/2/6/9/111?
10. Van Tiggelen R. Radiology in a French coat. Military radiology on the western front during the great war. Brussels: Academia Press; 2013.
11. Archives of the Roentgen Ray. 1903–4;8(12):224.
12. Edith A Stoney to Sir James Mackenzie Davidson, 7 July 1918. Mackenzie Davidson papers 40. Royal Society archives.
13. Collum VCC. The common cause. 1918 Dec 27. p. 444.
14. Skia (VCC Cullum) A hospital in France. Blackwood's Magazine. 1918 Nov. p. 632.

References

15. Florence Stoney to Mrs Laurie 17 June 1918 ML. TD1734/2/6/9/100b.
16. Crofton E. The women of Royaumont. East Lothian: Tuckwell Press; 1997. p. 264.
17. Crofton E. The women of Royaumont. East Lothian: Tuckwell Press; 1997. p. 163.
18. U.S.Army x-ray manual. London: Lewis. 1919. pp. 178–9.
19. Hirsch IS. Principles and practice of Roentgenological technique. New York: American X-ray Publishing Co; 1920. p. 53.
20. Edith Stoney to Mrs Laurie (undated). ML. TD1734/2/6/9/109a.
21. Stoney FA. Chronic congestion treated by electricity. Arch Roentgen Ray. 1906;10:325–9.
22. Skia (VCC Collum) p 621.
23. Edith Stoney to Mrs Laurie 30 Nov 1918 ML. TD1734/2/6/9/113.
24. Edith Stoney to Mrs Laurie 13 May 1919. ML. TD1734/2/6/9/124.
25. Crofton E. The women of Royaumont. East Lothian: Tuckwell Press; 1997. p. 206.
26. Crofton E. The women of Royaumont. East Lothian: Tuckwell Press; 1997. p. 204.
27. Scottish Women's Hospitals. Decoration of Officers: Account of the Ceremony. The Common Cause. 1919 Jan 17;482–483.
28. Crofton E. The women of Royaumont. East Lothian: Tuckwell Press; 1997. p 206. Quoting Florence Stoney to Mrs Laurie 23 April 1919.
29. Crofton E. The women of Royaumont. East Lothian: Tuckwell Press; 1997. p 138. Quoting Dr Erskine to Miss Kemp 22 Nov 1917.
30. Crofton E. The women of Royaumont. East Lothian: Tuckwell Press; 1997. p. 207.
31. Crofton E. The women of Royaumont. East Lothian: Tuckwell Press; 1997. p. 185.
32. Leneman L. In the service of life. The story of Elsie Inglis. Edinburgh: Mercat Press; 1994.
33. Guy JM. Edith (1869–1938) and Florence (1870-1932) Stoney, two Irish sisters and their contribution to radiology during World War I. J Med Biogr. 2013;21:100–7.
34. For example: Karbo K. In praise of difficult women: life lessons from 29 heroines who dared to break the rules. Random House. 2018.
35. Dowson R. George Gerald Stoney 1863–1942. Obituary Notices of Fellows of the Royal Society. 1942. pp. 183–96.
36. Edith Stoney to Mrs Laurie 12 May 1919. ML. TD1734/2/6/9/124.

Chapter 16
Return to Civilian Life

Awards and Decorations

The summer of 1919 was one of anticlimax. The war was over, and, for many in the country, the feelings were not of triumphalism but that such a tragedy must never be allowed again. Both Florence and Edith were exhausted. The military use of the Fulham Military Hospital came to an end in 1919, and Florence returned to her medical practice. Edith returned home from France to an uncertain future.

Following her distinguished service, Florence received many medals and honours (Figs. 16.1 and 16.2). It seems curious that some of Florence's obituaries regret that her war work was not honoured more, such as seen in the notice in *The Vote* on 28 October 1932. The suffragist movement contained significant anti-war elements, and if she were to continue in that movement, Florence probably felt a need to downplay her heroic and significant war record, with no reason to publicise the honours that she had received.

On 18 February 1919, it was announced in *The London Gazette* that Miss Florence Ada Stoney M.D., B.S. was to be an Officer of the Civil Division of the Most Excellent Order of the British Empire [1]. The OBE had been instituted by King George V on 4 June 1917 with an aim to honour those who had served in non-combatant roles during the Great War. The motto is 'For God and the Empire'. Initially the OBE had a single division, but in 1918 it was split into military and civil divisions, and Florence received her award in the civil division. Florence received the OBE primarily for her work at the Fulham Military Hospital. She took her place alongside three other women, all doctors, in a list of 56 recipients of the OBE announced on that day. Two were surgeons, Mary Forbes Liston, honoured for setting up an X-ray department in Glasgow, and Winifred Margaret Ross, who helped to set up the SWH unit at Royaumont. The fourth woman doctor, Mary Ethel Jeremy from Bournemouth, had worked in the British War Hospital in St. Malo.

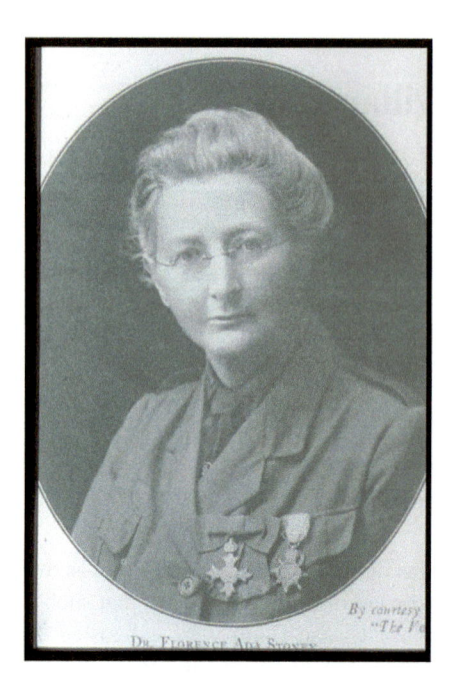

Fig. 16.1 Dr. Florence Ada Stoney wearing uniform and medals. (From 'The Voice') (location of reference not found)

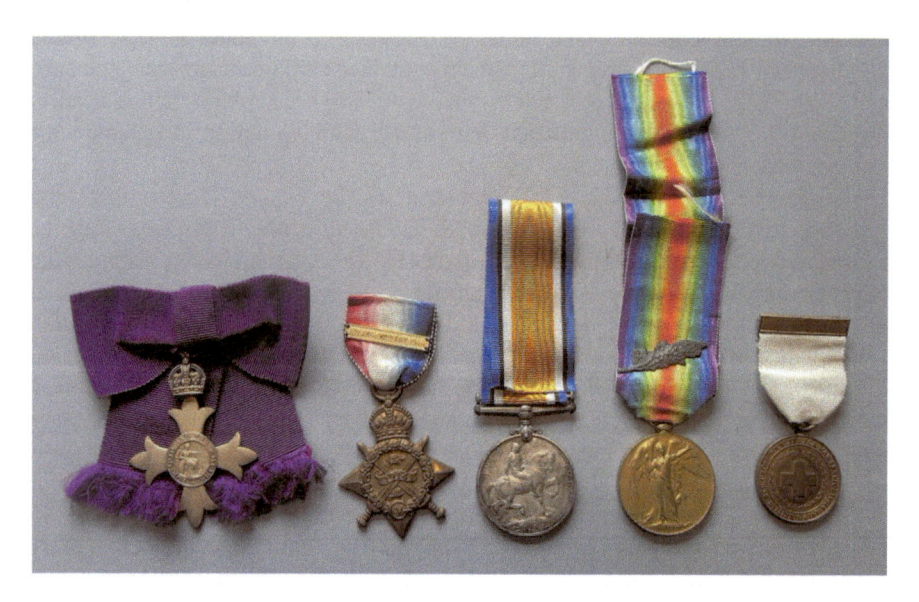

Fig. 16.2 Florence's World War I medals. L to R: OBE, 1914 Star 5 August to 22 November 1914, with bar given for service under fire; British War Medal, Victory Medal with oak leaf for mention in dispatches; British Red Cross Medal for war service, 1914–1918. (Held by Newnham College Cambridge)

Florence's second award was the 1914 Star for military service undertaken between 5 August and 22 November 1914. This medal was awarded to those who landed in France soon after the outbreak of hostilities and was nicknamed the 'Mons Star', depicting a four-pointed star. In October 1919 the King awarded a clasp to the medal for those who had given service under fire during that period, and Florence received this for her service in Antwerp.

Like her sister, Florence was awarded the British War Medal, which was given to members of the imperial forces who had served in the Great War and depicts an image of King George V as King of all the British Isles and Emperor of India. She was then awarded the Victory Medal (United Kingdom), which was issued to those who had received another war medal such as the British War Medal or the 1914 Star. Florence was mentioned in despatches, and as such she was entitled to wear a bronze oak leaf spray on her ribbon. The Victory Medal depicts on its obverse a full-length representation of 'Victory' as a winged woman and on the reverse has written 'The Great War for Civilisation 1914–1919'. In a typically irreverent manner the British soldier or 'Tommy' nicknamed the Stars, War Medal and Victory Medal as Pip, Squeak and Wilfred after three contemporary comic book characters.

Finally, in 1920, Florence received the British Red Cross Society Medal for War Service, which was granted to all members of the British Red Cross Society, for war work. The medal displays the classic Geneva cross of the Red Cross and was inscribed 'British Red Cross Society: For War Service 1914–1918'.

The British Association Meeting in Bournemouth, September 1919

'We are gathered together at a time when, after great upheaval, the elemental conditions of organisation of the world are still in flux, and we have to consider how to mould and influence the re-crystallisation of these elements into the best forms and most economic arrangements for the benefit of civilisation.'

These words were spoken by the Hon. Sir Charles A. Parsons KCB MA LLD DSc FRS. Edith and Florence were in the audience in the Winter Gardens Pavilion at Bournemouth. It was the evening of Tuesday, 9 September 1919. The occasion was the opening of the 87th annual meeting of the British Association for the Advancement of Science. Charles Parsons was the president for that year, and he was giving his presidential address [2].

As Charles Parsons spoke, the sisters remembered the past British Association meetings that they had attended with their father. Florence had been the last to become a life member, in 1908. They knew Sir Charles well. It was Parsons' father who had given their father his first job, discovering new nebulae using the Leviathan telescope back in Parsonstown. Florence recalled the beginning of the war, when Charles Parsons' wife Katherine so kindly donated the induction coil after her first one had to be abandoned during the retreat from Antwerp. The sisters both knew how important the speaker had been to their brother Gerald, giving him his first job as a draughtsman and promoting him to become the most senior engineer in his company. Gerald was now Vice President of the Engineering Section having been President of the section at the Newcastle BAAS Meeting of 1916, the last one convened before the war intervened.

They listened carefully, side by side, to what he had to say. Some of Parsons' militarism seems rather depressing to modern ears. Parsons reviewed the contribution of engineering and science to the recent war in a rather affirmative manner. Not surprisingly, he discussed his marine turbines that powered the new generation of battleships of which HMS Dreadnought was the first of the class and helped in the arms race that lead up to the Great War. Parsons declared the British Navy has led the world for a century and more. Lord Fisher had recently said 'many of the ships are already obsolete and must soon be replaced if supremacy is to be maintained; and there can be no question that, to guide the advance and development on the best lines, continuous scientific experiment, though costly at the time, will prove the cheapest in the long run'. Charles Parsons was promoting the post-war continuation of the Department of Research, the committee he had led when it was formed in the first summer of the war, the committee onto which he had drafted Gerald as a consultant. He also emphasised the extraordinary growth in military aircraft, from 272 at the outbreak of war to over 22,000 at its close.

Florence was particularly taken with his enthusiasm for airships for transatlantic transport. At a time when aircraft were still small and limited in range, he foresaw an important future for 'special commerce where time is a dominant factor and the demand is sufficient'. She wrote to her engineer nephew Archie in Australia about it, describing the photographs she had seen of a forest in France where lanes in different directions had been cut so that the airships could settle whichever direction the wind was blowing [3].

Nevertheless, Sir Charles foresaw clouds on the horizon. 'The possibility of the uncontrolled use on the part of a nation of the Power which Science has placed within its reach is so great a menace to civilisation that the ardent wish of all reasonable people is to possess some radical means of prevention through the establishment of some form of wide and powerful control'. The particular example he had in his mind is included in a footnote: 'For instance, it might some day be discovered how to liberate instantaneously the energy in radium, and radium contains 2½ million times the energy of the same weight of TNT'. Scientific knowledge grew, uranium replacing radium as the focus for atomic energy research. The foundation of the League of Nations the following January was insufficient to control the development of atomic weapons, leading to the final, dreadful fulfilment of his prediction about a quarter of a century later, at Hiroshima.

Other talks were of interest to the sisters. On Friday, Sir Arthur Eddington (1882–1944), the Quaker scientist, described his observations of the solar total eclipse that took place on 29 May of that year, where the bending of the rays of light proved Einstein's theory of relativity. When Archie wrote for an explanation of this new physics of relativity, Florence replied that he would have to ask his Aunt Edith, who understood these things. On the same day, Sir Charles Bright spoke on the development of radio communication, stimulated in part by the severance of the transatlantic cable by German action during the war. The sisters had always enthusiastically grasped new technology, and they expected to 'live to see (1) an all-British wireless chain put into effect without much further delay (2) every inter-Imperial cable connection supplemented by wireless and (3) a highly-developed wireless news service' [4]. The first broadcasts commenced in 1922, and Edith soon had both a valve and a crystal set working. In Florence's 1928 Christmas letter to Australia, she wrote how they had listened to a concert broadcast from the Albert Hall, on Armistice Night, 'most clearly and vividly', and gained 'great enjoyment from the music and talks' [5]. No doubt they attended the economics section contribution on 'The replacement of men by women in industry'. The Bournemouth Workers' Educational Association organised a citizen's lecture on astronomy by Herbert H. Turner from Oxford. He used lantern slides to illustrate the development of modern telescopes from Lord Rosse's Leviathan to the 100 inch telescope recently erected on Mount Wilson in California.

Votes for Women

A notable milestone had occurred before the end of the war. The electoral roll for October 1918, for 20 Reynolds Close in the Garden Suburb Ward of the Urban District of Hendon, listed for the first time the names of Edith Anne Stoney and Florence Ada Stoney as voters in national parliamentary elections. Florence was identified as an occupational voter, whilst Edith had the letters NM against her entry, meaning that she was still a naval or military voter. Their sister Gertrude, too, became a voter. After their father's death, she had purchased a flat in Kingsley Mansions, Queen's Club Gardens, West Kensington, and this ownership gave her the right to vote. The Victorian development of 33 blocks of well-appointed flats, where she had moved at the beginning of the war, was close to the famous Queen's Tennis Club and had its own tennis courts where the sisters could play when they had spare time.

The fight to achieve votes for women was partially won. In 1928 the government eventually passed the Representation of the People (Equal Franchise) Act, finally giving votes to all women over the age of 21 on equal terms with men. Nevertheless, the battle for equality remained, and, during the post-war period, both Edith and Florence remained actively committed to a range of issues to do with women's place and condition in society. Immediately after the end of the war, Florence contributed to a fund to press for Regulation 40D of the Defence of the Realm Act (DORA) to be revoked, and Florence is recorded as contributing one guinea [6]. This amendment, passed during the last year of the war, allowed the state to imprison a woman for the transmission of a venereal disease to an acting serviceman. The opposition to retaining it in force during peacetime was sufficiently robust that it was soon revoked.

Not all wartime advances for women were retained. By 1918, seven of the London medical schools had opened their doors to women in response to the wartime need for doctors. By 1919, these doors had largely been closed again, leaving only University College Hospital Medical School to maintain 12 places for women entrants each year, in addition to those women still being trained at the London School of Medicine for Women and the Royal Free Hospital.

Florence Moves to Bournemouth

Shortly after their visit to Bournemouth to attend the British Association meeting, Florence heard of the sudden death from pneumonia on 26 October of Frank Fowler M.D., a distinguished and well-respected Bournemouth radiologist with a national reputation, at the young age of 54. He ran a specialist radiology practice in the district of Westbourne and was medical officer in charge of the Electrical Department of the Royal Victoria and West Hants Hospital in Bournemouth (Fig. 16.3). Fowler had been elected to the Röntgen Society in 1900 and to the British Association of Radiology and Physiotherapy (BARP) in 1919, not long before his untimely death. He was an experienced radiotherapist and had spoken at the Electro-Therapeutical Section of the Royal Society of Medicine in 1911 and at the Annual Meeting of the British Medical Association held at Liverpool in 1912.

Fowler's death gave Florence the opportunity to leave London, where she was finding that her health was too shaken for her to continue her medical practice. Bournemouth was described by Barraclough in *The Book of Bournemouth* [7] as 'a mild, sheltered resort for all seasons; the invalid's winter resort and the holiday health resort in summer' and as such was an ideal place for her to live and work. The many medical indications and health benefits from residence had been recommended

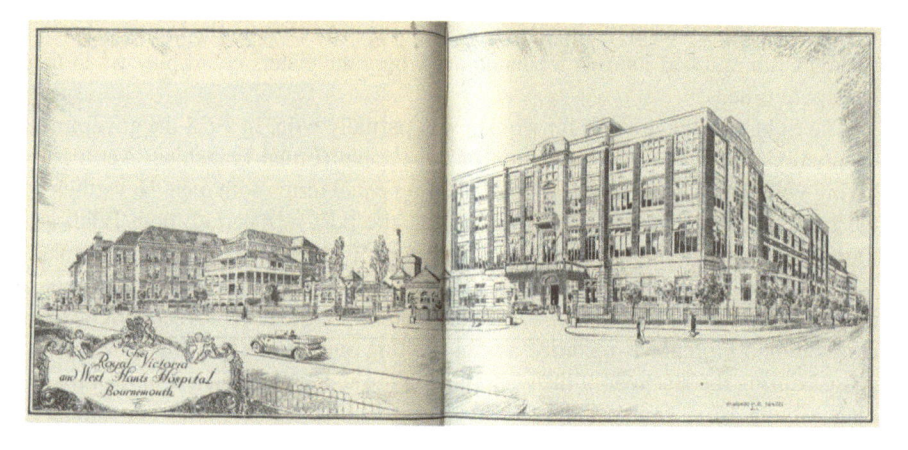

Fig. 16.3 The Royal Victoria and West Hants Hospital. (From Watson Smith S (Ed) The Book of Bournemouth 1934. Bournemouth: Pardy & Sons)

since the early nineteenth century [8]. Fowler was widowed by the time of his death, so Florence was able to lease his house and take over his practice at Ardvoulan, 29 Poole Road [9]. The district of Westbourne where Florence now lived and worked was affluent and mainly devoted to suburban residences and shops.[1]

Just before she moved to Bournemouth, from 6 January to 7 February 1920, Florence exhibited photographic examples of her radiographic work at the Royal Photographic Society. The photographs were shown by members of the Röntgen Society, and it was said that nearly 200 prints were 'tastefully hung' in the meeting room of the Royal Photographic Society in South Audley Street, London. The exhibition was popular with the public and was well reviewed in the press. It showed both contemporary and historical images and displayed the first radiograph taken in Britain by Alan A. Campbell-Swinton on 13 January 1896. This image was published in the *British Medical Journal* of 25 January 1896 [10]. Florence displayed six radiographs, which illustrated a congenital shoulder abnormality, old disease of the hip, a case of acromegaly, a wired knee cap fracture, a kyphosis of the spine and finally a plated forearm fracture. Florence therefore showed a mixture of common and less common abnormalities.

Florence took Fowler's place as the Honorary Medical Officer, and then Honorary Physician, to the X-ray and Electro-Therapeutic Department of the two, merged, local hospitals. In the Boscombe district, there was the Royal Boscombe Hospital, which had opened in 1877, and the Royal Victoria Hospital was in the Westbourne district [11]. The Royal Victoria Hospital was opened in 1890 and was in 17 Poole Road, close to where Florence was to have her house and practice. It was a voluntary hospital, and the building costs were met by public subscription. These two hospitals merged in 1911 as the Royal Victoria and West Hants Hospital, or it was simply known as the Royal Victoria Hospital. It was just 30 years old when Florence was appointed to the medical staff and was described as comprising all that is newest and best in hospital planning and construction. The hospital looked after all types of patients apart from those suffering from infectious diseases or with acute psychiatric disorders.

Florence also worked at the Victoria Home for Crippled Children in Bournemouth where she was Honorary Consultant in Actinotherapy.[2] The Victoria Home was located in Burnaby Road, Alum Chine, and had been opened in 1898. It was a branch of the Shaftesbury Society and Ragged School Union and cared for 73 crippled children (now called children with special needs) aged from 2 to 10 years. The children suffered from various paralyses, and also diseases of the bones and joints, rickets and various deformities, and were admitted for long periods of time varying from 3 to 12 months. They were given electrical, sunlight and massage treatments.

---

[1]The most famous resident of Westbourne was the author Robert Louis Stevenson (1850–1894), who wrote *Kidnapped* and *The Strange Case of Dr. Jekyll and Mr. Hyde* whilst living there.

[2]Actinotherapy: the use of chemically active (actinic) radiation for treatment. The term included ultraviolet radiation therapy but could also refer to light therapy and even the use of soft X-rays for skin radiotherapy.

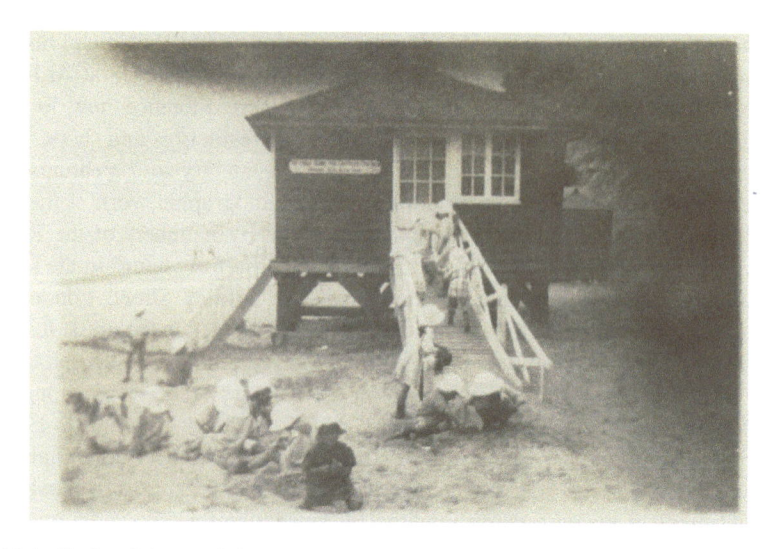

Fig. 16.4 The beach house of the Victoria Home for Crippled Children in Bournemouth at Alum Chine in 1927. (Unidentified photographer. Original photograph in author's archives)

Florence was ideally placed for this position and was able to obtain an ultraviolet unit for use at the home. It was said of her that she was 'a great believer in sunshine and scant clothing for children' [12]. Bournemouth was an ideal location for the home with its mild climate and local parks. The home had a permanent beach hut, and the children could enjoy the sea, sand and most of all sunshine and fresh air (Fig. 16.4). Actinotherapy was very popular in the 1920s, and many types of apparatus were produced. Treatments were recommended for tuberculosis, rickets and nutritional disorders and a variety of medical conditions [13] (Fig. 16.5).

Florence continued to be active in both local and national meetings, as well as in clinical work. Bournemouth was active in education and culture, with many museums, art galleries, clubs and societies, and this would have attracted the sisters [14]. Florence joined the Bournemouth Natural Science Society (BNSS) as soon as she moved to Bournemouth and was elected as a member in 1920. The society had been founded in 1903 and was flourishing. In February 1920 the society opened its own house at 39 Christchurch Road and offered its members lectures, field meetings and the reading and discussion of papers and had sections reflecting different areas of science. Although there is no record of either of the Stoney sisters presenting a talk, the programme would have attracted Florence's enquiring mind. The BNSS remains active today.

Florence remained an active participant with medical meetings in London and elsewhere. The Clinical Section of the Royal Society of Medicine (RSM) met on 11 February 1921 jointly with the Sections of Medicine and Surgery in a meeting on

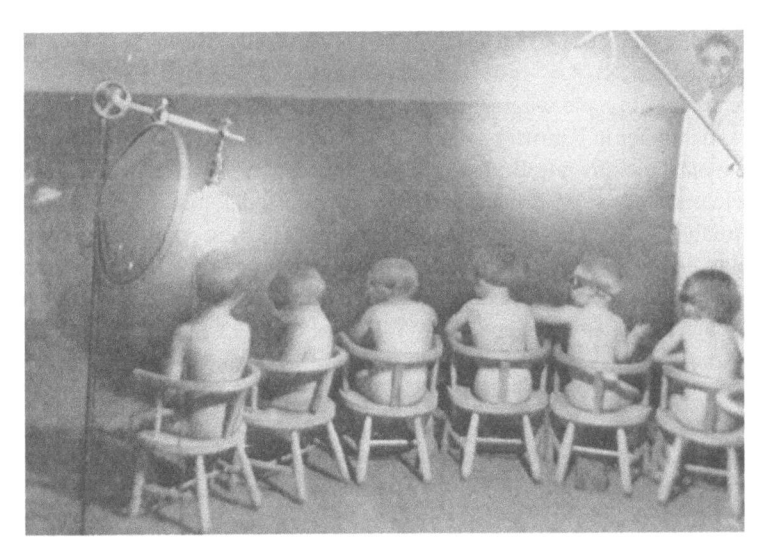

Fig. 16.5 Children being irradiated in an East London Clinic with a 'KBB' mercury-vapour lamp. (From Russell EH, Russell W Kerr. (1927) Ultra-Violet Radiation and Actinotherapy. Edinburgh: E&S Livingstone)

the medical and surgical treatment of Graves' disease.[3] Florence had been interested in treating Graves' disease since 1908 and by the meeting had seen 200 patients, all of whom were tabulated [15]. At this time there were various theories for the cause of Graves' disease, including the presence of bacterial toxins and intestinal stasis. It would not be until 1956 that Adam and Purves showed the presence of a thyroid-stimulating immunoglobulin in the patients that has a similar effect to the thyroid-stimulating hormone [16]. The medical treatment of the period involved rest and mental quietude, the removal of sources of infection such as pyorrhoea (dental sepsis) and the treatment of intestinal stasis.[4] Florence thought that the disadvantages of radiation were the length of time needed for treatment and the production of telangiectasia (prominent blood vessels) in the overlying skin and in scarring.[5] The induction of delayed malignancy had not then been appreciated. In the general discussion, Florence was commended for her work, and the relative merits and complications of medical, surgical and X-ray treatments were discussed. The overall conclusion was that 'that the outlook for patients with exophthalmic goitre was very much better now than at any other time'. The distinguished Manchester radiologist Alfred Barclay (1876–1949) noted that Florence's results were comparable to his own and to a further group of patients treated with X-rays and radium [17]. In

---

[3] Graves' disease is a common cause of an overactive thyroid gland and is often accompanied by bulging of the eyes, hence its alternative name of exophthalmic goitre.

[4] Pyorrhoea otherwise known as periodontitis is chronic dental infection. There was much interest at this time in chronic infections as the cause on many diseases.

[5] Radiotherapy may result in chronic inflammation with abnormal blood vessels and fibrosis.

reviewing the subject in 1937, Poulton and Watt were still speaking favourably of Florence's work [18].

Florence had to have what she described as 'a sudden bad operation in January (1922) and another in February'. The cause of Florence's surgery is unknown. Edith took time off to go down to Bournemouth to care for her. Her recovery was slow. By April, Florence was still off work and was being nursed at home. Having helped her sister through the first part of her convalescence, Edith went down with another chest complaint and went to the South of France for a rest.

By 12 February 1923 Florence was well enough to attend the London Association of the Medical Women's Federation (MWF). The MWF developed from the ARMW and its Articles of Association had been signed in 1917, and by 1925 there were over 1000 members. The London meeting would have been of great interest to Florence since a paper was read by Louisa Martindale on 'Modern Technique in the X-ray Treatment of Gynaecological Conditions'. Martindale spoke as President of the MWF. Florence contributed to the discussion that took place following the presentation.

The British Medical Association

Florence was an active member of the British Medical Association (BMA) throughout her career, and she continued to attend both national and local meetings. When she moved to Bournemouth, she joined the Bournemouth Division of the Dorset and West Hants Branch of the BMA and immediately took part in the activities of the division, attending her first meeting on 19 May 1920. The meetings were commonly held at St. Peter's Hall and at the Royal Bath Hotel in Bournemouth. On several occasions the minutes record Florence taking part in discussions, including the meeting on 10 October 1923 when Dr. F. H. Rodier Heath, the radiologist from Weymouth and District Hospital, gave a paper on 'X-ray Work in General Practice'. Florence herself gave a paper on 21 October 1925 on 'Ionisation with Reference to Septic Wounds', and it is recorded that afterwards 'a vote of thanks was passed for a most interesting and instructive paper'. Florence continued to attend meetings after her retirement and is last recorded being present on 1 October 1930 [19].

In 1920 Florence attended the 88th National Annual Meeting of the BMA, which was held in Cambridge from 30 June to 2 July. She took part in the Section of Electrotherapeutics and presented three radiographs illustrating tumours in the chest in the discussion of the paper presented by Robert Knox (1868–1928) on the diagnosis of lung tumours at the Cancer Hospital [20]. Knox was recommending for lung tumours the use of 'radioscopy (fluoroscopy) as a preliminary investigation' and that 'the patient should be screened in as many positions as possible' even though, by this date, it was well understood that fluoroscopy could contribute significantly to operator exposure and wartime experience had led to major concerns about radiation injuries.

Florence also attended the combined meeting of the Sections of Obstetrics and Gynaecology and Electro-Therapeutics on the treatment of uterine fibroids by radiotherapy. Lectures were given by Robert Knox at King's College Hospital and Louisa Martindale from Brighton. Florence had described her fourth patient that she had treated in the BMJ in 1917 and now presented details of eight cases [21]. She described the technique and the safety of the procedure. The patient had an induced menopause, and the uterus was reduced in size, avoiding the need for surgery. At this time the associated risk of inducing malignancy was not fully appreciated. The use of radiology for non-surgical treatment of fibroids continues today with the development of techniques such as image-guided focused ultrasound surgery and therapeutic uterine artery embolisation.

In 1923 the 91st Annual Meeting of BMA was held in Portsmouth, and Florence attended the Section on Radiology and Electrology. A session on diathermy included a long presentation by Francis Howard Humphris (1866–1947) who was a recognised expert on light or heliotherapy. Florence commented on the use of diathermy in chilblains and on the use of ultraviolet light to obviate the use of surgery in infections of the tonsils. The 93rd Annual Meeting in 1925 was in Bath, where Florence gave enthusiastic support to Dr. Eleanor Bond, who had just been elected as the first woman president of the Dorset and West Hants branch of the BMA [22].

Even in the year before her death Florence was writing to others proposing a physical medicine group within the BMA. The group, which included Florence, were practitioners of electro-therapeutics and physio-therapeutics and believed that the growing numbers of practitioners were not represented fully by their branches and divisions of the BMA. Many of the co-signatories of the letter were well known in the field of radiology.

When the division met on 14 October 1932, following Florence's death, the chair was taken by the Bournemouth physician Sydney Watson Smith (1882–1950) who referred to the loss, which the division had sustained through her death, and to all the work that she had done. It is poignant that the Annual Meeting in 1934 was held in Bournemouth with Watson Smith as BMA President and that Florence would not be attending.

The Wessex Branch of the British Institute of Radiology

The British Association of Radiology and Physiotherapy (BARP) was formed in April 1917 by a group of radiologists in London as a purely medical body unlike its successor, the multidisciplinary British Institute of Radiology. There was a concern that many who were in charge of radiology departments outside of the teaching hospitals were untrained in image interpretation although they were able to take good radiographs, and the aims were 'to promote the advancement of Radiology and Physiotherapy on scientific lines under the direct control of the medical profession'. Both Florence and Edith were elected to the BARP in 1919, and Florence is recorded as making a donation of five guineas to cover the initial expenses of the society. Although the BARP was only for clinicians it was possible for the council to elect scientists to both honorary and ordinary membership, and it would be on this basis that Edith was elected. Such non-medical members were in a very small minority, however. The only other physicist was the pacifist hospital physicist from the Middlesex Hospital, Dr. Sidney Russ, who was also on the council.

Florence was instrumental in setting up the Wessex Branch of the BARP in Bournemouth, and the preliminary meeting of the branch was held at Florence's house at 29 Poole Road at her invitation on 22 May 1921. The first branch meeting was held on 26 June that year. Dr. Gerald Earl Thornton from Salisbury had convened the preliminary meeting and became the first secretary. The first President was Dr. Beverley Steeds-Bird from Southsea. Meeting about three times each year, the 100th meeting of the Wessex Branch in 1949 again met at 29 Poole Road, when Florence's contribution was remembered. This meeting welcomed three of the five founding branch members, and note was made of the death of Florence Stoney. Florence was elected President of the Wessex Branch of the BARP in December 1924 [23].

As yet there was no specific examination for radiology or electrotherapy. In 1917 the BARP approached both London and Cambridge universities for the support of a diploma course [24]. A positive response was obtained from the University of Cambridge, and in particular Ernest Rutherford (1831–1937), who was shortly to follow J. J. Thompson as the Cavendish Professor of Experimental Physics, was supportive. There was a concern that there will be only one diploma and not multiple ones from many universities. The Cambridge diploma, the Diploma in Medical Radiology and Electrology (DMRE), was approved in March 1919 with teaching in Cambridge, with additional teaching in London organised by the BARP. There was always a difficulty in providing adequate practical and clinical experience for the increasing numbers of candidates. It is noteworthy that the DMRE treated X-rays work and electrotherapy as one profession. This was not to continue, and the two disciplines were to separate as the years progressed. For the first 5 years, the diploma was awarded to establish radiologists on the presentation of a thesis, and therefore in 1920 Florence was awarded the Cambridge DMRE honoris causa.

There had been a concern for some time about forming a proper institute for radiology with library and research facilities [25]. The object of the institute would be to 'house, co-ordinate, and to extend the work of, existing radiological societies', and its foundation was also intended to be a memorial to the radiation pioneers and martyrs. The British Institute of Radiology was therefore incorporated in 1924 with the alteration of title from BARP. Florence was actively involved in the new BIR from its inception and was one of 27 ordinary members of council in the 1924–1925 session, being a member in her own right and not as a representative of the Wessex branch even though she had just been elected president [26]. There were two female council members, the other being the remarkable Justina Wilson DMRE (d1950) [27]. Justina Wilson was interested in physical medicine and physiotherapy and had set up 'The Swedish Institute' in Cromwell Road to teach physiotherapy. She was

Physician in Charge of Electro-therapeutic Department at St. Mary's Hospital in London and, like Florence, practiced actinotherapy.

The new BIR arranged teaching for the new DMRE and also the certificate for the members of the recently formed Society of Radiographers (MSR). The BIR also organised the First International Congress of Radiology which took place in London at the Central Hall in Westminster from 1 to 4 July 1925 under the presidency of the great Liverpool pioneer Charles Thurstan Holland (1863–1941). Florence attended this congress as a nonspeaking delegate. Considerate as ever for Gertrude, she invited her sister to accompany her as her partner to one of the conference garden parties, which was held in the suburban outskirts of London in Esher [28].

The Wessex Branch of the BARP, which Florence helped to form, continues to be active today as the Wessex Branch of the BIR, although now meeting in Southampton.

Edith Returns to Education

When Florence left for Bournemouth in 1920, Edith stayed in Hampstead. She had returned home in February 1919 with little idea what to do next. By now Gerald had become Chair of Mechanical Engineering in the College of Technology at Manchester, a post he took up in 1917. His wife Isabella was chronically ill and remained in their house in Newcastle, whilst he spent his termtimes in Manchester, devoting most evenings to teaching engineering skills to adult evening classes. Whilst Florence was still engaged with her medical practice in London, she was planning to leave. Edith knew that her own experience in military radiography would not allow her to pursue a civilian career in radiology and that her BARP membership was not a licence to practice. Her other career, as a teacher and educator, remained a real option. She could not afford to retire without a pension.

Undaunted by her pre-war dismissal from the LSMW, Edith soon secured a lecturing post in physics in the Household and Social Science Department at King's College for Women in London, her satisfaction a little diminished by being unable, any longer, to share her news with her father. She took up her post in September 1919. The dean who appointed Edith was Dr. Janet Lane-Claypon, a graduate from the LSMW. In 1912 she had carried out a study which showed that babies fed on breast milk gained weight more rapidly than those fed on cow's milk, using modern epidemiological methods of cohort design and statistical analysis. She went on to develop a case-control study of 500 patients with breast cancer, concluding that cancer risk increased for childless women, women who married later and women who did not breast feed.

King's College for Women had been separately incorporated from its parent college into the University of London in 1908, and the course in the Household and Social Science Department had been set up in 1912. Many senior academic women were deeply sceptical of this plan to elevate women's work in the home to the level of intellectual recognition. Before the war, at Edith's first BFUW Executive meeting as treasurer, she had heard Lane-Claypon's predecessor Hilda Oakeley's views when she took part in a discussion of the matter. No matter how much one argued that an intelligent woman working in the home needed to reach a high degree of understanding of physiology, hygiene, physics and so on, cautious academics feared for the integrity of their positions especially in the eyes of their male peers. Viewing events in London from the intellectual heights of Cambridge, Ida Freund, a chemist from Newnham College, was especially critical. She quoted Lord Rayleigh's doubts as to 'whether technical subjects (applied sciences?) should or should not be studied under the supervision and fostering care of Universities'. She expressed concern that the men who would have to take the decision on 'the *existence* of a *science* of the home (Freund's italics)' would be without the necessary scientific qualifications for testing the claim and would have to take on trust the word of women that it was true. More prosaically, she stated that the time assigned for the six basic sciences taught during the first 2 years of the course, chemistry, physics, biology, physiology, hygiene and economics 'must make it impossible to reach anything approaching academic standard'. This standard, in her eyes, was that which she had set during '25 years of experience of teaching chemistry to students preparing for the Cambridge Natural Science Tripos'. It was an argument between two educational aspirations, and neither would give ground [29].

Nevertheless, the King's experiment proved to be very popular and attracted embarrassingly large amounts of money. Bequests flowed in, and by 1912 over £100,000 had been raised. Shortly after Edith was appointed in 1919, Dr. Lane-Claypon wrote a short popular article of explanation about the course that Edith had joined [30]. She pointed out that whilst there were several technical colleges that offered training in the domestic arts, the University of London was the only university that recognised Household Science as a subject for higher education. She explained that 'the Senate have agreed to receive an application for the degree of B.Sc. to be awarded to successful students'. She described the purpose of the course 'designed to teach the student the science which lies behind the ordinary features of daily life'. Quite unlike the Cambridge women students of Edith's day, 'matrimony, sooner or later claims a great proportion of past students. Trained women as wives and mothers, daughters and sisters, are an urgent national need, and the Household and Social Science Department is taking an important share in supplying the demand'. These were pragmatic words, responding to the perceived needs to reconstruct a shattered social infrastructure, and the seismic demographic changes as soldiers returned from the war, to be absorbed into civilian employment.

The ensuing debate about the place of women and their educational needs in postwar Britain polarised opinion, the militant faction arguing that the jobs gained by women during the war should not be released without a fight. Edith's personal experience was exactly the opposite. The vacancy she filled had been occupied by a man, William Wilson, during the war, and it would have been doubly satisfying to have replaced him. She had been present at the executive meeting of the BFUW in February 1914 when it had been pointed out that all the head science posts in the Home Science Department of King's College for Women were then male, but a decision had been made at that time not to raise the matter officially. Now, by her own ability, she helped to change this. Wilson himself had strong credentials as an academic physicist, and the vacancy had been created by his appointment as Reader in the Physics Department at King's College. By working hard, Edith had built up the skills, competence and experience that enabled her to compete successfully for this academic vacancy. Of course she had selected an opportunity in a women's institution, increasing her chance of success, but that was only sensible. She would leave it to others, now, to fight in the male-dominated arenas and concentrate her efforts where there was a chance of winning. Her task was now to show her students what could be achieved through hard work and dedication.

King's College for Women was housed in a new building in Campden Hill Road, a stone's throw from Chepstow Crescent where the Stoneys had lived until their father's death. Edith was expected to give 90 h of lectures to her first year students, followed by 120 h of laboratories. Edith was familiar with the style and content of the course, because it was of a similar design to those that she had seen during her visit to colleges in the United States in 1907. She inherited a syllabus that was conventional and unimaginative, although the emphasis on electricity and magnetism linked physics into the home. A staff photograph shows her slightly detached, with a calm, kind, strong face (Fig. 16.6).

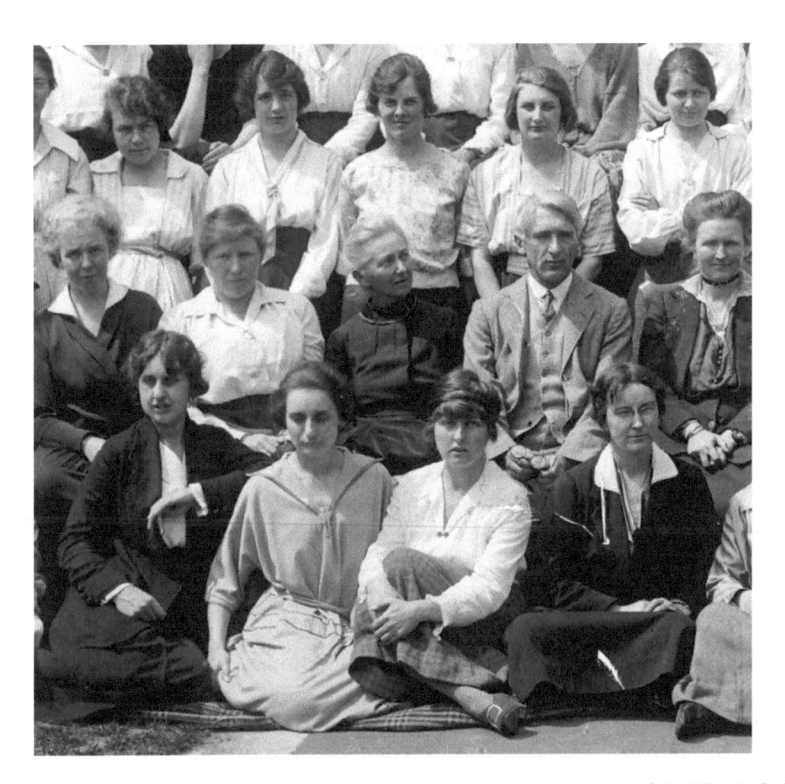

Fig. 16.6 Edith Stoney (second row, third from left) with staff and students of the King's College for Women, Household and Social Science Department c.1924. (King's College, London)

Edith was aware that, as a university lecturer, her publication record was thin. Her predecessor in this post, William Wilson, had continued to publish scientific papers in physics during the war, at a time when Edith was away in Salonika and France. He had worked on the photoelectric effect and the theoretical implications of relativity and quantum theory. She did not pretend to be in this league. Nevertheless, she was still motivated to contribute to the science literature and she returned to the work that had been stimulated by their visit to the cave in the Harz Mountains back in 1900. In the summer at the end of her first year at King's College, she developed her ideas about the way in which tiny hairs on the surface of lycopodium spores, barely seen at the highest magnification of Florence's microscope, alter their movement in air and inhibit Brownian motion. She concluded by noting the usefulness of a physical measurement to verify a difficult observation in botany, in this case the measurement of terminal velocity confirming the presence of these microscopic surface hairs [31].

Nevertheless, she had emerged from her war experience with a greater appreciation of the ignorance of many women about the developing world of technology in which they now lived. Matters of pure science may be fascinating, but her task now was to bring an appreciation of science to women who were working in the home. She developed this theme in a letter in which she extolled women to gain an understanding of the way in which modern domestic labour-saving devices worked. In doing so she aligned herself with several of her contemporaries, including Caroline Haslett, an engineer who was managing the newly formed Women's Engineering Society. Haslett saw 'a great opportunity for women to free themselves from the shackles of the past and enter into a new heritage made possible by the gifts of nature which Science had opened up to us' [32]. Edith encouraged the use of thermometry in the kitchen, to supplant the advice found in cookery books to 'see that your oven is hot enough, but not too hot'. She added other examples, including the operation of the pressure cooker, and the importance of knowing the boiling point of butter when cooking an omelette, to make her point [33].

Edith knew that some of her students wished to earn their own living when they graduated, so she set out some specific career advice. There were expanding opportunities, she believed, for women to act as laboratory assistants in schools, colleges and commercial laboratories, and, during her second year at King's, she wrote an article of explanation [34]. A survey she had carried out of some 400 science mistresses revealed that only about 10% had the help they needed in their laboratories. The introduction of experimental science into school and university curricula had brought with it the need to manage laboratories and workshops, and these required trained staff. During the war, she said, many 'lab boys' were replaced by girls, who had since successfully retained their positions. She included a list of skills, including typing and keeping accounts, soldering and brazing, glass blowing, cutting biological sections, caring for experimental animals, developing photographs, assisting with class demonstrations and lantern slides, being a fair carpenter and electrician and repairing scientific apparatus. She pointed out that women needed to continue to develop their technical and workshop skills, as men did, in order to justify continued employment. She estimated that a junior laboratory assistant might expect to start at about £1 per week and eventually earn £4–£6 a week or more. Edith urged those who had been employed in engineering works during the war to consider such a career. She used several personal examples in her article, including a remark that she had acted for many years as 'a sort of private part-time "laboratory boy"' for her father and a rather critical recollection of having to deal with ten untrained laboratory boys in 4 years when she was at the LSMW.

Women and Engineering

Edith published her article in *The Woman Engineer*, the journal of the Women's Engineering Society (WES). Edith was not alone in wishing to promote a continuing technical role for women in post-war Britain. So did Katherine Lady Parsons, Charles Parsons' wife. On Saturday, 15 February 1919, Katherine Parsons was present as the Women's Engineering Society was inaugurated at a meeting in London, the society that she had helped to form. The first president was Rachael, the Parsons' only daughter, who declared 'We do not wish to take men's work away but there are not enough skilled men to fill our factories, to carry on our industries, and stem the tide of foreign competition'. Rachael Parsons had been yet another successful student from Newnham, one of the first three women to study mechanical sciences at Cambridge. When her brother went to the front, only to be killed in action in France, Rachael took over his management of the Parsons' Heaton turbine factory. Katherine knew how women had taken on many engineering roles there during the war, where the proportion of women in her workforce had increased from 2% in 1914 to about 20% at the end of the war, a local growth that was broadly matched throughout the country. She was not thinking of the estimated 800,000 unskilled women who had filled the munitions factories; however important they had been to the war effort. The women employed at the Heaton works had been trained and skilled, evaluating alloys, testing model boats in their experimental tank and in checking electrical instruments. She knew that elsewhere women had undertaken a range of skilled workshop tasks including cutting crankshafts, forging, drilling and tool manufacture. There were an estimated 134,600 women working in general engineering works by the end of the war [35]. Katherine wrote that the investment in their training would be wasted if this work were to be unavailable after the war. 'It has been a strange perversion of women's sphere—to make them work at producing the implements of war and destruction and then to deny them the privilege of fashioning the munitions of peace. Women are merely told to go back to what they were doing before, regardless of the fact that they.... wish to have their economic independence, and freedom to make their way without any artificial restrictions' [36].

The WES had been set up as a reaction to the 'Restoration of Pre-war Practices Act' that had given legal force to the replacement of women by returning servicemen. Even those bastions of women's hard-earned freedom, the medical schools largely closed their doors to women. The King's College for Women course in home science accepted that many women would inevitably resume domestic lives and leave the world of paid work. The WES asserted that women should be trained and should take their place in the wider world of skilled employment, specifically in engineering. Edith saw both sides, believing in the worth of scientific knowledge in its own right whilst at the same time supporting the right of women to enter the skilled workplace as scientists and engineers.

References

1. The London Gazette. 1919 Feb 18. p. 2426.
2. Parsons CA. Address. British Association for the Advancement of Science. Bournemouth 1919. Science Museum Library PAR 92.
3. Florence Stoney to Archie Stoney. 21 Sept 1919. AS. Florence's letter does not mention Gerald, who presumably was unable to attend the Bournemouth meeting with his sisters.
4. All Red Wireless. Bournemouth Daily Echo. 1919 Sep 12.
5. Florence Stoney to Isobel Stoney. 1928 Nov 21. AS.
6. D.O.R.A. 40D Protest Fund. The Common Cause. 1918 Dec; 6.
7. Barraclough A. Geographical aspects of the Bournemouth area. In: Watson Smith S, editor. The book of Bournemouth. Bournemouth: Pardy & Sons; 1934.
8. Gordon SH. Bournemouth: the health resort. In: Watson Smith S, editor. The book of Bournemouth. Bournemouth: Pardy & Sons; 1934.
9. Sidney J. Mate's directory of Bournemouth, from 1921 to 1932.
10. A new kind of radiation. Br Med J. 1896;1:238.
11. Watson SS. The hospitals and benevolent institutions. In: Watson Smith S, editor. The book of Bournemouth. Bournemouth: Pardy & Sons; 1934.
12. Bournemouth Echo. 1932 Oct 12.
13. Russell EH, Russell W. Kerr. Ultra-violet radiation and actinotherapy. Edinburgh: E&S Livingstone; 1927.
14. Parry JE. Education and culture. In: Watson Smith S, editor. The book of Bournemouth. Pardy & Sons: Bournemouth; 1934.
15. Stoney FA. Discussion on the medical and surgical treatment of Graves Disease. Proc R Soc Med. 1921;1(14):18–61.
16. Adams DD, Purves HD. Abnormal responses in the assay of thyrotrophin. Proc Univ Otago Med Sch. 1956;34:11–2.
17. Barclay AE, Fellows FM. Hyperthyroidism treated by X-rays: a record of three hundred private cases. Br J Radiol. 1927:252–6.. BIR Section 32 (324)
18. Poulton EP, Watt WL. Treatment of exophthalmic goitre by deep x-rays. Proc R Soc Med Sect Ther Pharmacol. 1938;31:371–8.
19. Bournemouth Division of the Dorset and West Hants Branch. BMA Wessex branch Minutes and Papers 1906–1973. A400 Volume 5 Dorset and West Hampshire.
20. Knox R. X rays in the diagnosis of tumours of the thorax. Br Med J. 1920;ii:392–5.
21. Joint discussion of the treatment of uterine fibroids. Br Med J. 1929;ii:541.
22. Gertrude Stoney to Archie Stoney. 1925 July 25. AS.
23. Women in the Medical Profession. The Common Cause. 1925 Jan 2.
24. Barclay AE. The passing of the Cambridge diploma. Br J Radiol. 1942;15(180):351–4.
25. Thomas AMK, Jordan M. Radiological organisations in the United Kingdom. The invisible light. 100 Years of medical radiology. AMK Thomas, Isherwood I, Wells PNT. Blackwell Science. 1995. p. 101–4.
26. The Common Cause. 1925 Jan 2. p. 394.
27. ADW. Obituary Anna Justine Augusta Wilson. Br Med J. 1950;I:132.
28. Gertrude Stoney to Archie Stoney. 1925 Jul 25. AS.

29. Freund I. A degree standard in home science. The Common Cause. 1912 Feb 19. p. 195–7.
30. Lane-Claypon JE. The science of housewifery. The Graphic. 1919 Dec 20. p. 940.
31. Stoney EA. The carrying power of spores and plant-life in deep caves. Nature. 1920;105(2650):740–1.
32. Fara P. A lab of one's own. Oxford: Oxford University Press; 2018. p. 70.
33. Stoney EA. Labour-saving cooking. The Common Cause. 1923 Jul 20.
34. Stoney EA. Women laboratory assistants. Woman Engineer. 1922;1(2):165–7.
35. Pursell C. "Am I a lady or an engineer?" The origins of the women's engineering society in Britain. Technol Cult. 1993;34:78–97.
36. Parsons K. Women's work in engineering and shipbuilding during the war. Trans NE Coast Inst Engineers Shipbuilders. 1919;35:227–36.

Chapter 17
Family, Retirement and Travel

Life in Retirement

With the return of peace in Europe, family visitors arrived from Australia and from South Africa. But not everywhere was peaceful. Maurice and Anna FitzGerald, now frail and in their 70s, still living in Dublin, came to stay in June 1922. What they told Florence made her very concerned for their welfare. They were very doubtful that the Irish Free State, just established under the Anglo-Irish Treaty of December 1921, would end the violence in their country, and they were fearful for their future. Already the FitzGerald family home near Dublin had been broken into three times, and they were very frightened by these events. They brought news, too, that Classon's Bridge over the River Dodder had been blown up by the Irish Republican Army the previous year. This was where Edith and Florence had cycled as girls and where their father's funeral had passed only 10 years before. Its destruction was an act of symbolic, parochial vandalism rather than one of major strategic importance, there being several other bridges over the Dodder not far away, including the seventeenth-century packhorse bridge less than 5 minutes walk downstream. It was somehow characteristic of the protracted agony of the Irish conflict that it had taken 3 months of repeated explosions before the central span finally collapsed into the river. Florence persuaded Maurice that it would be wise to rent a house in Bournemouth for the following winter, for their peace and safety. Florence and Edith were very fond of their cousin Maurice. He reminded them of their brother Robert, and of their father.

Back in London, Gertrude made a point of keeping in touch with family and friends. She met George FitzGerald's youngest sons, John and George, when they visited London, both in training following war service. She popped over to meet her brother Gerald in the hotel where he was staying for a meeting of an International Electrotechnical Commission committee. A distant cousin arrived from America.

The emigration of aunts and cousins from Ireland continued. Their Aunt Constance, their mother's sister-in-law, had moved to Devon in 1917. Their Aunt

© Springer Nature Switzerland AG 2019
A. Thomas, F. Duck, *Edith and Florence Stoney, Sisters in Radiology*, Springer Biographies, https://doi.org/10.1007/978-3-030-16561-1_17

Frances, Bindon's widow, had left Dublin. She had spent some time with her married daughters overseas, Lilla in Cairo and Laura in Gibraltar, and was now living in a hotel in London, near Gertrude. During his visit to England, Uncle Robert, the Canon Stoney who had conducted their father's funeral, took Aunt Frances to stay with Florence in Bournemouth. Frances liked Bournemouth, and Florence eventually persuaded her to take a flat there, which she did in the summer of 1925. Mastrick Hall, a large mid-Victorian house in Branksome Park, had been divided into four flats, and Frances took number 2 on the second floor. She lived there until she died in February 1933, aged 77. Gertrude helped her to settle in and thought her old tall furniture suited the rooms well. But she was of the opinion that her daughter Anne, now divorced, should have helped by going to live with her. Nevertheless, she was pleased that her old Irish maid, 'rather a treasure', was there to look after her [1].

Gertrude was also pleased to make the acquaintance of Edith's eminent friends. In particular she met the botanist Edith Saunders, who was later described by J.B.S. Haldane as the mother of British plant genetics. Edith knew of Edith Saunders from Newnham, where she had been codirector of the Balfour Biological Laboratory for Women, a research facility staffed by Newnham and Girton students. Edith's study of the transport of lycopodium spores demonstrated her own interest in the overlap between the biological and physical sciences. Edith was also very pleased when Edith Saunders became the president of the botanical section of the British Association in 1920 having been a council member since 1914 [2].

Gertrude was in no financial position to ride out the post-war recession. Her finances were never as robust as those of her sisters. She never had a job and had financed her life largely through the support of her family. As she told Archie, there was not the remotest possibility of her affording the fare to visit them in Australia. Towards the end of 1922, she was obliged to downsize, leaving her flat in Kingsley Mansions and moving into a bedsit in a women's residential club. This club, at 30 Philbeach Gardens Earls Court, was run by the Ladies' National Clubs Ltd., an organisation that provided accommodation throughout London for educated women with limited means [3]. Putting a brave face on it, she described her new accommodation as 'one room of your *very* own and a dining hall in common which answers very well'. There were numerous such women's club houses, three in Philbeach Gardens alone, cheap, safe accommodation primarily intended for young independent women. The residents were referred to colloquially as 'latch-key ladies' [4]. A cheap, small room could be had for about 12s. 6d. a week, but the best could cost over £3. This included rates, electric light, baths, papers and box room space and, of course, the latch-key. The metered gas fire was extra. Meals could be taken in the dining room or served in the room. Guests could take meals, but there was an extra 6d. per meal if the guest was a man. When Gertrude wanted to meet a friend elsewhere, she could always go to the Halcyon Club in Cork Street, Mayfair, where she was a member at the preferential rate charged for Irish residents. Entertaining there, she could disguise her somewhat straightened circumstances. Luncheon for members cost 1s. 6d., and a three-course dinner could be had for 2s. 6d. [5]. But, as she pointed out to Archie, she could always spend the winter by the seaside with Florence.

Edith Retires

Edith was finding that her lectureship at King's College for Women was, to use Gertrude's phrase, 'knocking her up'. The stress was making her ill, and her absences from work were becoming a concern. By the beginning of 1924, she was obliged to withdraw from her lecturing post, and her position was taken by Miss T. J. Dillon, who remained until the 1950s. Soon afterwards, Edith suffered a major accident, which resulted in a badly broken leg. It was never set properly, and over the next few years she had to return to hospital on several occasions as attempts were made to correct the damage. The accident left her permanently lame, finally needing an orthopaedic boot to correct her gait. It was ironic that she had survived the war intact, only to be permanently disabled back home.

Gertrude continued to observe the world quietly from her latch-key room, surrounded by her furniture, paintings, sculptures, easel and paints from an earlier life, commenting on events as the world changed around her.[1] Like her brother Gerald, whose political view was 'Whichever party is in power I'm agin 'em'. Gertrude was not a particular fan of politicians, but took more notice now that she had the vote. Mr. Baldwin, she wrote, was 'a great muddler and has done a lot of harm and then there is Labour and that erratic Ramsey Macdonald'. Macdonald became the first British labour prime minister when he was appointed to lead the coalition government with the Liberals in January 1924. Gertrude remembered that she had met him when they had attended British Association meetings with their father [6, 7].

Florence was now 'full of energy' again, and she and Gertrude went away on holidays together, to Ireland and to Cornwall. After a whilst in a nursing home, Edith's leg was sufficiently mended for her to set off on a 2-month recuperation cruise to South Africa in December 1924. Soon after her return, however, she was back in hospital for more surgery.

With time on her hands, and retaining a wry sense of humour that was rarely evident, Edith wrote a letter to *The Times* newspaper:

> Sir—The great economic value of silk for electrical purposes is represented in your issue of today. But also the various cellulose fibres called artificial silk etc. have physical properties, which make materials made from them of special economic value. The smooth slipperiness of artificial silk materials makes them a cheap and healthy comfort as underclothing for far wider classes than can afford real silk.

She then added, remembering the mainly male readership 'Men are much more conservative than women in taking to new forms of dress, but time will persuade them too of this new benefit' [8].

They sold their house in Reynolds Close and Edith moved to join Florence in Bournemouth. Clearing out, she sent some scientific papers to Archie in Australia. Her father's papers from Queen's University went to Queen's College Belfast,

---

[1] 'She (Gertrude) always had watercolour painting equipment with her wherever she went'. A. J. Stoney interviewed by Edith McKinnon. Alex Stoney family archive.

where they remain to this day. In her letter to the vice-chancellor on 29 September 1926, she wrote:

> Last week I sent off the seals and minute books of Queen's University of Ireland.... I also sent some other materials, documents and books, which I thought you might like to have in your University Library should you not already have copies. Keep such as may be cared for; there is no need to return the others .... I have ventured to add a copy of the obituary notice of my father written by Prof. Joly, F.R.S., F.T.C.T. (1911) for the Royal Society in case there may be any wish to have one in the library.

She used polite, measured words, passing her father's memory into the care of another. The letter concludes:

> On behalf of my brother and sisters as well as myself, may I request you to convey to the Queen's University of Belfast our grateful appreciation that they are willing to accept these momentos, knowing that it would have been my father's wish that they should rest where the traditions of the old Queen's University are most nearly carried on.

His memory was being kept alive in Cambridge too. The following lines were published in the Cavendish Laboratory Supplement of Nature for a song entitled *The Jolly Electron*, sung to the tune of *The Jolly Miller*, at the Physical Society Club on 18 December 1926:

> There was a jolly electron—alternately bound and free –
>   Who toiled and spun from morn to night, no Snark as lithe as he;
>   And this the burden of his song for ever used to be
>   'I care for nobody, no not I, since nobody cares for me
>   Though Crookes at first suspected my presence on this earth,
>   'Twas J.J.Thompson found me—in spite of my tiny girth.
>   He measured first the "e by m" of my electric worth;
>   I love J.J. in a filial way, for he it was gave me birth!
>   'Twas Johnstone Stoney invented my new electric name,
>   Then Rutherford, and Bohr, too, and Moseley brought me fame;
>   They guessed (within the atom) my inner and outer game,
>   You'll all agree what they did for me, I'll do it for them, the same! [9]

The sisters were delighted to hear from Australia that Archie was to be married to Isabel Round. Soon, there was a new generation of the family. First Dorothy was born in April 1925, soon followed by two sisters and, at last, a boy, Alex, to maintain the family name. What was particularly pleasing was their choice of names. Their second great-niece was given the name Edith, and when a third daughter was born in July 1930, she was called Florence. Great Aunt Florence wrote from England on 7 October 1930 that she had put the name in her birthday book and that she felt 'quite proud at having a small namesake on the other side of the world to carry on the name of Florence Stoney into the next generation' [10].

Florence in Retirement

When Florence retired from her medical practice in 1927, the sisters left their home in Poole Road and moved to Heathercliffe, 12 Burnaby Road, a new house overlooking the sea at Alum Chine. Her practice was taken over by G. Lieba Buckley (1891–1956). Edith knew Lieba Buckley well from their time together in France. During the war, Buckley had shared her time between her medical studies at the LSMW and the X-ray department at Royaumont. When the radiographer Vera Collum was obliged to stop radiographic work as a result of radiation injury, it was Lieba Buckley who had taken over running the department at Royaumont until she too had to take time off. She returned to France in August 1918 and had worked with Edith until Royaumont closed as a hospital at the end of the year.

Florence and Edith made a visit to Ireland that summer. Civil war had erupted in 1922, as Maurice had feared, and had lasted 2 years. Eventually, following the election of 1927, some semblance of order had been restored. Westminster had yet to cede total authority to Ireland, but they still felt safe to travel. Florence described her trip in her Christmas letter to the Australian relatives, 'the country looking very lovely with the heather on all the hills, we went across to Kerry and Killarney, and over the places in Wicklow which we knew when we were children' [11]. They found that Classon's bridge had just been replaced with an ugly concrete structure enveloping the remains of the cobbled bridge of their youth, a sad indication of the profound changes being experienced in the country of their birth. When Florence went back with Gertrude a couple of years later, they limited their trip to the north.

More Distant Travel

The sisters had an adventurous streak and continued to combine this with their lively interest in the relationship between physics and medicine. Early in 1929 they set off together for a trip to India, following in the footsteps of a number of early graduates of the LSMW, where there had been an interest in women's health in India since the early days. For example, Mary Scharlieb had initially trained as a midwife in Madras. The first graduate from LSMW who went to India was Fanny Butler (1850–1889) who was a medical missionary [12]. There was a high death rate in India in childbirth, and Muslim and Hindu women were reluctant to see male doctors. A Medical Women for India Fund, Bombay, had been set up in 1882 with the aim of recruiting women doctors.

During their stay in Bombay, they were hosted at the annual dinner of the Bombay branch of the British Association of University Women by Dr. Margaret Balfour CBE, the President, who was on a return visit to the country to which she had devoted most of her life as a doctor. She had, that year, become a Fellow of the Royal College of Obstetrics and Gynaecology. They learned of her work with teenage pregnancies in Bombay, and of Dr. Kathleen Vaughan's work in Kashmir in which one in four deliveries were by Caesarean section, as a result of poor pelvic bone development. They returned to England in February 1929, sailing from Bombay on the SS Ranpura of the P&O Steamship Company, calling at Port Said, Aden, Malta and Marseilles, arriving in London on the 1 March. As they steamed through the Suez Canal on their way home, the boat illuminated its path using searchlights with focused beams that Edith had helped to design. It was rather pleasing that the reporter of *The Times of India* felt this worthy of note [13].

In January 1930 they were off on their travels once more, this time returning for a long trip to South Africa. They were away for 4 months, not arriving back in Southampton until the 10 May, sailing on the SS Balmoral Castle, stopping in Madeira on the way home. As always, their trips were part recreational and part serious. Whilst they were in Cape Town, they joined the audience of others in the women's movement for the visiting President of the Women's Freedom League, Mrs. Pethick-Lawrence, at her public meetings in support of establishing voting rights for women in South Africa. In May of that year, following an election pledge, white South African women were finally given the right to vote [14]. The different timings of women's suffrage in various countries in the Empire are interesting and curious. In 1893 New Zealand had enfranchised all women including Maoris, whereas in 1902 Australia had enfranchised only white women [15].

A *Cape Times* reporter took great interest in hearing Florence's views of the therapeutic uses of radium, following the launch of a local appeal by the Cape Hospital Board to set up a radium unit. Interviewed the day after she arrived in Cape Town, she was keen to stress that 'there must be special training quite beyond the usual medical training'. The appeal by the Cape Hospital Board, for £12,000 for 1 gramme of radium, matched the activity and cost of the radium available to the Marie Curie Hospital back in London.

The Marie Curie Hospital had been set up following a co-ordinated evaluation of the radium treatment of uterine cancer in three London Hospitals and the New Sussex Hospital in Brighton, under the lead of the Canadian gynaecologist Elizabeth Hurdon. The London hospitals were the South London Hospital for Women, the Elizabeth Garrett Anderson Hospital and the Royal Free Hospital, and the study were co-ordinated by the London Association of the Medical Women's Federation [16, 17]. By this time cancer treatment using radium was being carried out in London at all of these hospitals, using radium on loan from the British Empire Cancer Campaign and the King Edward's Hospital Fund. By the beginning of 1928 nearly 200 patients had been treated, and a decision was made to co-ordinate this fragmented service under one roof. The Marie Curie Hospital at 2 Fitzjohn's Avenue, Hampstead, fully staffed by women, had only just started taking patients when the sisters set off for their trip to South Africa, opening its first 25 beds on 16 September 1929 [18]. Several of the founders of this hospital were well known to Florence. For example, the surgeon Maud Chadburn had been an anaesthetist at the Royal Free Hospital and surgeon and senior obstetrician at the London Hospital for Women during Florence's association there. She took out an annual subscription of one guinea (£1.1s) to support it.

Florence was keen to point out to the reporter the importance of working as a team when treating cancer using radium. Her career as a radiologist, with Edith at her side to give technological and scientific guidance, had given her a profound sense of the importance of co-operative working in modern medicine. One commentary at the time used the following words to describe the working environment at the Marie Curie Hospital. 'It was essential to have a centre where radium treatment—the success of which depends on careful dosage and technique—could have the facilities of the co-ordination of the surgeon, physicist, radiologist, and pathologist' [19]. When Florence gave her opinion to the *Cape Times* reporter about radium treatment that 'there must be team work, otherwise a great deal of mischief can be done', she was expressing her very general understanding about the seismic changes that had occurred during her medical career and would continue to profoundly alter the practice of medicine. She had been trained at a time when the individual authority of a doctor or surgeon was absolute, when he was viewed as omniscient and omnipotent in all his medical decisions. She saw a future in which the doctor took her place at the interface with her patient, already supported and advised by specialist colleagues with skills and knowledge in biochemistry, physics, engineering and statistics. This co-operative working would eventually grow to include experts in cytogenetics, artificial intelligence, robotics, epidemiology and the raft of other sciences and technologies that comprise twenty-first-century medicine. It was a view that she could trace back to setting up the X-ray department at the Royal Free Hospital with her sister 30 years before, knowing that, however competent an individual doctor might become, she would be all the greater by working in a team with one or more experts with other skills, for the ultimate benefit of her patients [20].

Heliotherapy and Osteomalacia

Florence was an enthusiast for the therapeutic value of sunlight, even rigging up cubicles for heliotherapy in her own garden. By the 1920s a scientific rationale for the value of ultraviolet radiation in the treatment of bone disease, especially rickets, was developing. Vitamin D had been discovered in 1918, and by the end of the 1920s, the part played by ultraviolet light in its synthesis was understood. Florence spent some time investigating the causes and effects of osteomalacia (bone softening) during their visit to India in 1929, which she attributed to limited exposure to ultraviolet rays from the widespread custom of Purdah. She gave advice to various hospitals on the installation of ultraviolet light in hospitals for the treatment of rickets, osteomalacia 'and other diseases of darkness.'

During the sisters' visits to Cape Town in 1930, Florence gathered enough further data on which to base her last published paper, on "The Pelvis and Maternal Mortality" presented in March 1930 to the BIR [21]. This paper described pelvic deformities and showed historical specimens, using cases from her observations in Africa and India and also locally in Bournemouth. Florence emphasised the desirable rounded or gynaecoid shape of the normal female pelvis and observed that the oval pelvic shape, more typical of European races, could cause difficulties in childbirth. She associated the rounded pelvic shape with races who 'had *plenty* of ultra-violet light (vitamin D)', an assertion at the cutting edge of understanding at that time. The value of this paper was soon recognised and was emphasised by Noel Hypher in 1931 [22].

One patient she looked after was a 32-year-old married but never pregnant woman in Bournemouth who was poor and spent her life as caretaker in empty houses. She seldom went out into the daylight before she was bedridden, so that even her face and hands received no sunlight, so she was entirely dependent on dietary vitamin D. She attended the hospital by ambulance for 9 months before a skiagraph (radiograph) was taken which led to correct diagnosis (of osteomalacia). She had the four typical fractures through the obturator foramina, with tri-radiate beaked pelvis. Also the neck of each femur had fractured. She was treated with ultraviolet light for 12 months, and she recovered her power of walking, and the six fractures had all firmly united.

In this paper written towards the end of her career, we can feel Florence's concern for the health of mothers and young girls. It was known that lack of vitamin D produced decalcification of the bones and that lack of sunlight results in overactivity of the parathyroid glands. This results in deformity of the pelvis and the presence of rickets in children and osteomalacia in adults, and both will deform the shape of the pelvis. Florence emphasised the need for sunlight and good bone health in growing girls, and this is as important today as it was in Florence's time. She finishes by saying 'Maternal mortality in this country is partly due to want of sunlight on the whole skin surface (or its equivalent in other forms of vitamin D.)' and exclaims 'If preventable—why not prevented?'

Towards the end of 1930, the Electro-Therapeutic Section of the RSM had a discussion on the uses of diathermy, and Florence mentioned her patient who had six pelvic fractures caused by osteomalacia. Florence initially treated her with diathermy for 9 months with no success, and therefore the treatment was changed to ultraviolet light, and after 12 months the patient, who had previously had to be carried, was able to walk to the hospital for further treatments, and 'When she (Dr. Stoney) last saw her she was engaged in scrubbing floors.' The accepted rationale for the use of diathermy using high-frequency electric fields was to stimulate healing perhaps by deep heating. The ultraviolet light would stimulate the formation of vitamin D.

Healthy childbirth was a concern for both Florence and Edith. They were interested in what the Bishop of Birmingham said in his Lloyd Roberts Lecture of 1930 where he 'pleaded for further research into feeblemindedness' or learning difficulties as we would say today. In response, they wrote a letter to The Woman's Leader in *The Common Cause* [23] in which they emphasised the need for sunlight, calcium and vitamin D to promote healthy childbirth. They were particularly concerned with fashions in women's clothing in both India and England that covered the skin and restricted exposure to sunlight arguing that the resulting pelvic deformities could result in difficulties in labour and injuries in childbirth, with potential consequences for the subsequent mental development of the newborn child.

Edith and Women's Issues

Following her retirement, Edith renewed her concern with promoting the rights of women. In a letter to *The Vote* she drew attention to a report in *The British Worker* in which a magistrate had referred to the right of every Briton to work. She pointed out that this should equally apply to married women workers and be directed 'towards any other restrictions against women as women' [24].

She continued to promote the cause of women in the workplace, attending the 1930 meeting of the National Council of Women in Portsmouth as a delegate of the British Federation of University Women. Edith had been unable to drive after her leg was damaged, but by now she was sufficiently recovered to take their 'little car' for the 50-mile drive to the conference. Florence accompanied her on the drive along the south coast from Bournemouth. As she told Archie in her Christmas letter, she was concerned that Edith was now dependant on the car to get about, but that her crippled leg limited how far they could go. Florence thought that perhaps it was time for her to learn to drive. The only other member of their household was no good at driving. This was their young cousin, Audrey Brew, Uncle Hugh's daughter, who was living with them and helping with the cooking.

Perhaps stimulated by discussions in Portsmouth, Edith went back to the issue that had been central to the purpose of the Household and Social Science degree, the education of women in the science and technology of the domestic workplace. She wrote an informative popular article on the impact that electric devices were having in the home [25]. She starts with a social comment: 'The "Domestic Problem" means that many small middle-class households must now manage without a maid, or with one who is young and untrained'. Much domestic drudgery is now in the past: 'Lamps needing cleaning have gone, and coal ranges with their daily lighting and weekly cleaning are obsolete'. On the other hand, 'girls of classes likely to become maids are now given some education in the elements of physics and chemistry, and other women (including those of University education) have to see to their own household work'. With Gertrude in mind, too, she added 'Life in a flatlet can be made immeasurably better through the facilities afforded by gas and electricity' and, recognising the only-too-real experience of many young women at the time, 'Still more grateful is their help to a so-called 'working woman' with small children'. Using her own life as a yardstick, and recognising that the readership of *The Woman Engineer* would understand, she wrote that 'We all know much more about mechanics now; the use of wireless, bicycles and cars secures this'.

The main theme of Edith's article was that all modern electrically heated domestic appliances, such as cookers, irons and domestic water heaters, should be fitted with a calibrated thermostat and a thermometer as means to control the temperature. Her concern was that these controls, which were found on high-specification and expensive cookers, were rarely included on moderately priced ovens. She included other necessary requirements: a heatproof glass door, a light with an external switch, an internal windscreen wiper to clear condensation, and more than one thermometer to show the temperature at different levels in the oven. She expressed the opinion that chefs using large expensive ovens, such as those installed in a castle or hotel, whose apprenticeship allows the temperature to be judged by hand and eye, needed the assistance of technology less than the novice but technically educated housewife or maid in the kitchen of her cottage or flat with its smaller, cheaper cooker. In a way, she was only making a comment on changing times and encouraging her readers to adapt their lives for the better. Commercial interests could be relied on to introduce these innovations to a wider market once any fear of change had passed. Even in her 60s, Edith continued to embrace each new technology as it emerged and encouraged other women to do so as well.

The British Association meetings remained of interest. The 1931 meeting in London was particularly important since it marked the centenary of the founding of the Association. Edith bought a copy of commemorative edition of the 'The Retrospect' only to be disappointed to find no reference to the contributions that her father had made over so many years. At least Charles Parsons' bequest that helped defray the costs of publication was noted with thanks. Edith eventually donated her copy to the British Federation of University Women [26].

The Death of Florence

During the sisters' visit to South Africa, the reporter from the *Cape Times* noticed in passing that Florence was still suffering from the effects of her early work with X-rays. This visit was 2 years after she had fully retired from radiological practice, and her hands were still carrying visible signs of previous radiation exposure.

Florence was being treated in Bournemouth by Sydney Watson Smith (d1950), who was an honorary consulting physician and dermatologist to the Royal Victoria and West Hampshire Hospital. His name is preserved in the funded Sydney Watson Smith Lecture of the Royal College of Physicians Edinburgh. He was chairman of the Bournemouth Division of the BMA and wrote of her saying 'It is now notorious that those pioneers in X-ray work and those exposed unduly to unprotected rays usually die very painful deaths, and Dr. Stoney was no exception: she suffered greatly and bravely, and she knew quite well what would be the manner of her death' [27]. Florence had met and knew many of the radiology pioneers, and knew fully well what fates they had succumbed to, and that she would most probably die herself from cancer. In 1921 there was a very well-publicised death of the young London radiologist William Ironside Bruce (1879–1921) [28]. Bruce's name is one of the initial 14 British names on the Radiation Martyr's Memorial that was erected in the grounds of St. Georges Hospital in Hamburg in 1936. It was following the shock of Bruce's death, and the resulting public outcry, that issues of radiation protection were finally taken seriously. A letter from Robert Knox appeared in *The Times* of 29 March 1921 with the purpose of reassuring the public. The radiology community was small, and Knox would have known all of the radiation martyrs individually. The Röntgen Society had published its first British code of practice in 1915, and this was to be implemented, and there was to be a new standing committee of recognised experts. This committee, the British X-Ray and Radium Protection Committee, was set up that year, lasting in that form until 1952 and giving excellent service over 31 years. That Florence suffered from the adverse effects of radiation is to be expected for someone practicing radiology when she did; however, that she lived as long as she did is a testimony to her care in giving treatments and examinations.

Unfortunately Florence developed cancer of the spine. Modern cancer therapy was still in its early days, and radium or deep X-ray therapy was not introduced into Bournemouth until 1937. Florence was moved back to London for treatment, which was at the Cancer Hospital in Fulham Road.[2] She died there on 7 October 1932 at the age of 63. She had lived in Bournemouth for 12 years. The cause of Florence's death was given on her death certificate as being the result of a fibrosarcoma growing from the transverse process of the seventh cervical vertebra. She had no post mortem, and therefore the diagnosis will have been made from a surgical biopsy. Although Florence suffered from the effects of a chronic radiation exposure, there is no direct evidence that her death was caused by radiation, and so her name is not included as one of the radiation martyrs on the memorial in Hamburg. Her occupation is recorded on the death certificate as 'Physician. Daughter of George Johnstone Stoney DSc FRS (Deceased)' reflecting the very high esteem in which both sisters held their father's memory. No record of Florence's burial or cremation has been found.

Florence was deeply mourned by her large circle of friends and colleagues, and many obituaries appeared in professional journals and newspapers both at home and abroad, including *The Times* [29], *The British Journal of Radiology* [30] and *The Bournemouth Daily Echo* [31]. Helen Chambers, the pathologist at the Marie Curie Hospital, remarked that she was blessed with exceptional ability and intellect. Agnes Savill wrote of her 'knowledge of suffering humanity, wide sympathy, and rare gift of whimsical humour in conversation'. She added that 'Her charming and welcome smile, her eyes with the bright twinkle behind the glasses, her amusing and entertaining comments—at radiological gatherings we shall all miss that quiet pioneer, that little figure with a great heart'. Mabel Ramsay, a physician who had accompanied her to Antwerp, remembered her to be 'British to the core, she will yet always remain in my memory as a very courteous and kindly Irish lady' [32]. *The Times* obituary remarked on her health, 'good though never robust... she accomplished much by steady application and conserving her strength'. Of her personality: 'She had a good deal of quiet humour. She had gentle kindliness and rich sympathy for suffering, and showed courage in her last, long and painful illness'.

At probate her estate was valued at £10,505 19s. 5d. In her will, she made provision for Gertrude, leaving her £1500 in bonds and shares, presumably trusting that the interest would enable her to continue an independent life. She also made bequests to her Australian nephews and niece and left £10 to her cousin Dora Stoney,

---

[2]The Cancer Hospital was founded as the Free Cancer Hospital in 1851 by the surgeon William Marsden who had also founded the Royal Free Hospital in 1828. It later became the Royal Marsden Hospital.

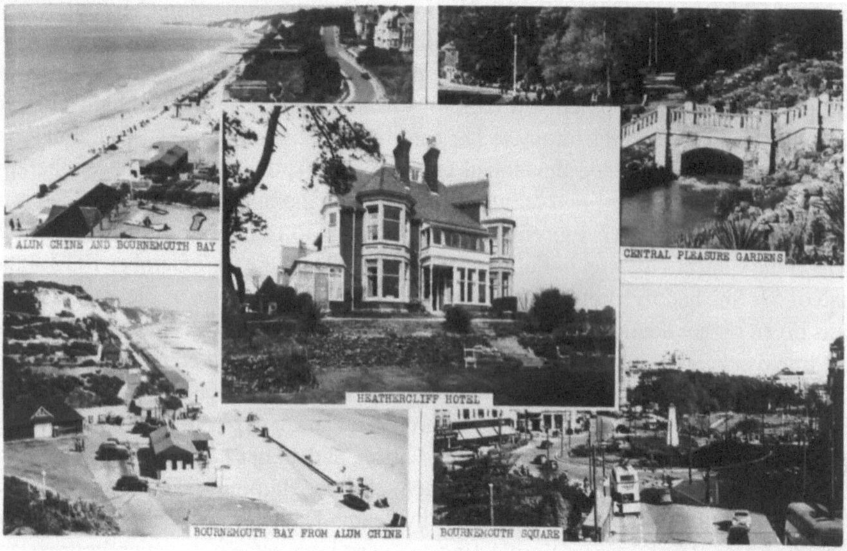

Fig. 17.1 Heathercliffe Hotel, 12 Burnaby Road, Bournemouth. A postcard sold at the hotel which is shown centrally, with surrounding pleasant images of its environs. (Unidentified publisher)

who had served in the Territorial Force Nursing Service during WW1 and had left Ireland after the war to live in London. Florence left the main part of her estate to Edith, who continued to live in the Burnaby Road house until her own death. The house subsequently became a hotel, the Heathercliffe Hotel (Fig. 17.1). Neither of their two Bournemouth residences exists today.

References

1. Gertrude Stoney to Archie Stoney. 1925 July 15 and Sept 18. AS.
2. Gertrude Stoney to Archie Stoney. 1922 Jun 28. AS.
3. Gertrude Stoney to Archie Stoney. 1923 Feb 25. AS.
4. Peel CS. Where "latch-key ladies" live. The Common Cause. 1922 May;12:117.
5. Halcyon Club pamphlet (undated). WL. 367-942132 HAL.
6. Gertrude Stoney to Archie Stoney. 1924 Nov 23. AS.
7. Gregory RA. James Ramsay Macdonald 1806–1937. Obituary Not Fellows R Soc. 1939;2(7):475–82.
8. Stoney E. The Times. 1925 May 9;10.
9. Paget RAS. Nature 1926 Dec 18.
10. Florence Stoney to Archie Stoney. 1930 Oct 7. AS.
11. Florence Stoney to Archie Stoney. 1928 Nov 21. AS.
12. McIntyre N. How British women became doctors. London: Wenrowave Press; 2014. p. 141–4.
13. Clever sisters. Irish Times. 1929 Apr 6.
14. The Vote. 1930 Mar 21.
15. Mukherjee S. Sisters in arms. Hist Today. 2018;68:72–83.

16. Chambers H. The Marie Curie hospital. Medical Women's Federation Newsletter. 1930 Mar;19–23.
17. Dickson RJ. The Marie curie hospital 1925-68. Br Med J. 1968;4:444–6.
18. Platt K. The Marie Curie hospital. The Common Cause. 1930 Feb 28;28.
19. 'M.E.C.' Women are doing great work in cancer research. Aberdeen Press and Journal. 1930 Feb 5.
20. Radium Fund Appeal. Cape Times? c. 1930 Jan. CK.
21. Stoney F. The pelvis and maternal mortality. Br J Radiol. 1930;3(33):426–9.
22. Hypher N. The diagnostic value of radiology in obstetric practice. Br J Radiol. 1931;4(40):171–7.
23. Stoney EA, Stoney FA. Difficult childbirth and the mentally unfit. The Common Cause. 1930 Dec 26;352.
24. Stoney EA. The right to work. The Vote. 1926 May 21.
25. Stoney EA. Thermometers and heat-control in domestic apparatus. Women Eng. 1931;3(7):111–2.
26. Howarth OJR. The British Association for the advancement of science: a retrospect 1831–1931. Centenary. 2nd ed. London: BAAS; 1931.
27. Watson Smith S. The Late Dr. Florence Stoney. Br J Med. 1932;ii:777.
28. Thomas AMK, Banerjee AK. The history of radiology. Oxford: Oxford University Press; 2013. p. 14–5.
29. Dr. Florence Stoney – Medical Women in the war. The Times. 1932 Oct 8;14.
30. Obituary. Florence Ada Stoney, O.B.E., M.D. (Lond), D.M.R.E. (Camb). Br J Radiol. 1932;5(59):853–8.
31. Obituary. Dr Florence Stoney O.B.E Bournemouth Daily Echo. 1932 Oct 2.
32. Ramsay M. The Times. 1932 Oct 12.

Chapter 18
Legacy

Edith's reaction to her sister's death was later summed up by her close friend Dr. Lisa Potter: 'She was devoted to her sister Dr Florence Stoney, and never really recovered from the shock of her death' [1]. After her bereavement she needed a complete break and booked herself on another winter cruise, a holiday to the Caribbean. She came back to her empty house in Bournemouth on 11 March 1933, wondering how to fill the void left by the loss of her sister.

Neither Florence nor Edith had ever visited their nieces and nephews in Australia. Now she was determined to remedy that and, while she was at it, take the opportunity to sort out some of the family heirlooms that should be better cared for by the next generations of Stoney family.

She had sailed on the P&O steamship Mongolia from England, delighted to inspect this vessel that had been built in Newcastle upon Tyne by Armstrong Whitworth, with its twin Parsons' marine turbine engines. She had planned this as simply a holiday. But, during the voyage, she was contacted by cable with a request for her to break her journey in Adelaide so that she could speak at the forthcoming conference of the National Federation of University Women in Australia on the subject of 'Electricity in the Home'. Australian Women had gained access to university education and had been awarded degrees earlier and more easily than had occurred in Britain. The University of Melbourne graduated its first women in 1882, and this was followed by the Universities of Sydney and Adelaide in 1885. Each state had set up its own federation for the growing group of women graduates, and, in 1922, a National Federation had been established. A sense of the size of the country emerges from the newspaper reports anticipating the conference. 'News has been received of the Brisbane delegation, which left last Friday on the long motor journey from Queensland... The party hope to arrive next Friday'. Three women had registered from Tasmania and a single delegate from Western Australia.

Edith was surprised and delighted to find that her nephew, named Gerald after her brother, was waiting on the quayside to meet her when the Mongolia berthed in the Outer Harbour on Saturday 6 January 1934, 2 days before the start of the conference. This first family meeting was supposed to have been on her arrival in Melbourne, and he had travelled the 160 miles from Wilmington, where he was working as a country doctor, to welcome her. This was the first time they had met.

She also found herself to be a celebrity, at the centre of media attention, giving numerous interviews during her stay in Australia. One headline trumpeted: 'Woman Has Won Five War Medals'. Nevertheless, the headline writers were confused about what sort of person she was. One declared her to be an 'engineer/nurse', another described her as a 'woman electrician and mathematician' and a third was sure she was an 'engineering pioneer'. The *Worker* publication respectfully called her a scientist whilst another headline presented her a 'distinguished mathematician and radiologist'. Whatever were her credentials for eminence, however, she charmed the female reporter from the Adelaide Advertiser: 'Very gentle and sweet, with her silvery hair and kind blue eyes, she looks as if she might have been engaged all her life in studying Celtic literature and making point lace' [2]. Elsewhere during her visit, she was described as 'small and slight almost to the point of fragility, she names running a motor car, bicycling, and gardening as her favourite hobbies' [3].

There was great interest in her activities, and in those of Florence, with much emphasis on their contributions to wartime radiology. Edith's discovery of the X-ray signs of gas gangrene was widely reported. Her contributions to the design of marine turbines and searchlights were noted, although the assumed application during Zeppelin raids was a journalistic extension. Her talk on home electricity made little impact. More notably she gave an address on the engineering work done by women during the war. She reminded her audience that 90% of the munitions workers in England during the war were women who, before 1915, had been charwomen, seamstresses, artists, ladies' maids and so on. Edith recounted how these women had to leave the engineering works at the end of the war to make way for the returning soldiers. She also recognised the more skilled engineering work of some women, setting their own tools, repairing guns, making accurate gauges and so on, estimating that, by the end of the war, over 1.3 million women had been trained to carry out some form of engineering work. Edith gave credit to Lady Parsons particularly, for her work to secure recognition for women engineers.

Edith was happy to give her opinion to reporters on a number of topics, from the place of women in medicine to the place of cinema in society. She expressed the view that women had made more progress as doctors in Australia than in Britain but pointed to some notable and outstanding British women doctors, in particular the surgeon Lady Florence Barrett, who was by then president of the London School of Medicine for Women.

She told one woman reporter that, in Britain, university women were concentrating, amongst other things, on the elimination of noise in modern life. Was she pulling her leg? The reporter was delighted to learn about this effort, writing that 'there is something about this modest ideal that takes one very pleasantly out of academic fields to wander among the possibilities of a tranquil future, where the steam sirens shall hoot no longer and motor bicycles shall be stilled'. Nevertheless, it says something about Edith's practical character that she considered this to be a research objective worth aiming for.

She was critical of the place of cinema in modern society, which she described harshly as 'dope for the masses', no more than an antidote for the monotony and boredom of mass production factories. She expressed regret that the modern factory worker seemed to prefer the escapism offered by the cinema rather than looking for education in their leisure hours.

One reporter confused arithmetic with mathematics. She spun a story that 'because the early women at Cambridge were weak in arithmetic it was declared that it was useless for women to take mathematics!' [4]. Over 50 years on and she could still remember the hurt embarrassment when her father learned of her failure to pass her first public examination in arithmetic. The memory was only slightly softened by recalling that her marvellous sister had suffered a similar failure.

Ten days after first reaching Australia she arrived in Melbourne. This had been her original destination, her travel interrupted by the Adelaide conference. Having completed her obligations to the Australian Federation, Edith then continued her journey on the steamship Ormonde to meet the family. On arrival she was surprised, and a little annoyed, to find that her nephew Archie had brought all his family down from Brisbane to meet her. She had planned to meet them later so they need not have bothered. Nevertheless, Edith's visit was a good excuse for a large family gathering, with her nephews, nieces, with their spouses and children, all gathered round two huge dinner tables in Glamorgan, the McComas' home town [5]. A visit to the University of Melbourne allowed her to make a presentation on behalf of Florence. Then she was off to see her nephew Gerald again and to stay with him in Wilmington for a few days. With an English view of the way in which the daughters of a doctor should be educated, she wanted to buy a pony for her two grandnieces, Diana and Pru, so that they could ride to the private school instead of attending the local state school.

She travelled the 1000 miles or so to Brisbane by train, amused to have to change trains at the state boundary at Albury where the broad gauge from Melbourne met the standard gauge onward to Sydney. She arrived in Brisbane on 19 February and remained for 10 days, staying in the Hotel Canberra, where she met several of Archie's colleagues from the University of Queensland. Her membership of the International Association of Lyceum Clubs opened the way for her to be entertained at the Lyceum Club in Brisbane, for which she wore her 'black picture hat and black lace gown'.

Edith visited Archie and his family in their home in Prospect Terrace. She had been delighted when she had heard that Archie had named two of his daughters after her and Florence. This gave her a special interest in them, and especially in her namesake, who was by then a tall 6-year-old. Little Florence was nearly four. Edith remembered the joy she had felt in Dublin, cycling up and down outside their house in Palmerston Park, and wanted to share that experience with her great nieces. Before she departed she left money for each girl to have a bicycle, Edith's being specially made because of her height. Edith's daughter rode this same bicycle as she grew up, and it survives to this day (Fig. 18.1). Another gift was Florence's lovely Leitz microscope that she had as a student, which Edith had brought with her in its custom-built wooden case all the way from England to present to her nephew.

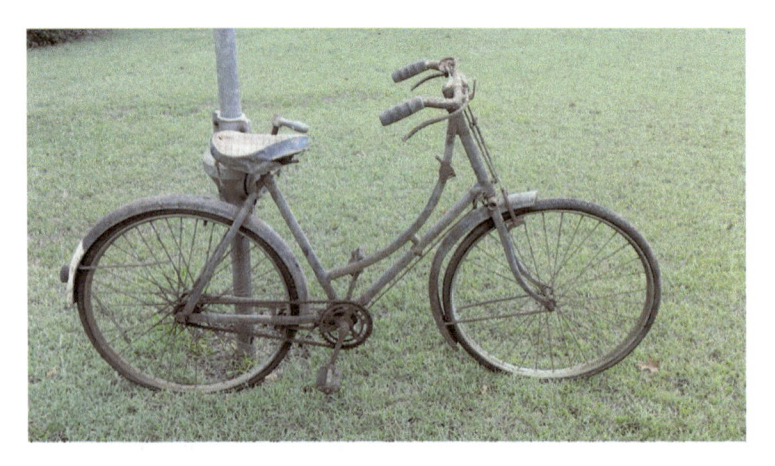

Fig. 18.1 The bicycle given by Edith to her grandniece Edith in February 1934 (Frances Smith)

Edith bade her relatives farewell at Brisbane railway station on 1 March, retracing her rail journey to Melbourne, sailing on the Otranto on 6 March. But she still had another commitment. During her visit to Adelaide, Edith had been approached by the sole representative of the West Australian University Women's Association, asking her to meet in Perth on her way home. The stop on 12 March gave just sufficient time for the local hosts to collect her at Freemantle port, to show her over the University at Crawley and then to join others for lunch at the Francatelli Lounge. Amongst those she met there was the Glaswegian Dr. Roberta Jull (née Stewart) who, in 1897, had been the first woman to establish a medical practice in Perth, the lawyer Margaret Battye who had been the first woman barrister to defend a client in Western Australia, the biologist Alison Baird and the ornithologist and writer Pauline Reilly [6].

Benefactress

Edith had become financially secure, inheriting the most part of her sister's estate. As a result she started to consider ways in which she might distribute her money for the benefit of others. By this time the BFUW was a much larger and more forceful group than it had been in its formative years when Edith had been the treasurer before the war. By 1930, 3000 academic women had joined, all concerned about the difficulties in getting funding for research, about gaining parity with their male colleagues and about income and opportunities for promotion. In early 1936 she offered £250 to fund scientific travel through the British Federation of University Women. The money was to be used for a studentship for 'research in biological, geological, meteorological or radiological science', to support a woman graduate of a university of Britain or Ireland, no more than 27 years old, to spend at least 6 months research in Australia. It was to be called the Johnstone and Florence Stoney Studentship in memory of her father and sister. The offer was taken to the Executive of the BFUW at its meeting on 7 March 1936 by the biochemist Ida Smedley MacLean, another Newnhamite. Thereafter, in each successive year until her death, Edith offered further studentships, extended to include other destinations in the Commonwealth. In all Edith gave £1500, sufficient for six studentships, the final funding for a student to visit South Africa being offered only a month before she died. She left an additional bequest of £3000 from her will.

These were significant sums of money, and the Executive Committee minutes became increasingly effusive in their appreciation of Edith's generosity, expressing their 'deep gratitude to Miss Stoney for her magnificent gifts'. Whilst the BFUW offered other grants for travel and study, none reached this level of funding, the others being only worth at most £100 each.

The recipient of the 1936 studentship was Mary Elizabeth King, a botanist from Girton. She spent her time in the Women's College in Sydney and studied bacterial diseases of citrus fruit ('citrus blast') and beans ('halo blight'). The second studentship in 1937 was awarded to Miss Joyce Laing PhD from Newnham, who went initially to continue her work on insect parasites (fruit flies) on sugar cane, working at the University of Queensland, Brisbane from November 1937 to May 1938. Her report suggests that she changed her topic to the marine zoology of Moreton Bay. On her return to Cambridge, Joyce married the parasitologist George Salt. The next award was made, shortly before Edith died, to Miss MCA Cross, a biochemist who worked in the Animal Nutritional Laboratories in Adelaide. On 24 June 1938, the day before Edith died, Rachael McAnally, PhD, a student of Ada MacLean, was awarded a studentship to carry out work in biochemistry in the Onderstepoort Veterinary Institute in Pretoria, South Africa. The final award before the war was offered, on 30 June 1939, to Miss L Alice Baker, a geography graduate, to work on land utility in parts of New Zealand. This arrangement failed, however, partly because of the outbreak of the war and partly because Miss Baker moved to India, and she withdrew in June 1940. There is no record of any further award being placed, although the studentship was, until quite recently, still being offered [7].

Edith retained a close connection with the Marie Curie Hospital. Rather surprisingly, when the hospital was first opened in 1929, it had no radiological equipment. Shortly after Florence died, the hospital launched an appeal for funds to purchase and install X-ray equipment for both diagnostic and therapeutic use. Soon the hospital had raised sufficient funds to buy the next-door house, and by June 1934 the new high-voltage X-ray equipment was installed. This gave the hospital the additional capability to treat fibroids and menorrhagia. It became immediately obvious that the facility was too small, attracting so many patients that some had to be refused treatment. Further funds were raised, supported by a letter to *The Times* from Maud Chadburn, chairman of the hospital, signed by the physicist Sir William Bragg and the politician Stanley Baldwin [8]. With full franchise, women's issues were well up the political agenda. Not to be outdone, the Prime Minister, Ramsay MacDonald, offered some radium bromide to the Marie Curie Hospital that had been originally acquired to illuminate gun sights during the war [9].

Nevertheless, the hospital still did not have any diagnostic X-ray equipment or darkroom. An additional £1000 was still needed. Edith offered to pay, in memory of her sister. On 16 September 1935, she attended a small reception to inaugurate this new X-ray diagnostic suite. The department was named after Florence, 'the pioneer woman in medical X-ray work'.

In spite of her increasing frailty, in the autumn of 1936, she was off on her travels again. She first prepared her garden for next spring. On 18 November she signed her will. Two days later she set off on the Arundel Castle for a 2-month cruise and holiday in South Africa. This visit seems to have been associated with her offer of a further £250 for another BFUW scientific fellowship, this one in South Africa. On her return there was plenty to attend to, and in the next couple of months, she visited either London or Cambridge four times. Dorothy Round, her great-nephew Archie's sister-in-law, was visiting London, and they met briefly at a big dinner at Crosby Hall, the headquarters of the British Federation of University Women. Edith was pleased to introduce her to the heads of two colleges whom she knew. Spring arrived and her daffodils and wallflowers came out [10].

At the end of March 1937 Edith was again invited to attend a large reception at the Marie Curie Hospital, when the enlarged pathology research laboratory was opened by Queen Mary. It was named after Helen Chambers. She was another Newnham student, who had studied natural sciences at Cambridge before moving on to enter medicine at the London School of Medicine for Women, where she arrived at the same time as Edith had joined as lecturer in physics. After the war, Chambers had taken a full-time appointment with the Medical Research Council to study radiobiology and immunology and had led the drive to establish radium treatment of cancer of the cervix, which had resulted in the founding of the Marie Curie Hospital.

The event was held under a large marquee in the garden of the hospital. It now had 39 beds, of which 29 were devoted to the treatment of cervical and uterine cancer. The team was very pleased to report that 85% 5-year survival rates had been achieved for those whose cancer had been diagnosed at an early stage. Edith had accepted the invitation to attend, and had made the effort to travel up to London, an effort that now always tired her, especially to meet Eve Curie, Marie Curie's daughter, who attended as a special guest. It was less than 2 years since Marie Curie had died, and Eve's biography of her mother was about to be published. Edith listened with great interest to the account of Marie Curie's life and work from someone who, though not a scientist herself, had been so close to her [11].

Edith remained the main reference point for those who remembered her father and his work. When she received a request from the Royal Dublin Society to send them a photograph of her father, she chose the one of him standing by the heliostat that he had invented. Her father's new heliostat, originally intended for Archie in Australia, was given by Gerald to the Science Museum in South Kensington, in Edith's name.

Edith's health deteriorated during the next 12 months. When she attended the meeting of the Academic Committee of the BFUW at Crosby Hall on 18 June 1938, her friends and colleagues found her to be obviously very ill. She was to be elected as a vice president at the annual meeting the following weekend. The business of the meeting included the award of the latest Johnstone and Florence Stoney travelling fellowship. This would be her last professional meeting.

Edith Stoney died, aged 69 years, a week later on Saturday 25 June 1938, at her home in Bournemouth. Her death certificate recorded the cause of death as uraemia and chronic interstitial nephritis.[1] Following the instructions she left in her will, there was a private cremation at Bournemouth Crematorium where her ashes were scattered. Amongst the many floral tributes was a wreath from the Victorian women graduates, sent on their behalf by the Australian haematologist Dr. Lucy Bryce who was visiting England at the time [12]. There was no memorial stone. As with her sister, even in death she was tied to her father: on her death certificate is entered, under the heading 'occupation' 'Spinster of independent means, daughter of Johnstone Stoney D.Sc. (deceased)'. Her Australian relatives learned of her death, by post, 3 weeks later.

There can be few whose obituary notices appeared in such a wide range of publications and geographical locations. Notices of her death were placed in *The Times*, *The Daily Telegraph* and *The Irish Times*, using the precise words specified in her will as 'the eldest daughter of the late G Johnstone Stoney DSc FRS', devoted to her father to the end and still conscious of her senior position of family responsibility. Obituaries were published in *Nature* [13], *The Times* [14], *The Electrician* [15] and *The Lancet* [16] and also in Australia where her brother's family had settled [17, 18]. *The Lancet* emphasised her teaching role for medical students. *The Times* noted that she had just been elected as one of the vice presidents of the BFUW and spoke at length of her service during the war. The obituary in *Nature* described her as a mathematical physicist and noted that she was pleased to have just presented a further travel award. The three-page 'In Memoriam', written by Ida Smedley-Maclean in the University Women's Review, emphasised her work for the Federation of University Women. In it, the writer recalled that she had arrived at the London School of Medicine for Women as a student at the same time as had Edith and that she had worked under Florence, then Demonstrator in Anatomy. 'The high standard of intellectual work shared by both of them made a deep impression on their students' [19].

Edith's will was considerably longer and more detailed than her sister's. A copy is still held by the Newnham College archives and was summarised in *The Times* [20]. It included several interesting bequests. Notably, for Newnham, she left £3000 to establish a second studentship under the title 'The Johnstone and Florence Stoney Studentship'. This opened a career pathway for other women that had been closed to her. It was 'to be held at the London R.F.H. (Royal Free Hospital) School of Medicine for Women by some student of Newnham College who has taken a Mathematical Tripos or has taken Physics in the Final of a Natural Science Tripos and who proposes to go on to medical qualification'. She added 'I ask Newnham College to undertake this since I am impressed with the need for women doctors who have more knowledge of Physics or Mathematical Physics than comes into the

---

[1] That is, she died of kidney failure.

ordinary medical qualifications'. The first recipient of this studentship, Mary Townsend, completed her Part II Tripos in Physics in 1940. The studentship helped to support her medical training at the LSMW from 1940 to 1944 where she was also the Bird Scholar. She became MRCP in 1948 and worked at the Birmingham Children's and the Burney and District Hospitals before being appointed to be the senior Medical Officer for Maternal and Child Welfare for the Dorset County Council in 1961.

However, Mary Townsend appears to have been the only student to have received support under the strict terms of Edith's will. These were certainly too restrictive in their scope. It was awarded again in 1949, but not taken up. In 1957 the conditions were loosened so that it was tenable 'at any Medical School, with a preference for the London School of Medicine, by a member of the College who has obtained an Honours Degree of Cambridge University'. As a result, many medical students during subsequent years benefitted from the support from this studentship, mostly those studying in Cambridge. More than 20 names are recorded in the College records as recipients during the 1960s and 1970s. One was Jean Guy (née Aldridge) whose biographical paper on Florence and Edith Stoney gives extensive detail on their war years. These days, the studentship has become part of the Stoney and Balfour Travelling Scholarship, to assist Newnham medical and veterinary students with the cost of clinical electives during the second year of training, and former Newnham students training elsewhere. Edith may not have totally approved of the defocusing of her original intentions.

A few other aspects of Edith's will may be noted. A further £100 was made available to enable an Australian girl to come to England to study. The Marie Curie Hospital received a further £3000 for their diagnostic X-ray department, anticipating that this 'will cover the cost of renewal and bringing up to date the present apparatus in a few years time'. As a further contribution to radiological training, she gave £1000 to the London School of Medicine for Women for prizes along the lines of the present 'Florence Stoney' prize. And in what must be possibly the only example of academic instructions in a will, she added suggestions for topics for essays: (1) the treatment of cancer by methods primarily not surgical, (2) on laboratory work associated with the influence of radiations (X-ray, radium, UV light, etc.) on tumour or allied growths and (3) on the treatment of hyperthyroidism by methods primarily not surgical. Her father's Boyle medal was returned to the Royal Dublin Society. Two pictures of her father made by her sister Gertrude were offered to the Art Galleries of Melbourne and Brisbane.

She left small bequests to her three Australian nephews, Archibald, Gerald and William and to her niece Margaret East, to whom she left what she called the "Stoney annals", since lost. She exhorted them to use their bequests for university education of their children. Otherwise, the residue of the estate was to be divided between Archibald's children, for their education. Her brother Gerald received those instruments and books of her father's which had not been disposed of otherwise. Her nephew Gerald got her father's grandfather clock. Gertrude was bequeathed any of her jewellery, clothes, books and household effects that she wished, together with a bequest of £250. Her cousins Frances and Dora, Charles' daughters in Yelverton, received £100 each.

Lisa Potter's recollections of her friend are perhaps the closest we can get to understanding Edith's enigmatic personality:

> She took nothing for granted, and was astonished by nothing. She was perfectly aware that two and two made four, but if anyone could suggest a method of making it something else she was all out to try it. She was full of contrasts, amazingly energetic, and capable of a vast amount of work. Her active spirit was encased in the most fragile body... Though perhaps old maidish and fussy in some of her ways, she was extraordinarily broad-minded about big things. Above all she had an immense tenacity of purpose with which she drove her body to the last minute... The world is a poorer place by (the loss of) someone who was different from other people in a ready-made age.

References

1. Potter L. Obituary for Edith Stoney. CK.
2. War adventures of a woman scientist. Adelaide Advertiser. 1934 Jan 9;14.
3. Brisbane Courier-Mail. 1934 Feb 20;15.
4. Miss Edith A. Stoney. Melbourne Argus. 1934 Jan 17;15.
5. Personal communication from Edith McKinnon.
6. University Women's Luncheon. The West Australian. 1934 Mar 14;4.
7. Johnstone and Florence Stoney Studentship. WL. 5BFW/06/056, 066, 068. Executive Committee minutes. WL. 5BFW/02/18,19,20.
8. Chadburn MM, Runciman H, Mellanby E, Bragg W, Baldwin S. The Times. 1934 July 20.
9. Radium for cancer fight. Aberdeen Press. 1934 Dec 7.
10. Edith Stoney to Miss Round (probably Archie's sister-in-law Dorothy). 1937 Mar 29. AS.
11. Cancer research. The Times. 1937 Mar 20.
12. The Melbourne Argus. 1938 Jul 19.
13. Stoney E. Nature 1938 Jul 16;103–104.
14. Cullis WC. Miss Edith Stoney. X-ray work during the war. The Times. 1938 Jul 5;16.
15. The Electrician. 1938 Jul 8.
16. Stoney E. M.A. Lancet. 1938 Jul 9;108.
17. Benefactor of research. The Argus (Melbourne). 1938 Jul 19;7.
18. Miss Edith Stoney's aid to science. Brisbane Courier-Mail. 1938 Jul 30;2.
19. Smedley-Maclean I. In memoriam. Edith Anne Stoney. University Women's Review. 1938 Oct 26;22–24.
20. Wills and Bequests. The Times. 1938 Aug 23;13.

Correction to: Edith and Florence Stoney, Sisters in Radiology

Correction to:
A. Thomas and F. Duck, *Edith and Florence Stoney,*
*Sisters in Radiology***, Springer Biographies Series**
https://doi.org/10.1007/978-3-030-16561-1

This book was inadvertently published with the following errors:

On page 64, Figure 3.7 has been replaced with a new figure, which has been included in this errata.

On pages 184 and 185, Figures 11.2, 11.3, and 11.4 were displaced from their legends, which has been corrected.

The chapters have now been updated.

The updated online versions of the chapters can be found at
https://doi.org/10.1007/978-3-030-16561-1_3
https://doi.org/10.1007/978-3-030-16561-1_11

© Springer Nature Switzerland AG 2019
A. Thomas, F. Duck, *Edith and Florence Stoney, Sisters in Radiology*, Springer Biographies, https://doi.org/10.1007/978-3-030-16561-1_19

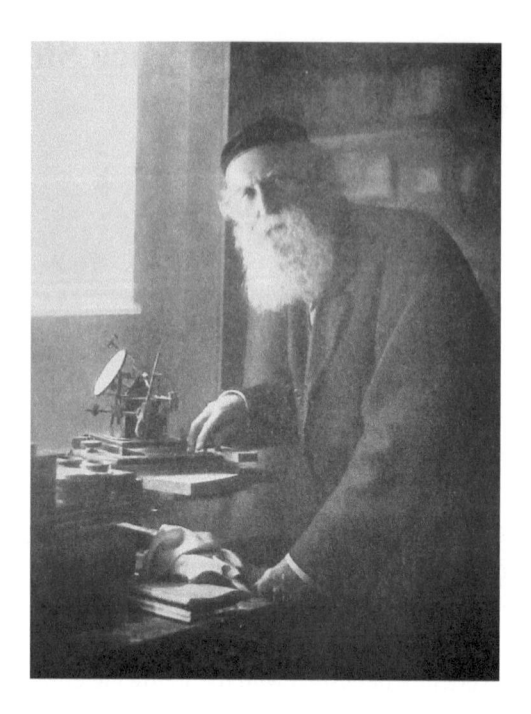

Correction to: Edith and Florence Stoney, Sisters in Radiology

Appendix: Wartime Uses of Radiology and Medical Electricity

There is a unique document in the archives of Royaumont Abbey. On the face of it, it is unremarkable. It is a blank request form for Edith's radiology department (Fig. A.1). This seemingly simple document represents a complete change in the relationship between the radiological service and the doctors who used it. Here is the evidence that the Royaumont department was advanced, organised and independent.

The most important part of the form lies in the list of services on offer. These were radiography, localisation, electrical treatment and nerve testing. In this appendix, the methods used by Edith and Florence Stoney under each of these headings are described in detail. Wherever possible, the personal experience of the two sisters is made part of the story when the evidence is available.

War commonly stimulates the use of new techniques in medical diagnosis and treatment, and WWI was no exception. These advances arise from a combination of causes: the large numbers of casualties, the unusual nature of many injuries, the availability of military funding for new equipment and the specialist expertise of one or two leading medical staff. Florence and Edith both exploited these advances in their military radiological practice.

Radiography: X-ray Diagnosis of Gas Gangrene

Plane radiography was the main use of X-rays during the war. It showed skeletal damage and the presence of foreign bodies. Generally the soft tissues, liver, muscle, kidney and so on, are not easily distinguished from one another. There was one new use for X-rays that emerged during the war, however, and this was for the diagnosis of gas gangrene.

On 20 October 1916, two papers were presented to the Section of Electro-Therapeutics of the Royal Society of Medicine (RSM) on radiography in the diagnosis of gas gangrene [1, 2]. The first, by Agnes Savill, presented a series of 67 X-ray plates taken between 1 July and mid-September 1916 at Royaumont.

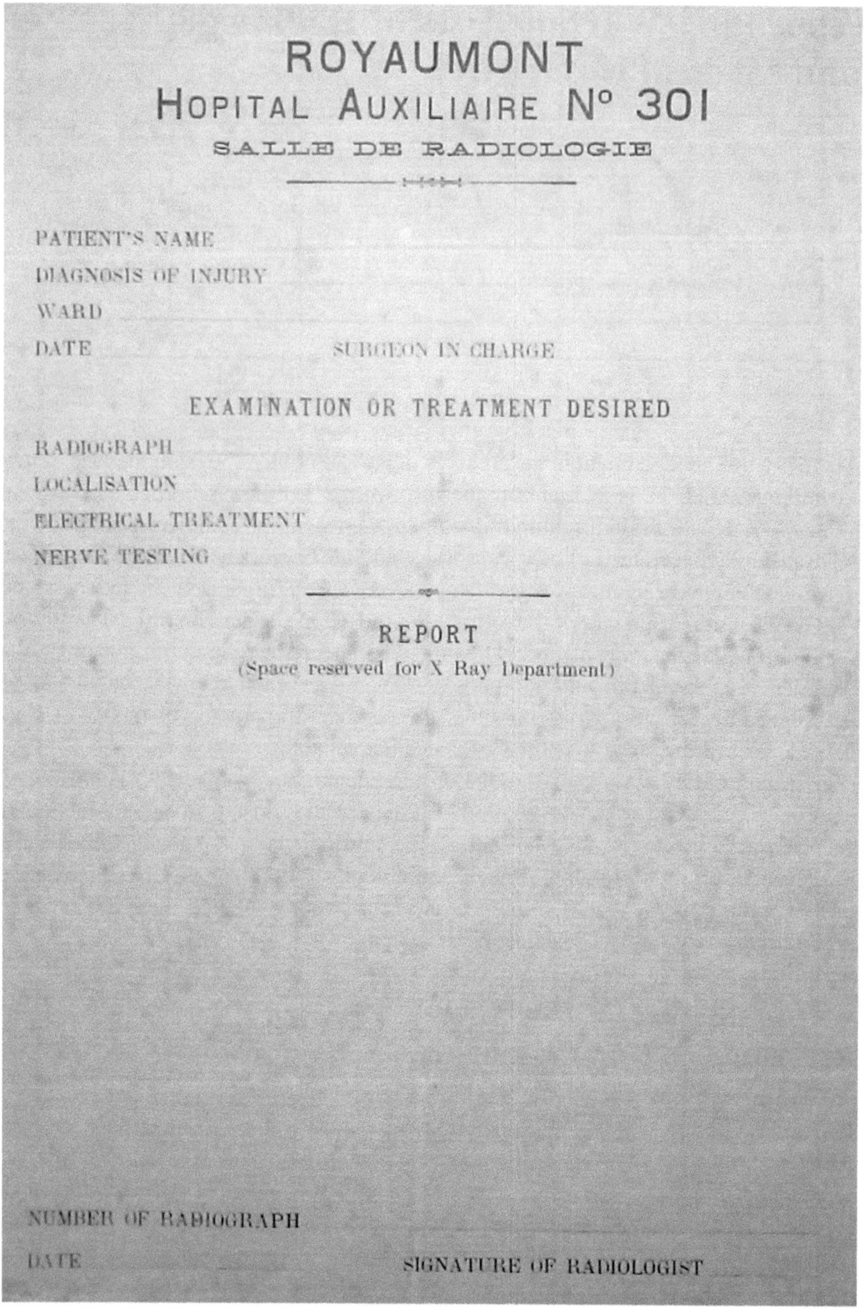

ROYAUMONT
HOPITAL AUXILIAIRE N° 301
SALLE DE RADIOLOGIE

PATIENT'S NAME
DIAGNOSIS OF INJURY
WARD
DATE SURGEON IN CHARGE

EXAMINATION OR TREATMENT DESIRED

RADIOGRAPH
LOCALISATION
ELECTRICAL TREATMENT
NERVE TESTING

REPORT
(Space reserved for X Ray Department)

NUMBER OF RADIOGRAPH
DATE SIGNATURE OF RADIOLOGIST

Fig. A.1 Request form for radiology, electrical diagnosis and electro-therapy used by Edith at Royaumont. (Archives of the Fondation Royaumont)

The second, by Dr. Martin Berry, radiologist at the Royal Herbert Military Hospital Woolwich, presented 28 studies performed within a similar 3-month period. These two series were the first to present the range of radiographic appearances that may be associated with gas gangrene. This infection was, at that time, a major cause of death of soldiers injured in France.

The previous year, Edith had also made radiographs that showed evidence of gas gangrene. This was during her first encounter with military radiography, seeing casualties with gas gangrene for the first time, in Troyes in the autumn of 1915. Florence and Edith understood the pioneering nature of her observations and later, in 1917, examples of her X-ray plates were donated to the War Collections of Medical Specimens at the Royal College of Surgeons of London. Amongst them were plates of gas gangrene dated 3 October 1915. The accompanying document, written before she left Salonika, states that these radiographs were 'probably the earliest record for X. Ray (*sic*) of Gas Gangrene' [3]. The images were also included in an exhibition of wartime radiology at the Royal College of Surgeons in August 1917, when again they were claimed to have been the earliest record of the use of X-rays to diagnose for gas gangrene. Sadly, these wartime radiographic records were lost when the RCS was in a bombing raid during the Second World War [4].

Edith may or may not have been the first to observe the radiographic appearance of gas gangrene. Almost certainly it was an observation that was made independently in many of the front-line X-ray units during the first part of the war. Neither were Savill and Berry the first to note that the gas released by the anaerobic bacillus responsible for gas gangrene altered the appearance of the soft-tissue X-ray shadow. Savill gives credit to Dr. Pech, from the nearby Creil Military Hospital, for teaching her about the radiographic signs to notice, although she reported that striations, his main diagnostic sign, were absent except in rare cases in her own series. This is perhaps not surprising, given the basic equipment that she was using.

Gas gangrene was not seen in Salonika, and so it would not be until Edith returned to France in the autumn of 1917 that her knowledge of this diagnosis became useful again. In London, a few cases infected with the gas gangrene bacillus would have arrived at the Fulham Military Hospital, where Florence would have observed the characteristic X-ray appearance. Nevertheless, it was predominantly a problem of front line hospitals in France, the soldiers requiring immediate surgery for there to be any chance of recovery.

Alexander Fleming had noted, working as a bacteriologist at the No. 13 General Hospital in Boulogne in the summer of 1915, that 'the flora of these infected wounds has been found to be very different from that met with in civil practice'. He and others were working to identify the most prevalent microbe likely to be responsible for causing gas gangrene [5]. Material from suspect tissue samples would have been taken to the bacteriology laboratory for culture, eventually to demonstrate the presence of the gas gangrene bacilli *Clostridium perfringens* with its characteristic stick-like appearance. This germ was widely present in the well-manured soil of northern France. Of more importance, uniforms were also widely contaminated. Shrapnel tore ragged holes in uniforms and flesh carrying the bacillus deep with the wound, making it very difficult to fully clean and disinfect. The subsequent infection created gas sometimes deep within the tissue.

A threefold attack on diagnosis developed. An experienced surgeon's observation was often sufficient, supported sometimes, as the infection took hold, by noting the characteristic and nauseating odour. Secondly, once the bacteriological appearance of the bacillus was known, cultures could demonstrate its presence in pus samples taken from the wound, although this might prove difficult if the wound was deep, compromising bacteriological confirmation. To these two was now added radiography which, used judiciously, had the potential to stage the progress of the disease, to determine the extent of the infected tissue, and to discover unrecognised deep-seated infections. Fast diagnosis was essential, so that any infected limb could be amputated immediately to prevent spread to the rest of the body and probable death.

Savill reported that, in her series, 304 cases contained (presumably bacteriological) evidence of gas gangrene of which 100 presented clinical evidence of interstitial gas. As Edith had realised, radiographic demonstration of gas in the tissue was possible because of its low X-ray attenuation coefficient, in a similar way to the contrast that delineates the air-filled lungs. Savill identified three radiographic appearances, simple swelling, swelling with a cloud-like outline, and striation. The attraction of a radiological diagnosis was undoubtedly its speed, leading to early treatment: the diagnosis was, in principle, immediate, whilst bacteriological incubation would take a while. The difficulty with Savill's interpretation was that the appearance of the striations was unusual, appearing only after the infection was well developed, and the more common appearance of swelling could easily have arisen from other causes.

By 1918 the management of gas gangrene was well advanced in Royaumont and Villers-Cotterêts. Edith had no problem in playing her part in the well-organised multidisciplinary approach to the disease, and knew that her own understanding and skill was being highly appreciated. Frances Ivens ensured that all clinical staff were trained to understand the radiographic signs of gas gangrene and how to recognise the variety of ways in which it might manifest itself. Vera Collum, orderly turned radiographer, was as knowledgeable as any:

> Since the early days of the War the X-ray plate has had its share in detecting the lurking enemy. As a rule, with gas infection, the radiographic plate merely confirms the examining surgeon's diagnosis. Occasionally, in rush work such as ours was, when the cursory examination of the wounded man on his admission gives no hint of the gas infection, the plate reveals the fact that the anaerobe is at work in the soft tissues lying deeper in the wound; or that gas, perhaps at some distance from the entrance to the wound, is beginning to track along the muscle sheaths. It is when the radiographer gets such an indication,—say in the case of a wounded knee, with gas tracking up the thigh—that the plate is of supreme value; for it is in such a case that it is the radiologist's report, and not the grading of the examining surgeon, that the man is sent straight in to the operating theatre, that the knife and the Pasteur serum may between them arrest the mischief before it has gone too far.

> The aim of the radiographer then, is to produce negatives in every instance of such fine quality that the slightest indication of the presence of gas in the soft tissues may be clearly visible; and secondly, in order that his reading of the plate may not be confused by the

shadows of gauze or wool, or uniform fabric in the wound itself, ... to radiograph wounds wherever possible without a scrap of dressing on them. [6]

By the end of the war, the doctors of Royaumont had made enormous advances in the treatment of gas gangrene. As indicated in Collum's report, they had made contact with the Pasteur Institute in Paris where Professor Michel Wienberg (1868–1940) had developed anti-toxin sera for the treatment of gas gangrene [7]. Frances Ivens had used the early anti-toxin sera experimentally in 1915 and 1916, treating ten very seriously infected cases that would not have been expected to live. Five of her patients survived. Then, during March to September 1918, all 433 detected cases of gas gangrene infection were treated. Only 38 died and in only 7 was the death attributed to gas gangrene. This was an astonishing and dramatic achievement: left untreated, the mortality rate for gas gangrene was about 75% [8].

Before moving on from radiology, there is one other radiological sign to be mentioned that was also noted in Chap. 11. When bone was shattered it was often difficult for the surgeon to determine which fragments were still supported by a blood supply and so might have a chance of re-growth, and which were dead and needed to be removed. Florence realised that these two had different radiological appearances. The dead bone, or sequestra, gave a denser shadow, and this diagnosis gave the surgeon confidence when deciding which bone fragments needed to be excised and which left in place [9].

X-ray Localization of Foreign Bodies

The main challenge, for army surgeons, was the localisation and extraction of bullets, shrapnel, and other foreign bodies embedded in the tissues of wounded soldiers. Without good localization, surgeons had to probe blindly within tissues, sometimes unsuccessfully, and often causing as much damage as did the projectile. Radiological techniques offered the only effective means by which surgical extraction could be guided.

By the First World War, 20 years after the discovery of X-rays, it was estimated that over 200 slightly different methods for localization had been developed. Simple methods to take and view stereoscopic pairs of radiographs were well established. Biplane radiography, for which the X-ray images were taken in two directions, often but not always at right angles, was also being used. Whilst both these approaches were an improvement over the plane X-ray image, neither gave the answer to the surgeons' questions "where should I cut, in which direction should I probe and how deep will I need to go?'

Which of the following methods was used depended on the competence, skill and commitment of the user and the availability of the appropriate specialised equipment. For many military applications it was estimated that localisation to within 5 mm would sufficient, although locating a small foreign body in the eye, for example, might need greater precision. There was another factor, however, which depended on whether the hospital was acting a casualty clearing hospital or a base hospital. For the conditions during the attack near Villers-Cotterêts in May 1918 and the subsequent months in Royaumont, localisation for as many casualties as possible was required and fine precision had to be sacrificed for efficiency. In the base hospitals, where there was sufficient time for careful preparation before and during operation, more sophisticated methods could be used. This would have been true for much of the time at the Fulham War Hospital, for example, where Florence gained a reputation for her high level of skill in localisation. Edith similarly was credited for the quality of her localisation, a skill most likely developed in the quieter times in Troyes and Salonika.

In the simplest and cheapest method of localisation, two X-ray images were made in which the X-ray tube was displaced by a few centimetres between the first and the second exposure. The resulting two X-ray plates were then viewed through an appropriate stereo viewer, to give the observer a three-dimensional view of the foreign body with respect to the surrounding bone and other landmarks. The inclusion of a stereo viewer in most of the lists of X-ray equipment, including that for the SWH X-ray ambulance, demonstrates this to be a very widely used method for a quick visual impression of the location of an embedded bullet or fragments. Many alternative viewers were available. Both Florence and Edith used the Pirie stereoscopic viewer, which included a prism to give the appropriate optical conversion from translational imaging to stereoscopic viewing [10–12] (Fig. A.2).

Another simple method that was often used in busy times was bi-plane fluoroscopy. Two X-ray views were made with the beams at right angles to one another, and the surgeon was given guidance by placing two skin marks, one for each view, above the position of the foreign body.

The simple stereoscopic viewer was very useful, but did not give the surgeon any more than a general view of the anatomical locations and distributions of metal fragments. The bi-plane view was better, but still lacked the ability to locate accurately. To be more precise about the depth of the foreign body below the skin, localization methods used measurements from the two X-ray views, taking the relative change of position of the shadows of objects on either a fluoroscopic screen or film [13]. Overcouch or undercouch tubes were standard in most X-ray departments by this time, allowing either fluoroscopy (undercouch tube) or film (overcouch tube) to be used. A plumb line was used to identify the vertical beam axis. When a fluoroscopic screen was used it was often mounted on a frame whose position could be adjusted and locked over the patient. In a darkened X-ray room, the image of the bullet was first shown on the screen, and the tube position was adjusted so that the shadow was on the vertical beam axis F_0P_0 (Fig. A.3). The skin was marked at this point either using the plumb line or through a perforation hole in the screen, so recording the entry point for the surgeon's knife. Then the tube was moved sideways by a measured distance to F_1, and the movement of the shadow on the screen was recorded. The vertical depth of the bullet could be determined from these two distances and a knowledge of the distance between the tube focus and the screen.

One widely used method for this determination was the Mackenzie Davidson localiser. This was a frame with crossed threads to show the geometry of the two

Fig. A.2 Pirie spectroscope preferred by both Florence and Edith Stoney for viewing stereoscopic X-ray pairs

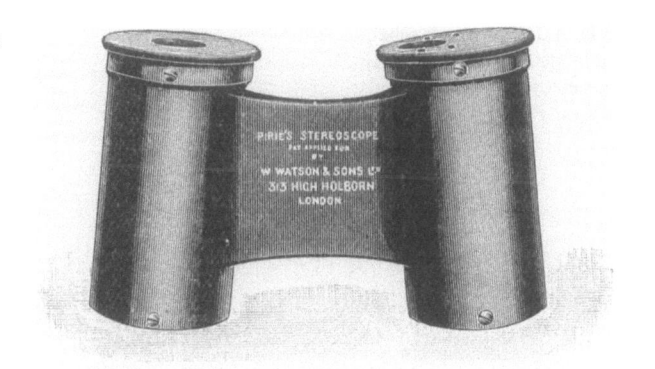

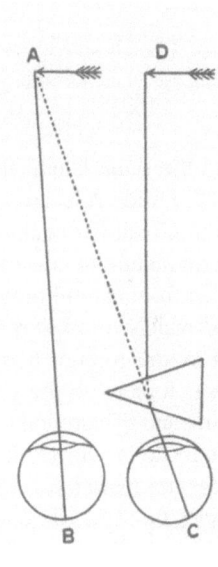

X-ray beams. Florence took such a localising stand with her to Europe, noting that she owed much 'to Sir James Mackenzie Davidson for his constant help as to the best methods of localising'. Florence noted, however, that in many cases the rough simpler method was sufficient, and in some cases more appropriate. Some of her worst cases were those in which the rifle ball burst to pieces inside the limb, and stereoscopic viewing was sufficient to aid the surgeon to determine the overall extent of the embedded fragments, rather than the localisation and quick extraction of a single bullet.

Agnes Savill also wrote up her own experience of localisation from her work at Royaumont. She used an alternative to the Mackenzie Davidson frame in which the depth was calculated using a nomogram rather than a physical embodiment of the crossed X-ray beams. This method had been described by William Hampson [14]. The nomogram method was made possible by using the same the tube-to-

Fig. A.3 The simple tube-shift method of foreign body localization.
$PP_0 = P_0F_0(1 - F_0F_1/QF_1)$

screen distance and the same lateral tube movement for all exposures (Fig. A.4). Edith's inclusion of a slide-rule amongst her equipment suggests that she, too, preferred calculation. Given her background as a mathematical physicist, it would have been more in her nature to consider the geometry from first principles, and to work out the position from careful measurement and calculation. Graphs and tables were also published widely to assist radiographers with these calculations.

Once the depth of the foreign body below the skin had been calculated, the surgeon would insert forceps to the estimated depth below the skin mark, in the direction of the beam, and fish around until she got hold of the bullet. In some cases, where the operation could be carried out on the X-ray couch, radiographic guidance was possible during the operation (Fig. A.5). Additional probes were inserted to reach the bullet under fluoroscopic control, the radiologist using a hooded screen because the operating room could not be darkened.

Tube shift methods were well suited to rapid evaluation of the location and depth of foreign objects, and could be developed to locate several targets in the same body. But they lacked the generality required for the development of true stereotactic surgery. Specifically, they assumed that the surgical approach would be along the axis of the X-ray beam. Sometimes this was possible but, not infrequently, critical organs and structures lay in the way, and when this occurred the information given to the surgeon was of limited value. Furthermore, it could be quite difficult to maintain a straight-line incision into deeper tissues along an arbitrary line. In response to these challenges a variety of mechanical pointers or "compasses" were developed, the precursors of modern stereotactic surgical techniques. Of these, the most widely used by French radiologists was the Hirtz compass, first described in 1910 by the French military radiologist Eugène Hirtz (1869–1934) [15]. Hirtz had originally intended to study science at the *École polytechnique* but ill health caused him to

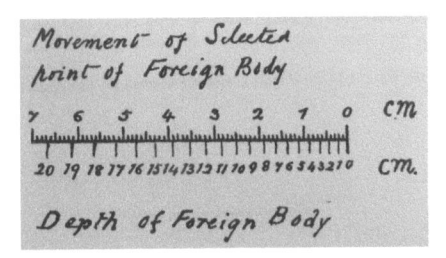

Appendix: Wartime Uses of Radiology and Medical Electricity 337

Fig. A.4 Hampson's nomogram for calculating the depth of a foreign body for a fixed tube to film distance, Q, of 50 cm with a lateral tube movement, $F_0 - F_1$, of 10 cm

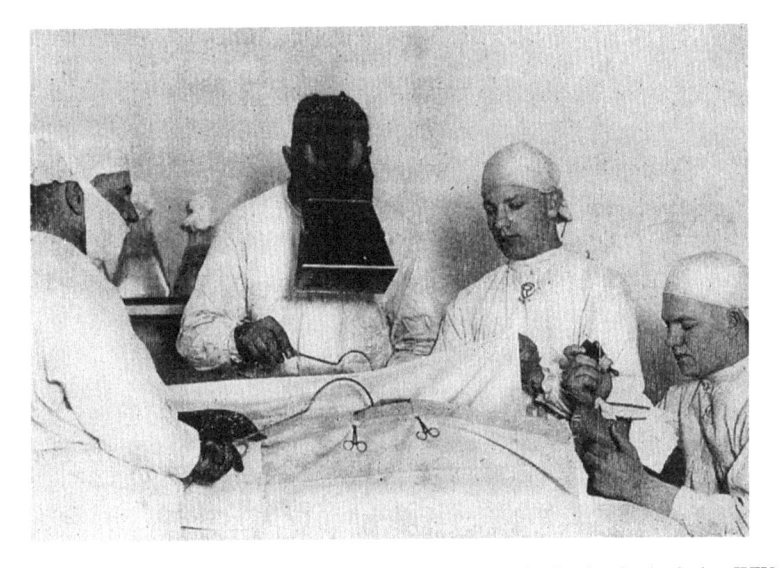

Fig. A.5 Fluoroscopic assistance during the surgical removal of a foreign body during WW1

change to medicine. During the war he worked with Marie Curie to promote the use of mobile X-ray vans. After the war he took the post of Head of Radiology, Electrotherapy and Physiotherapy at the *Val-de-Grâce* hospital in Paris and is credited with establishing the first non-military school of radiography there.

Localisation using the Hirtz compass was significantly more complicated than other approaches. Agnes Savill remarked that she had tried Behieren's compass, a simpler mechanical device, and was planning to master the 'somewhat alarming preliminary calculations and drawings' for the Hirtz compass [16]. Recalling her competence in operating the Newnham equatorial telescope, these calculations would have been child's play for Edith, who also had obtained a compass for her unit in Salonika [17]. The following is a detailed description of the equipment and its use. Readers less technically inclined may find the next few paragraphs challenging. They have been included in order to emphasise the degree of skill that users, including both Edith and Florence, would have needed to include the method into their radiological practice.

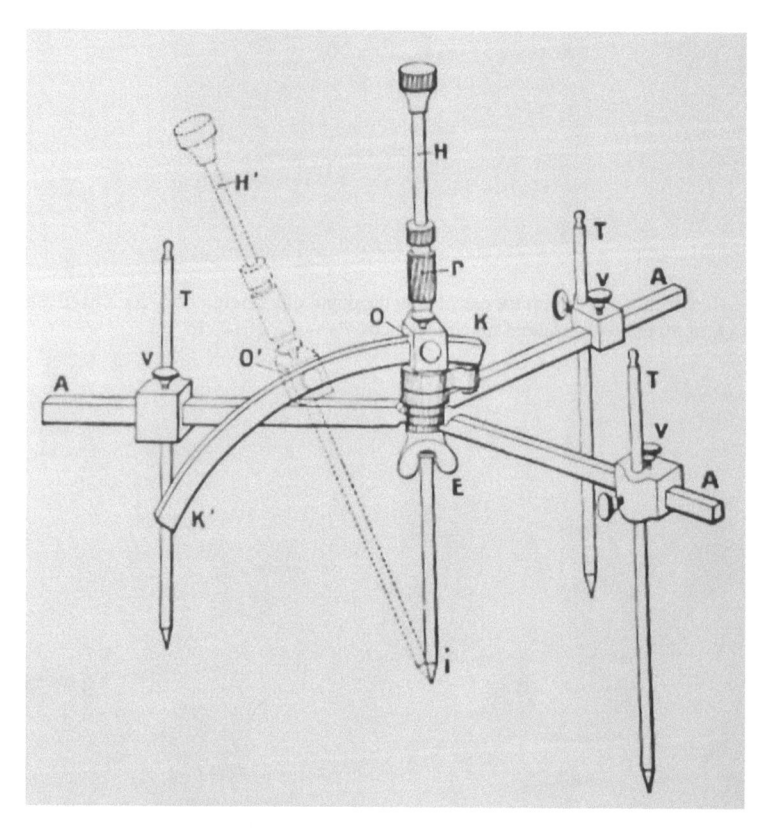

Fig. A.6 The Hirtz compass. The curved arm KK' is mounted so that its centre of curvature, i, is positioned at the foreign body to be removed. Insertion of rod H by a distance equal to the radius of curvature will always place its tip at the object

The design of the Hirtz compass may be understood by referring to Fig. A.6. The bullet to be removed was assumed to be at i, the origin of the frame of reference. The purpose was to mount the curved arm KK' in such a way that the rod H would always be aligned with this origin, no matter from which angle it was directed. In order to fix this position, the arm was mounted on a triangulation frame. This consisted of three coplanar horizontal radial arms, $A\ A\ A$, all free to rotate to, and be locked at, any angular position around a central spindle. A vertical leg T was mounted on each horizontal arm, free to be moved along the arm, be adjusted in height, and then to be locked in place by clamp V. In use, the lower ends of these legs rested on pre-marked places on the curved skin surface (Fig. A.7). By adjusting the leg heights, the arms A, A, A were brought into a plane that was exactly perpendicular to the beam axis, with the central spindle on that axis. By adjusting the height of the curved arm, the bullet could be bought to its centre of curvature. Then, no matter how the arm KK' was rotated, and no matter where H was positioned on it, insertion of the rod to a fixed distance would always reach the foreign body.

Fig. A.7 The Hirtz compass in position on the skin. The bullet is located at distance d below the vertical entry point S, and can be equally approached through entry point S'

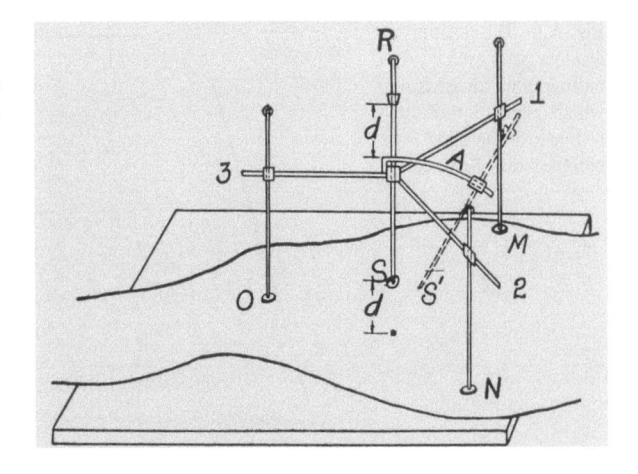

The practical application of the compass followed three phases: (1) localisation using X-rays, (2) mechanical adjustment of the compass and (3) its surgical use. The first phase, radiological localisation, did not use the compass itself. Three radiographic markers were placed on the skin, and their positions were established with respect to a measurement plane perpendicular to the beam axis, which could be either a fluoroscopic screen above the patient, or a film under him. The easier approach used a fluoroscopic screen. The depth of the bullet along the beam axis was measured using a tube-shift method such as that shown in Fig. A.3. Any vertical gaps between the skin and the screen on this axis and above each marker were then measured. This was done by direct measurement, centring the beam on each marker in turn and passing a measuring probe through the axial perforation in the screen. These five measurements were sufficient to adjust and clamp the compass (phase 2).

An alternative, but more complicated, method for phase 1 used film to determine the settings for the compass. In this case there was no need to align the radiographic axis precisely with the target, so long as the general location of the object had been determined by previous film or fluoroscopy. A film cassette was first placed on the couch, beneath an overcouch X-ray tube. A marker cross-wire was attached to the cassette, aligned with the beam axis using a plumb line. The film-to-focus distance Z was set. The patient was laid on the couch over the film cassette, and three skin markers put in place, as with the fluoroscopic method. Then the usual double X-ray exposure was made, once with the tube moved by a distance Y in one direction, followed by a second exposure once the tube had been moved to the opposite limit, $-Y$. The resulting film showed four pairs of shadows, three from the skin markers $M_1, M_2 : N_1, N_2 : O_1, O_2$, and one pair from the object P_1, P_2 (Fig. A.8). A single shadow was cast by the axial marker x.

Once the film had been developed, two further marks were made on it at F_2 and F_2'. These identified the positions of the axial ray for the two displaced beams (in the figure, $Y = 3$ cm). $F_2 F_2'$ was drawn parallel to $M_1 M_2$ etc. The heights above the couch were then calculated from geometric considerations. For example, the height of marker M, $d_m = Zm/(2Y + m)$ where m was the distance between M_1 and M_2.

Fig. A.8 The positions of shadow pairs on a radiographic image from which calculation of the settings for the Hirtz compass may be made

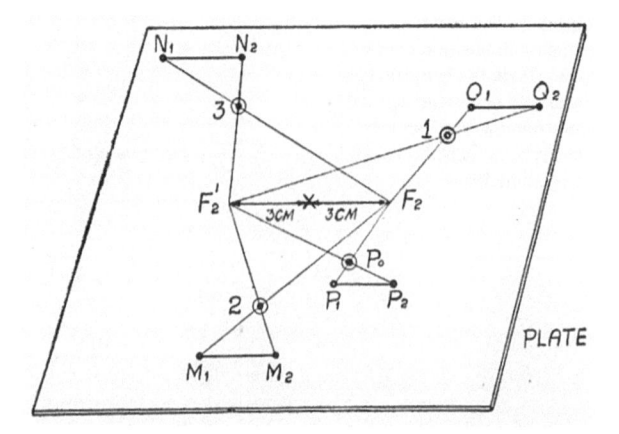

Finally, the relative positions of the three rods and the bullet (1, 2, 3 and P_0) were established as shown in Fig. A.8, and the positions of the rods and their heights were adjusted from these measurements and locked in place.

Once the compass was set it could then be placed on the skin with each leg on its skin mark (phase 3). The surgeon chose the most appropriate route for entry, using rod H as guidance for the direction and depth to reach the object.

Hirtz first described his compass 4 years before the onset of hostilities in August 1914. Once warfare started, the steady stream of wounded soldiers into military hospitals precipitated it into prominence and it was rapidly accepted into French radiological practice. As early as February 1915 a study of its use was presented to the French *Académie des sciences* reporting successful localization and extraction of foreign bodies in 88 of 90 cases [18]. It was never enthusiastically taken up by British military surgeons or radiologists. We can only speculate on its adoption by Florence at the Fulham Military Hospital, who certainly initially preferred the more simple Mackenzie Davidson method.

Electrotherapy

In the words of Dr. Ettie Sayer, reporting in 1915 to the Electro-Therapeutical section of the RSM on her recent visit to France 'The French War Office considers that the wounds of this Great War call for electrical treatment on a wholesale scale' [19]. At the base hospitals, rehabilitation of injured soldiers was a far greater challenge than during the initial acute management of injury. This was where the soldiers were rehabilitated either to return as soldiers to battle, or to be pensioned off to re-enter civilian life. Their medical management was derived, not from the methods used to treat acute illness, but instead from those techniques that, in times of peace, Florence had used for treating her patients with chronic disabling illnesses such as paralysis or rheumatism. As a result, the methods used in the middle-class health spas, widely established throughout Europe by the beginning of the twentieth century, were those that were adapted and developed as the main means to rehabilitate the wounded in wartime.

Ettie Sayer was another of the women science graduates who had gained access to higher education in the latter decades of the nineteenth century. She was awarded a science degree from University College, London and then trained as a doctor at the LSMW, graduating in 1899. Later, she was appointed as assistant medical officer to the education department of the London County Council, one of the first women to take such a position. Her report to the Royal Society of Medicine described her observations in a 500-bed military hospital in Bordeaux. This had four large rooms for physical therapy, one each for electrotherapy, thermotherapy, mechanotherapy and massage. Day-to-day management was under the guidance of a trained masseuse, the historical predecessor of the modern physiotherapist. As described by Dr. Sayer, 120 cases were each having two, 25-minute treatments each day, 15 men to a room, cycling through all four treatment methods every 2 days.

Such was common practice in French military hospitals and in the largest military hospitals in Britain including the Fulham Military Hospital. All military hospitals used electrotherapy as part of their programme of rehabilitation. Edith's challenge in Salonika, given that there was not a trained masseuse in the unit, was that of deciding how to select the best of these known techniques under the conditions in which she found herself. She was well aware of her own lack of medical training, saying that her sister would call her a "dilution quack". She may have known enough, though, to have been suspicious of one widely used method, in which a low electric current was passed through one or more limbs, by immersing them in a saline bath to which electrodes were connected. The method was often applied to treat the stumps of amputees, and in the treatment of trench foot. In both cases any value was most probably the result of regular hygienic irrigation, the electric wires adding a placebo effect for soldiers who would have been unlikely to have even had electric lighting in their homes.

One application with a better physiological and research basis was interrupted electrical stimulation. An electric current that was large enough to cause muscle contraction was switched on and off, applied using the saline baths as with the simpler method. During the war, with the vast experience from thousands of wounded, a consensus developed that interrupted treatment had real benefit in increasing the bulk and strength of wasted and damaged muscle. In this approach, a mechanical metronome was commonly used to interrupt the voltage about once every second (Fig. A.9). Henri Bordier, professor of medical physics in the faculty of medicine in Lyon, had reported as early as 1902 the outcome of a study on normal subjects using a programme of 10-minute sessions of interrupted electrical stimulation of arm muscles. After treatment every other day for 2 months an average increased girth of the arm of a little over 2 cm was reported. The induced repetitive muscle contraction helped to stimulate circulation and muscle bulk and strength, especially where motor nerve damage made mechanotherapy against weights, or using a static bicycle, difficult or impossible. Dr. Sayers described how, in the French electrotherapy departments she visited, galvanic and faradic supplies, each with its own metronome interrupter, fed six to ten resistance boxes set up about 1 m

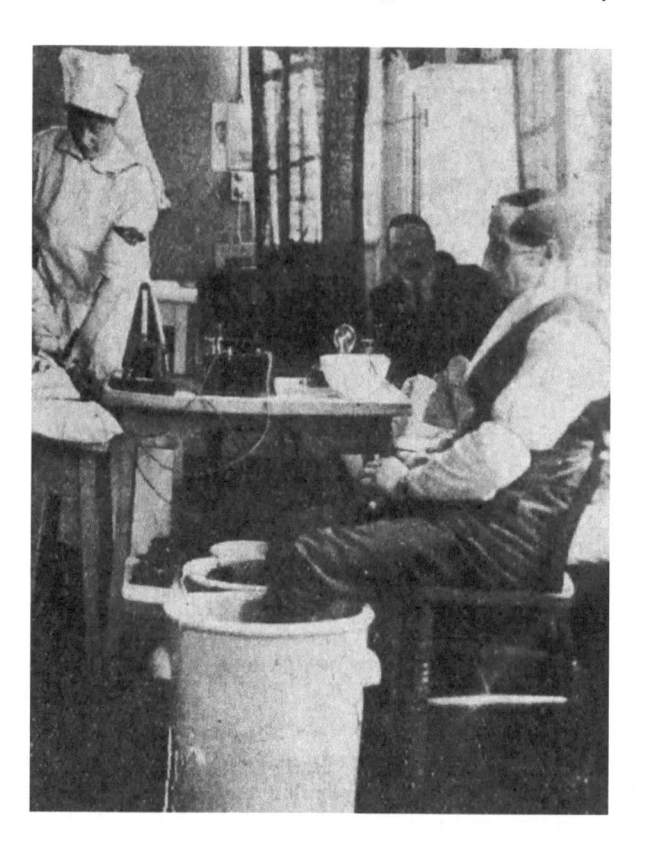

Fig. A.9 Casualty receiving intermittent electrical stimulation for paralysis of the legs. The controlling metronome is clearly visible

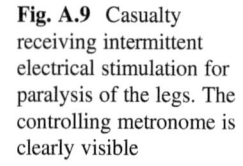

apart on each side of the treatment room. These were connected to arm-baths, leg-baths or waterproof chairs with wet pad electrodes. She went on, graphically;

> The faradics go to one side, the galvanics to the other; they sort themselves to their particular electrodes; the clinical assistants apply the pads; the main current is turned on; the resistance is adjusted to the particular needs of each patient.

But these methods of electro-therapy were not the only way in which electricity was being used, as Edith knew. By this stage, the use of high-frequency resonant oscillators for medical diathermy had passed through several stages of development. By the start of the war, instruments such as that bought by Edith in Paris in October 1915 were operating at frequencies of a few MHz at voltages up to about 800 V and currents of about 2 mA. In use, the electrodes were firmly grasped, until warmth was felt in the wrists and forearms. This new equipment had developed from the earlier high-frequency equipment that Florence had used for the treatment of varicose veins in 1905, for which short evacuated glass tubes held in an insulated handle directed sparks onto the region under treatment causing sparking and tingling. As early as the middle of February 1916, Edith reported that she was already treating a lot of rheumatism cases using her new Gaiffe high-frequency diathermy equipment. When the HF instrument was operated at the highest power using a very small electrode, the high frequency current was sufficiently high to destroy the tissue, and so the method could be used for very fine and accurate surgery. The very high temperatures created a fine cut, simultaneously cauterising the vessels to minimise blood loss.

Another widespread and popular use of therapeutic electricity was ionic therapy. Edith used this approach during her time in Salonika, and Florence used it to treat Edith's varicose ulcers during her brief respite in London in July 1918. The therapeutic purpose of ionic therapy was to enhance the transport of ionic therapeutic agents through the skin. A high DC current, slowly increased using a rheostat to somewhere between 50 and 100 mA, was applied over a large area for periods of up to 30 minutes. Metal electrodes up to 10 cm^2 were covered in several layers of felt, soaked in the appropriate ionic solution and applied to the region to be treated. The drugs most often used were the chlorides of sodium, ammonium and lithium (for scar softening), sodium salycilate (for pain relief), zinc sulphate (to treat wounds and ulceration) and cocaine hydrochloride (for local analgesia) [20]. Ionic medication slowly became less popular after the war, largely because burns from high local currents could occur if the skin was not prepared sufficiently well or the electrodes were applied badly.

There is no evidence that specific ultra-violet therapy had any applications in military medicine, although the more general use of sunlight to encourage wound healing was certainly used at Troyes, Salonoka and Royaumont. Historically, the first use of both ultraviolet therapy and high frequency therapy occurred in the same year that X-rays were discovered, 1895 [21]. In that year, the Danish Nobel Prize winner Niels Finsen (1860–1904) introduced ultraviolet treatment for lupus vulgaris, a disfiguring form of tuberculosis, and the biophysicist Jacques-Arsène d'Arsonval (1851–1940) established high-frequency electrotherapy in Paris after studying the effects on the body of electric currents of different frequencies.

Electrodiagnosis of Nerve Injury

Many war injuries resulted in temporary or permanent paralysis or in sensory loss. The injuries were as unexpected as were the realities of modern trench warfare. Jules Tinel, the head of neurology of the fourth French Military Hospital at Le Mans wrote, in 1916, 'The frequency of peripheral nerve injuries in this war is considerable. This has been a surprise'. In retrospect it is Tinel's surprise that is astonishing, given what we now know about the conditions at the front line. In addition, medical staff started to see neurological symptoms that were difficult to relate to the observed injuries. It soon became clear that many such symptoms could have a psychological as much as a physical cause.

X-ray techniques, whilst outstanding for the diagnosis of skeletal injury and the location of foreign bodies, had little to offer in the diagnosis of paralysed limbs or loss of sensation. A different diagnostic approach was required. Paralysis and sensory loss were commonly found in wounded soldiers, and surgeons needed a means to determine the location and severity of injury. The use of electricity to investigate nerves had been developed at the end of the nineteenth century, but this had been used mostly for diseases of the nerves and not for trauma. The war wounded brought very large numbers of bruised, torn and severed nerves before the doctors, with little or no means at their disposal with which to approach their diagnosis and treatment.

Electrodiagnosis was used only in major centres of excellence, under conditions where time could be spent in developing the skill required for its successful use. It was used by Florence to supplement her radiological work in London, Edith writing that 'she (Florence) is so skilled at muscle testing (electrically) that the surgeons at her present hospital always make her do all such work for injured nerves etc.' [22]. Edith herself offered nerve testing on her radiology request form at Royaumont, and recorded four occasions on which this test was carried out in Villers-Cotterêts, in late 1917 and early 1918 [23]. The timing suggests that Edith was introduced to the technique by her sister during her stay in London in September 1917.

Techniques for electro-diagnosis had been established during the latter part of the nineteenth century, pioneered particularly by the French doctor Duchenne de Boulogne [24] and introduced into Britain by Hughes Bennett [25] and De Watteville [26]. Maps of motor points for the placement of the stimulating electrodes were widely available, identifying the locations where the nerve or muscle to be examined is sufficiently superficial to be stimulated by an electric voltage applied to the skin. However, in these earlier texts, paralysis from traumatic injury is mentioned only in passing. Up to the outbreak of war, those involved with electro-diagnosis had very little experience with the investigation of the widespread and varied traumatic effects of modern warfare on those exposed to high explosives and high velocity arms.

For those wishing to introduce electrodiagnosis into their war practice, the main source of information was a book by the French radiologist Adolphe Zimmern (1871–1935) *Electrodiagnostic de guerre* [27]. The general British view to electro-diagnosis may well be characterised by the following quotation from a 1916 paper: 'Very skilled and experienced men have been able to claim a fair degree of success, but failures have been numerous, so much so that not a few surgeons and neurologists have stated that the method has little or no value' [27]. Electro-diagnosis was thus condemned by the words of senior clinicians who failed to gain the appropriate scientific understanding and technical support required for diagnostic success.

The electro-diagnostic techniques described by Zimmern were straightforward and were not original. A galvanic (DC) or faradic (AC) voltage was applied to the skin, either using a local sponge electrode of about 1 cm diameter and a large ground electrode, or between two small local metal electrodes (Fig. A.10). The thresholds of electrical current were recorded at which a small muscle contraction or twitch was first observed, these measurements being of primary diagnostic importance. For DC voltages, controlled using a rheostat, standard sequences of polarity switching were used and two pairs of thresholds were noted, using both positive and negative

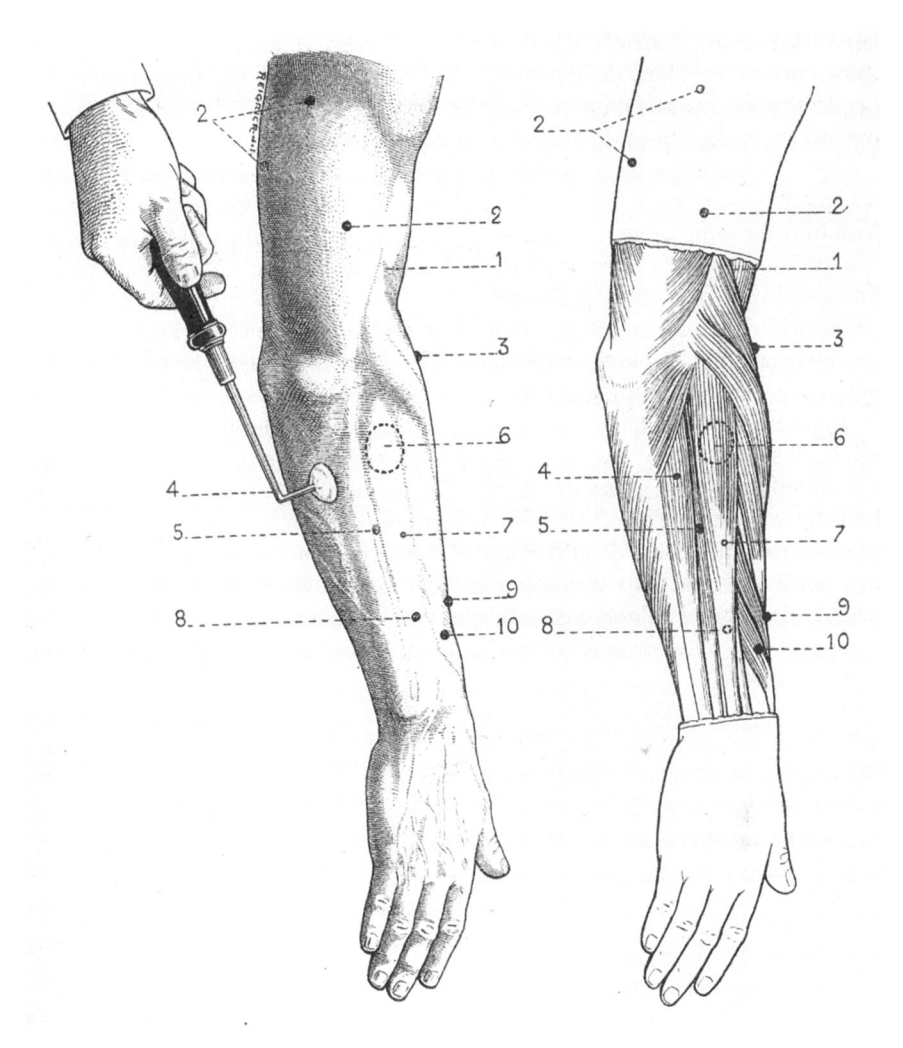

Fig. A.10 Diagram showing the correct electrode placements for local stimulation

polarity, and in each case on closing or on opening the circuit. Qualitative observations included an altered speed of contraction and the inversion of the normal response to altered polarity. For faradic (AC) stimulation, pulses were generated at a rate of about one each second using a battery, coils and automatic circuit breaker. The voltage was adjusted by changing the distance between a primary and secondary coil.

Zimmern discussed a variety of traumatic injuries that could result in motor paralysis and for which electro-diagnosis could be of value. Injury may have caused irritation, tension, compression, or complete division of a nerve and in each case he explained how the site and character of the traumatic injury might be examined.

Gunshot wounds frequently also caused the severance of muscles and tendons, and Zimmern described how these injuries could be investigated. He stressed the importance of repeat investigation, recognizing that some paralysis recovered spontaneously, even though this may take several months to occur.

Such studies had a clear medical purpose, but there was also another, military, agenda. Zimmern wrote 'The faradic coil is a valuable means of testing sensibility, both from the point of view of affections of the sensory system, and for the purpose of exposing malingers'. He continued 'When the secondary coil is moved slowly up towards the primary, a point is reached . . . at which the patient begins to experience a slight tickling sensation, which is at first disagreeable, and gradually becomes definitely painful'. The use of such a method to identify soldiers who simply desired to remove themselves from the front line is obvious.

Another technique that was easy to apply was "voltaic vertigo", arising from the electrical stimulation of the ear, in which a threshold for vertigo of over 4 mA was considered diagnostic of injury. The test for voltaic vertigo was compulsory in the French army, and the result was of considerable importance alongside radiological examinations in French Medical Board to advise on pension awards. The electrical examination was the only diagnostic test that would offer explicit evidence on the underlying cause of an observed paralysis, with a prediction of a possible partial or total recovery. An army pension was awarded only if a disability was both severe and incurable.

Paralysis might also arise from purely psychological trauma, the stress of days and weeks under bombardment. These electrical tests helped to differentiate between simulated, hysterical or functional paralysis. This would have helped in resolving the tension between the military, who wished to return soldiers to the front line as soon as possible, and the doctors, who were concerned with their medical care.

References

1. Savill A. X-ray appearances in gas gangrene. Proc R Soc Med. 10:4–16 (also Br Med J. 1917 Jan 13;1(2924):65–66).
2. Berry HM. The recognition of gas within tissues. Proc R Soc Med. 1917;10:17–24 (also Arch Radiol Electrother 1916;21:213–220).
3. Record of X ray work by a member of the Scottish Women's Hospital. ML. TD1734/2/6/9/130.
4. Record of X ray work by a member of the Scottish Women's Hospital. The Common Cause. 1917 Aug 31; 251.
5. Fleming A. The bacteriology of septic wounds. Lancet. 1915;186:638–43.
6. Skia (VCC Cullum). A hospital in France. Blackwood's Magazine. 1918 Nov; 613–640.
7. Weinberg M. Bacteriological and experimental researches on gas gangrene. Proc Roy Soc Med. 1916 Mar 10;119–143.
8. Crofton E. The Women of Royaumont. East Lothian: Tuckwell Press; 1997. Appendix 2 pp 335–339.
9. Stoney F. J R Soc Med (Elect Ther). 1916;9:93–4.
10. Pirie H. Observations on everyday X-ray and electrical work. J Rontgen Soc. 1910;6(25):105–10.
11. SWH List of equipment Troyes X-ray. ML. TD1734/6/2/3/8.
12. Stoney FA. The women's imperial service league hospital. Arch Roentgen Ray. 1915;19(11):388–93.
13. United States Army X-ray Manual. Ch 7 Localization. London: Lewis; 1919.
14. Hampson W. A localising device. J Rontgen Soc. 1915;11:10–5.
15. Hirtz EJ. Un appareil simple pour la location précise des corps étrangers a l'aide des rayons de Roentgen. J Belg Radiol. 1910:240–9.
16. Savill A. Some notes on the X-ray department of the Scottish Women's hospital, Royaumont, France. Archiv Radiol Electrother. 1916;20(12):401–10.
17. Scottish Women's Association. Minutes of the equipment committee. 1916 June 26. ML. TD1734/1/5/1.
18. Menard M. Localisation des projectiles et examen des blessés par les rayons X. CR Acad Sci. 1915;1:183–5.
19. Sayer E. The organization of electro-therapy in military hospitals. Proc R Soc Med. 1916;9:39–46.
20. Jones HL. In: Bathurst LW, editor. Medical electricity. 7th ed. London: Lewis; 1918.
21. Duck FA. Physicists and physicians, a history of medical physics from the renaissance to Röntgen. New York: IPEM; 2013. p. 232.
22. Edith Stoney to Mrs Laurie. 1917 July 6. ML. TD1734/2/6/9/68.

23. Villers-Cotterets Workload statistics. ML. TD1734/8/4/1/2.
24. Poore GV. Selections from the clinical works of Dr Duchenne (de Boulogne). London: New Sydenham Society; 1883.
25. Bennett AH. A practical treatise on electro-diagnosis in diseases of the nervous system. London: Lewis; 1882.
26. De Watteville A. A practical introduction to medical electricity. 2nd ed. London: Lewis; 1884.
27. Zimmern A, Perol P. Électrodiagnostic de guerre. Paris: Masson; 1917 and in English translation, (1918) edited by Elvin Cumberbach.

Index

A
Actinotherapy, 291–293, 297
'ad eundem gradum' degree, 128
Ada Johnson, 60
Adelaide, 319–323
Agnes Savill, 244–251
Alfred Keogh, 167
Ambulance Flottante, 230
Ambulance Volante, 230
American colleges, 130
Anaesthetist, 187
Anatomy demonstrator, 95–97
Anglo-French Hospital, 164–167
Animal Nutritional Laboratories, 323
Antwerp, 158–164
Aortic regurgitation, 173
Arabian Nights, 197
Archibald Reid, 226
Arithmetic examination, 17
Association of Registered Medical Women (ARMW), 117, 119, 157
Astronomy, 72, 74, 76
Atomic scale, 73
Austin, 226, 229–232

B
Bacteriology, 186
Belgian Red Cross Society, 158
Bicycle, 320–322
Bournemouth Natural Science Society (BNSS), 292
Brisbane, 319, 321–323, 326

British Association for the Advancement of Science, 37
British Association of Radiology and Physiotherapy (BARP), 290, 295–297
British Federation of University Women (BFUW), 322–325
  aims of, 148
  report, 149
British Medical Association (BMA), 79, 290, 294, 295
Budget management, 17
Butt and Co Ltd, 271

C
Calcutta Orthopaedic Centre, 220
Cambridge Higher Local Examinations, 17
Cambridge, student in, 55–61
Carey Coombs, 171
Catholic Apostolic Church, 29
Cavendish Electrical Company, 230
Celtic music, 134
Château Tourlaville, 164–167
Cheltenham Ladies' College, 67, 69, 70, 72, 74, 225, 226
Chepstow Crescent, visitors to, 134–137
Civilian organisation, 230
Coolidge tube, 156, 161, 165, 174
Countess Gleichen, 220
Croix de Guerre avec Etoile, 278–280
Croix de Guerre avec Palme, 278
Cycling, 1–4, 6
Cycling for Ladies, 3
Cycling, costume, 3

D

Defence of the Realm Act (DORA), 289
Diploma in Medical Radiology and Electrology (DMRE), 296
Disordered Action of the Heart (DAH), 171–174
Dorothea Beale, 67, 69
Dublin Mechanics Institution, 9
Dublin, port of, 10
Dundrum, 2, 6
Dynamo, 228, 232, 233, 235, 236

E

Edith Cavell X-ray van
   British Red Cross, 232, 234
   emotions, 234
   equipment, 233
   film radiography, 236
   film radiology, 233
   Florence's enthusiasm, 232
   foreign body localisation, 235
   light-proof, 236
   maintenance budget, 235
   medical care, casualties, 238
   mobile radiology, 232
   operational requirements, 239
   parochialism, 235
   publicity value, 233, 236
   RAMC, 239
   technical criticisms, 236
   vehicle's engine, 235
Eleanor Sidgwick, 47, 51, 53, 55, 63
Electrical diagnosis, 247, 256
Electrical massage, 216
Electrical vibrators, 195
Electrine, 40
Electrocautery, 186, 205
Electrocoagulation, 196
Electrodiagnosis, 344
Electromagnetic radiation, 10
Electro-massage, 195
Electrons, 10, 40
Electrotherapeutic equipment, 189
Electrotherapy, 167, 170, 195, 214, 340–343
   in Salonika, 203–206
Elizabeth Garrett, 13
Elizabeth Garrett Anderson, 79, 80, 82, 88
Engine/dynamo, 191, 193, 194

F

FitzGerald-Lorentz contraction, 12
Fluoroscopic technique, 168
Fluoroscopy, 225, 234, 235, 237, 239, 272
Force feeding, 152
Foreign Service Division, 156
Fourth Hague Convention, 160
Frances Ivens, 149, 244–247, 252–255, 258–260, 262
French army health service, 183
Fulham Military Hospital (FMH), 167–171

G

Gaiffe
   apparatus, 277
   equipment, 267, 268, 271, 277
   room, 267
   table, 272
Gas gangrene, 189, 329, 331–333
General Medical Council (GMC), 76
German advance, 259, 260
Girton and Newnham Unit, 179, 180, 186, 187, 189, 191, 192, 195
Graves' disease, 112, 113, 293
Gynaecological radiation, 131

H

Hampstead Garden City Belgian Relief Committee, 177
Hampstead Garden Suburb, 139, 140, 289
Heliotherapy, 189, 311
Hertha Ayrton, 149, 150
High-frequency electrotherapy, 203, 205, 206, 213, 217, 343
High-frequency therapy, 195
Hirtz compass, 336–340
'Hot-air douche' method, 206

I

International Electrotechnical Commission committee, 305
Interrupted electrotherapy, 341
Ionic therapy, 343
Irish famine, 31
Irish Home Rule, 153
Irvingite church, 29

J

Johnstone and Florence Stoney Studentship, 322, 325
Johnstone Stoney, death of, 137–139

K

'Kill Home Rule with kindness', 56

Index

L
Latch-key ladies, 306
Lead-lined gloves, 271
Ledoux-Lebard portable X-ray system, 274
Leitz microscope, 321
Leviathan, 33, 36
Liberal education, 8, 16
Localisation, 188
Logarithmic scale, 72
London meetings
 ARMW, 118, 119
London School of Medicine for Women (LSMW), 79, 80, 82, 83, 85–87, 91, 92, 94–97, 101
Louisa Aldrich-Blake, 143, 144
Louisa Martindale, 94
Louise McIlroy, 186–190, 195
Lyceum club, 131, 132
Lycopodium spores, 134, 300, 306

M
Mabel St Clair Stobart, 155, 156, 158–164
Macalister-Wiggin tube, 250
Mackenzie Davidson method, 340
Marie Curie, 225, 227, 228
Marie Curie Hospital, 310, 311, 315, 323, 324, 326
Martina Bergman Österberg, 98
Mary Murdoch, 93–95
Mary Scharlieb, 82
Mary Waller, 141, 142, 144
Mathematics Tripos, 46, 50–55
Medical electricity, 122
Medical laboratory science, 186
Medical physics, 194
Medical physics teaching, 121–124, 130, 131
Medical planning, 225
Medical technology, 225
Medical women, consulting rooms, 116
Medical Women's Federation (MWF), 294
Mental health physician, 186
Mesopotamia, 237
Metaphysical/theological idea, 11
Michelson-Morley experiment, 12
Microscopy, 4
Militant Suffragettes, 151–153
Military radiography, 190
Minnie Baughan, 199
Mitral stenosis, 173
Mobile X-ray units, 225
Mobilisation, 197
Modern telescopes, 289
Motoring, 140, 141

N
National Union of Women's Suffrage Societies, 178, 227
Natural Science Tripos, 325
Nerve Injury, electrodiagnosis of, 343–346
Nervous exhaustion, 273
New Hospital for Women (NHW), 88–91
Newnham College, 45–51, 286, 298
 astronomer, 61–66
Not Yet Diagnosed [Nervous] (NYDN), 173
Nunquam Non Paratus, 26

O
Oakley Park
 abandoned, 29
 catastrophic finances, 32
 estate management, 30
 financial state, 30, 31
 maids, 41
 residual viability, 31
 sale, 35
 straw, 28
Order of the British Empire (OBE), 285
Oscilloscope tube, 255
Osteomalacia, 311, 312

P
Paralysis, 340, 342–346
Parsons marine turbines
 design of, 125
 stability of, 125, 126
Parsonstown, 26
Penny-farthing bicycle, 1, 2
Pension, 340, 346
Philippa Fawcett, 50–55
Photography, 6

Q
Queen Alexandra's Imperial Military Nursing Service, 158
Queen's College Galway, 36
Queen's University, 6–8, 15, 16, 37, 38

R
Radiant heat therapy, 205
Radiation burns, 271, 272
Radiation monitors, 270
Radiation safety, 270, 271
Radiography, 157, 161, 165, 169, 174, 192
Radiology, 155–157, 167, 174

Radiology (*cont.*)
    at Villers-Cotterêts, 251–257
RAMC mobile units, 226
Red Cross VAD scheme, 158
Reflector telescope, 6
Resignation, 142–144
Restoration of Pre-war Practices Act, 301
Reynolds Close, 139–141
River Aisne, 257
Röntgen Ray apparatus, 106, 110
Royal College of Science for Ireland (RCSI), 8, 18, 19
Royal Dublin Society, 9
Royal Dublin Society's School of Drawing, 9
Royal Free Hospital (RFH), 80, 81, 83, 325
Royal Photographic Society, 291
Royal Society of Medicine (RSM), 290, 292, 329
Royal University, 6
Royal Victoria and West Hants Hospital, 290, 291
Royaumont, 227, 228, 231–233, 235, 239
    radiography, 278
    X-ray department, 309
Royaumont Abbey, 244, 246, 247, 260
Royaumont, closure of, 277

S
Schall X-ray tube, 203
Scottish Edith Cavell Fund, 232
Scottish Women's Hospitals (SWH), 225, 237
    all-women hospital service, 178
    clinical applications, 179
    diaphragms, 183
    familiarity and confidence, 182
    high-quality equipment, 182
    medical physicist, 180
    NUWSS, 178
    pre-packed system, 181
    wartime medical care, 179
    women's leadership, 178
    X-ray department, 179
    X-ray service, 180
Searchlight mirrors, function of, 126
Serbia, 199–202, 207, 211–213, 217
Sex Disqualification (Removal) Act, 150
Simple parallax technique, 168
Sir Alfred Keogh, 171
Sir Frederick Treves, 156–158
Skiagrams, 103, 105, 170
Skin complaints, 152
Soldier's heart, 171–174

Somerville Students' Association Report, 129
Sophia Jex-Blake, 79, 80, 85
Spectroscopy, 10
Spiritualism, 158
St Sava, 214, 215
Starvation, 28
Steamboat ladies, 129
Stereo X-ray photographs, 278
Stereoscopic photography, 41
Stobart Unit, 159, 167
Stoney Scale, 40
Stoney's stereographic process, 188
Subatomic scale, 73
Suffragettes, 147, 152
Suffragists, 147, 148, 152, 153
Sydney University, 8
Sydney Watson Smith, 314
Syphilis, 170

T
Territorial Force Nursing Service, 316
The Art and Pastime of Cycling, 1
The Great War, 155
Thermonuclear reactions, 10
Thyroid-stimulating hormone, 293
Tithes, 28–30, 32, 38
Transatlantic transport, 288
Trinity College, 8
Trinity College Dublin, 32
Troyes, 180, 183–191, 193, 195, 196
Tuberculosis, 177

U
Ultraviolet light, 311, 312
US Army Medical Corps, 225
Uterine fibroids, 173

V
Vera Collum, 265–270, 272
Victoria Hospital for Sick Children (VHSC), 91–95
Vital force, 11
Vitamin D, 311, 312
Voluntary Aid Detachment (VAD), 217
Votes for women, 289, 290

W
War Office, 156–158, 162, 167, 168, 171, 226, 229, 230, 255

Wartime medical applications, 204
Wartime medical staffing, 143
Wartime radiology, 320
Wehnelt radiometer, 183
Wilhelm Conrad Röntgen, 103, 105, 110
William Ironside Bruce, 314
Woman scientist, 275
Women in medicine, 79–82
Women in society, 41
Women lawyers, 150
Women's education, 12, 13, 15, 18, 19, 21
Women's Engineering Society (WES), 301
Women's National Service League (WNSL), 156–158, 164
Women's suffrage, 285

X

X-radiation, 193
X-ray ambulance, 231
    functions, SWH vehicle, 229
    generators, 229
    life-threatening illness, 227
    medical radiology, 227
    military radiology, 230
    mobile X-ray unit, 227, 228, 231
    national women's activities, 227
    peripatetic radiology units, 226
    peripheral radiology, 229
    radiological equipment, 229
    specification, 228
    suffrage movement, 228
    SWH project, 226
    War Office requirements, 230
X-ray computed tomography, 262
X-ray equipment, 124, 153, 177, 180, 181, 192, 200, 204, 225, 228, 232, 275, 279, 323
X-rays
    discovery, 70
    fibroids, 94
    first bibliography, 215
    first set, 70
    fluoroscopic screen, 272
    foreign bodies, 333–340
    goods, 221, 222
    investigations, 274
    in military, 214
    mobile set, 273
    new opportunities, 75–77
    non-malignant uterine haemorrhage, 94
    physical nature, 73
    remote hospitals, 202
    skin radiotherapy, 291
    transformers, 115
    treatment, 109
    United States, 113–115
    use of, 152
'Xtraordinary Challenge', 1

Z

Zander apparatus, 205
Zeppelin airships, 160
Zeppelin raids, 177

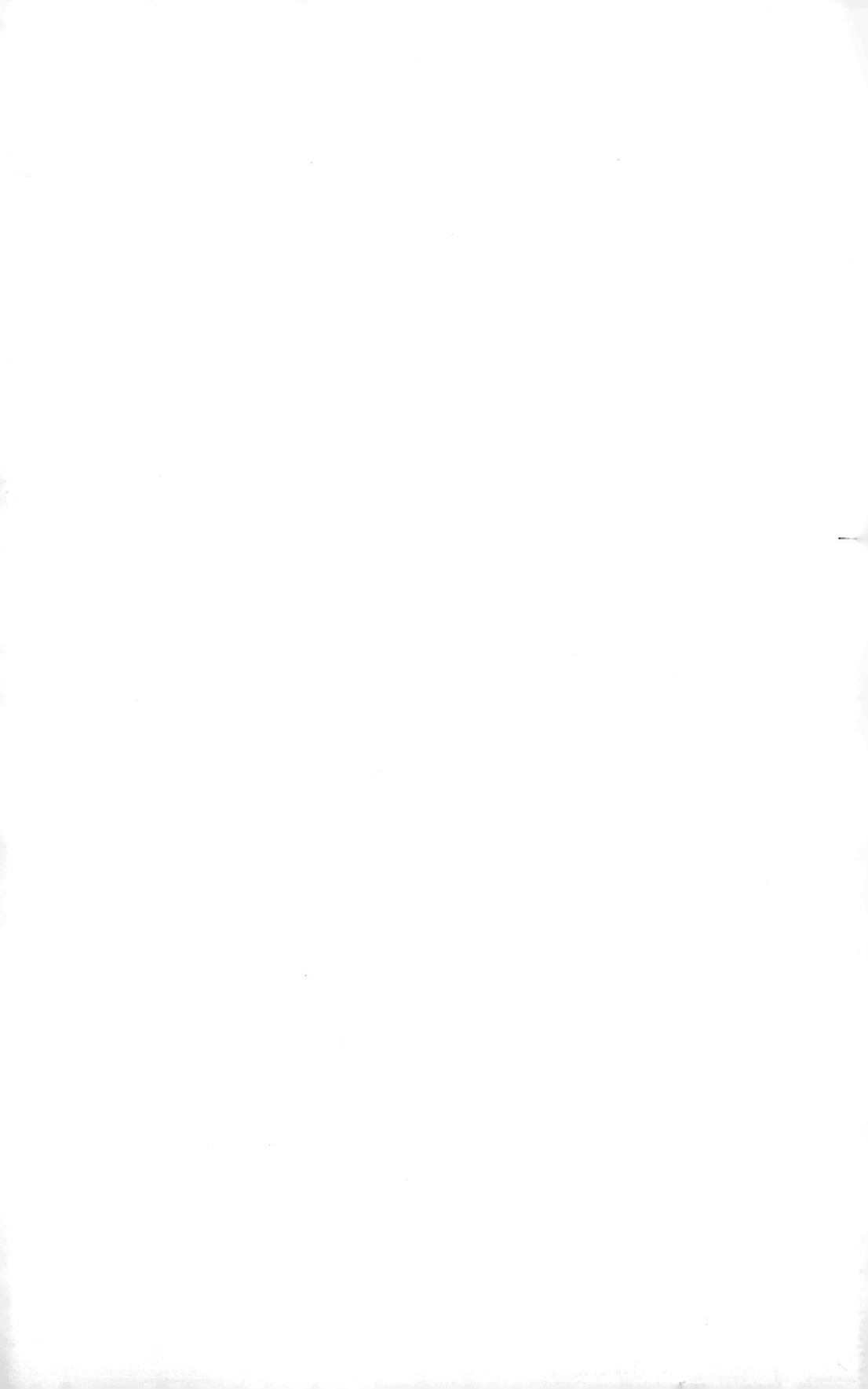